BEHAVIORAL MEDICINE

International Perspectives

Volume 1

Development in Clinical Psychology

Glen R. Caddy, series editor
Nova University

MMPI-168 Codebook, by Ken R. Vincent, Iliana Castillo, Robert I. Hauser, H. James Stuart, Javier A. Zapata, Cal K. Cohn, and Gregory O'Shanick, 1984

Integrated Clinical and Fiscal Management in Mental Health: A Guidebook, by Fred Newman and James Sorensen, 1986

The Professional Practice of Psychology, edited by Georgiana Shick Tryon, 1986

Clinical Applications of Hypnosis, edited by Frank A. DePiano and Herman C. Salzberg, 1986

Full Battery Codebook, by Ken R. Vincent, 1987

Developments in the Assessment and Treatment of Addictive Behaviors, edited by Ted D. Nirenberg, 1987

Feminist Psychotherapies, edited by Mary Ann Douglas and Lenore E. Walker, 1988

Child Multimodal Therapy, by Donald B. Keat II, 1990

Psychophysiology for Clinical Psychologists, by Walter W. Surwillo, 1990

Strategic Health Planning: Methods and Techniques Applied to Marketing and Management, by Allen D. Spiegel and Herbert H. Hyman, 1991

Behavioral Medicine: International Perspectives (Vol. 1–3), edited by D.G. Byrne and Glenn R. Caddy, 1992

In Preparation:

Language and Psychopathology, by Stephen Schwartz

The MMPI: A Contemporary Normative Study of Adolescents, by Robert L. Colligan and Kenneth P. Offord

BEHAVIORAL MEDICINE

International Perspectives

Volume 1

Edited by

D.G. Byrne, Ph.D., M.A.Ps.S., F.I.C.P.M.
Department of Psychology
Australian National University
Canberra, A.C.T.

Glenn R. Caddy, Ph.D., ABPP, AABM
Academy of Medicine and Psychology
and Nova University
Ft. Lauderdale, FL

ABLEX PUBLISHING CORPORATION
NORWOOD, NEW JERSEY

Printed in the United States of America.

Library of Congress Cataloging-in-Publication Data

Behavioral medicine : international perspectives / edited by D.G. Byrne, Glenn R. Caddy.
p. cm. — (Developments in clinical psychology)
Includes bibliographical references and index.
ISBN 089391620X (v. 1)
1. Medicine and psychology. 2. Medicine, Psychosomatic.
I. Byrne, D.G. (Donald Glenn) II. Caddy, Glenn R. III. Series.
[DNLM: 1. Behavioral Medicine. 2. Psychology, Medical.
3. Psychophysiologic Disorders. WM 90 B4194]
R726.5.B4256 1991
616'.001'9—dc20
DNLM/DLC
for Library of Congress 91-26136
CIP

Ablex Publishing Corporation
355 Chestnut Street
Norwood, New Jersey 07648

To Annie, with love and thanks
D.G.B.

To Thomas and Hazel Caddy,
whose love has sustained me always
G.R.C.

Table of Contents

Preface

There have been many landmarks in the history of clinical psychology. In the late 1950s and the 1960s, great progress in the theories and applications of behavior therapy signalled an inevitable but much welcomed shift in orientation from that of counselor and psychometrician to that of independent psychotherapist. The advent of behavior therapy gave the clinical psychologist, at last, a basis for the treatment of behavioral disorders and personal distress which was theoretically unique to the science of psychology. If there has been a professional landmark in the last decade, however, it must surely be seen in the arrival of behavioral medicine.

Behavioral medicine, as a distinct discipline, has existed for not much longer than 10 years, yet in that time it has made a considerable impact both on clinical psychology and on the practice of medicine. The course and magnitude of this impact are obvious in the amount of written material, both empirical and speculative, which has been generated in the past decade. In addition to a large array of text documenting important areas of behavioral medicine, the area has given rise to its own specialized journal (the *Journal of Behavioral Medicine*) and several complete issues of other clinical and research journals (see, for example, *British Journal of Clinical Psychology,* No. 4, 1982, and *Journal of Psychosomatic Research,* No. 5, 1982). The sheer prominence of material emerging in the area provides adequate testimony to the seriousness and interest with which the formative years of behavioral medicine have been greeted.

In the early years of any field, definitions are often rather diverse, and those attached to behavioral medicine are no different. Schwartz and Weiss (1978) defined it as:

> The interdisciplinary field concerned with the development and integration of behavioral and biomedical science, knowledge and techniques relevant to health and illness and the application of this knowledge and these techniques to prevention, diagnosis, treatment and rehabilitation.

Somewhat more succinctly, Surwit, Williams, and Shapiro (1981) wrote:

> Behavioral medicine is broadly defined to encompass the application of principles from all behavioral sciences to medical problems.

Along more rigidly behavioral lines, Pomerleau and Brady (1979) claimed behavioral medicine to be:

> The clinical use of techniques derived from the experimental analysis of behavior—behavior therapy and behavior modification—for the evaluation, prevention, management or treatment of physical disease or physiological dysfunction.

Whichever position one takes, whether it be rigidly behavioral or more flexibly biopsychosocial, the essence of these definitions is clear. Behavioral medicine concerns the use of psychological evidence and techniques, typically but not exclusively those deriving from behavior therapy, in the diagnosis, prevention, and management of physically manifest illness.

Behavioral medicine is frequently confused with its close cousin, psychosomatic medicine, and the practitioner of the former is often asked to distinguish between the two. Surwit et al. (1981) argued that, whereas psychosomatic medicine placed its emphasis on the pathogenic influence of personality traits leading, through neurotic conflicts, to physical illness, behavioral medicine was concerned with physiological responses arising initially through maladaptive environmental interactions, becoming established or learned by means of objectively testable chains of causal influence, and leading ultimately to physical pathology. In practice, behavioral medicine rejected psychodynamic labelling, emphasized the experimental principles of learning in treatment, and confirmed the importance of evaluation and replicability of treatment procedures.

If psychosomatic medicine takes its theoretical beginnings from the psychodynamic movement of Freud and his successors, behavioral medicine is firmly rooted in the stress theories of Selye and those who followed him, the learning theories of Skinner and those coming after, and the integrative work on biopsychosocial approaches to illness beginning with Levi and his colleagues.

Just as clinical psychology had developed scientifically to the point where it could legitimately give rise to a new area of practice, medicine too was demonstrating, by and large, a readiness to accept approaches more broadly based than those concerned with the strict application of technology. The recognition by both professions that the treatment of human disease required attention to the *environment* and the *psyche,* as well as the *soma,* created a fertile ground for the integration of knowledge and practice. This promise of growth, and the considerable body of evidence it had already produced, prompted the development of this series of books.

The intention of *Behavioral Medicine: International Perspectives* is not to supplant any of a number of excellent works in the field, but to provide, as far as possible, a total overview of contemporary thought and clinical wisdom. In doing so, it draws widely and diversely, mixing contributory chapters from North American, European, and Australasian authors, with invitations to contribute being dependent only upon the judgment of the editors that individual authors would produce the best possible overviews of the area. The deliberate diversity of sources is reflected in the title of the volumes. Any exercise involving such judgment is bound to attract disagreement; in recognizing this, the editors are aware that many who are eminent in their own areas are not represented in these volumes. Nevertheless, we are confident that the breadth of authorship of each of the volumes in this series more than adequately compensates for individual omissions.

Uppermost in our minds in the early stages of planning was the need for comprehensiveness within a systematic organization of material. Consequently, as the project progressed, it grew from one to two and then three volumes. The sheer wealth of material in the area demanded that size could only be reduced by sacrificing whole sections crucial to a complete overview of behavioral medicine. In the final construction, it was decided that breadth of coverage overrode other considerations.

The organization of the three volumes is traditional, and follows an "organ/system" approach. Importantly, however, we have attempted to preface each section with a chapter outlining the anatomy, physiology, pathology, and epidemiology of the set of medical conditions under consideration. While the set of volumes will have a wide application across professional boundaries, the essentially interdisciplinary nature of behavioral medicine means that many readers will not have a background in the medical sciences. For them, it is important that concepts and terminologies in the substantive chapters are understood, and quick reference to an introductory summary seemed the best way of achieving this. Similarly, in the opening section of each volume, certain key issues in the clinical psychology of assessment and intervention have been discussed in summary chapters designed to acquaint the reader not trained in psychology with the unique contributions of this science to behavioral medicine. These additions, while somewhat increasing the length of the works, seek to establish the utility of these works across professional boundaries.

It is our hope that this series of books will serve a wide audience. In guiding our large group of excellent contributors, we have attempted to encourage chapters encompassing the inextricably joined areas of empirical evidence and clinical skill and practice. It was our hope from the beginning that the series would be as useful to the clinical practitioner grappling with the problems of single patients as it would be to the researcher requiring contemporary and comprehensive reviews of the available evidence needed to guide further studies. In principle, we hold the view that the two areas cannot be separated; if this comes across in individual chapters, it is a tribute to the subject grasp and clear thinking of the many eminent scientists and practitioners who have contributed so ably to the series.

Enterprises such as these owe much to many people. In this respect, the contributing authors are most immediately deserving of our thanks. In spite of heavy teaching and research loads, and overwhelming clinical commitments, such contributor worked to the difficult deadlines imposed to produce chapters of both breadth and depth. To our contributors, then, we are inestimably grateful. The editing of a series of works, when editors themselves are separated by some thousands of kilometers of land and ocean, produces its own particular difficulties. One is inclined to thank the systems of international postage, but at times these have not proven the most reliable means of communication. Colleagues on both sides of the Pacific have, however, helped our task very considerably. Of course, families tolerate much from members who pursue such ephemeral activities as editing books, and for this tolerance we are distinctly grateful.

The task of putting this work together has brought to each of us unique rewards. If we share one, however, it is the feeling that the series will have contributed palpably to the promotion of behavioral medicine as an area so new but with so much promise for the future.

D. G. Byrne
G. R. Caddy

REFERENCES

Pomerleau, O. F., & Brady, J. P. (Eds.). (1979). *Behavioral medicine: Theory and practice*. Baltimore: Williams & Wilkins.

Schwartz, G. E., & Weiss, S. M. (1978). Behavioral medicine revisited: An amended definition. *Journal of Behavioral Medicine, 1,* 249–251.

Surwitt, R. S., Williams, R. B., & Shapiro, D. (1981). *Behavioral approaches to cardiovascular disease*. New York: Academic Press.

I

INTRODUCTION

1

Definitions and Constructs in Behavioral Medicine

Glenn R. Caddy
Don McCulloch

Nova University
Ft. Lauderdale, FL

Behavioral medicine has been described as a popular emerging field (Agras, 1982; Brownell, 1984), a frontier (Matarazzo, 1980), and a clinical revolution (Basmajian, 1985). It appears to represent both a revolutionary concept and a new frontier for the field of psychology. The conceptual framework of this emerging field is revolutionary in that it represents a change from the way both psychologists and physicians traditionally have thought about and approached disorders; it is a new frontier in that it is based on the emergence of a modern and effective technology whose boundaries appear virtually limitless.

The domain encompassed by the term *behavioral medicine* has witnessed phenomenal growth in the last several years (Matarazzo, 1980; Gentry & Matarazzo, 1981; Brownell, 1984; Wedding & Williams, 1983; Thoresen & Eagleston, 1985). Whether the field continues its growth and lives up to the bold predicative descriptors noted above may, in part, hinge upon the way psychologists in the behavioral medicine arena define their field for themselves and for professionals of other disciplines.

DEFINING BEHAVIORAL MEDICINE

Various prominent individuals, as well as the Society of Behavioral Medicine, appear to accept the definition that developed out of the Yale Conference on Behavioral Medicine (Schwartz & Weiss, 1977) and, thereafter, its modification (Schwartz & Weiss, 1978). According to this widely circulated definition, behavioral medicine is:

> The interdisciplinary field concerned with the development and integration of behavioral and biomedical science knowledge and techniques relevant to health and illness and the application of this knowledge and these techniques to prevention, diagnosis, treatment, and rehabilitation. (Schwartz & Weiss, 1978, p. 250)

This definition is both broad and inclusive. It avoids specific reference to any particular philosophic orientation or school of thought. In it the word *behavioral* is used in a generic sense, and, as Masur (1979) has pointed out, its usage does not necessarily refer to the behaviorism concept as commonly used by the psychological community. Indeed, the emphasis in this definition is on the word *interdisciplinary*, which communicates the working together of many disciplines on an essentially equal basis. This is in contrast to the word *multidisciplinary*, in which many separate disciplines make specialized contributions yet often without real communication or cohesiveness. Agras (1982) has commented on this issue in the following terms: "One way to conceptualize the development of behavioral medicine is to regard it as representing an emerging network of communication among an array of disciplines not previously well connected. These disciplines include the behavioral and social sciences and the biomedical sciences and medical specialties" (p. 797). This broad approach to defining the field of behavior medicine is not without its detractors, and one author, Heslegrave (1985), has pointed to the lively continuing debate in the literature concerning the most acceptable definition for the field.

Criticisms of the definition given by Schwartz and Weiss (1978) are that it is too broad and inclusive and that no specific technology is identified as distinguishing the field (Pomerleau, 1979, 1982; Weddington & Blindt, 1983). It may well be positive if the field continues to grow as rapidly as has been witnessed in the last decade. But if the unique and effective factors that presently characterize behavioral medicine are lost through lack of clarity and focus in the process of this growth, the revolution could be over before its important potential contributions can be made known. Owen (1983) addressed this issue in the following terms: "A danger is that an overinclusive definition may result in an identity so diffuse that the field will diversify excessively and lose its focus" (p. 88). This issue becomes especially critical in the setting in which behavioral medicine may have its most profound impact—the hospital. It is to be anticipated that medical doctors may raise their eyebrows when a provider without a medical degree announces that he or she is engaged in activities that are defined with a title including the term *medicine*. Without a definition that communicates clearly the scope and the limits of behavioral medicine, it is likely that interdisciplinary activity with the traditional medical specialists will be difficult to achieve.

Reviewing the history of behavioral medicine, Inglis (1983) makes the following observation concerning medical physicians at behavioral science and medicine conferences in the early 1970s: "for the most part ordinary physicians had no idea at all about what behavioral scientists are, far less about what they actually may be expected to do in the medical field" (p. 306). A decade later, Inglis believed that things were probably not that much different. Of course, the revolutionary message that those in behavioral medicine want to communicate is that a new evolving and effective set of technologies now exists which can be applied in the treatment of many physical disorders heretofore thought only to be the appropriate concern of physical medicine. The publication of works such as the present volume, as well as many other recent publications in the field, serves to amply illustrate the emergence of this new technology.

The technologies which distinguish the practice of behavioral medicine consist of a variety of empirically validated techniques that developed mainly out of behavioral psychology (Pomerleau, 1979, 1980; Brownell, 1984; Redd & Rusch, 1985). A message that the proponents of behavioral medicine desire to communicate to other established disciplines is that these techniques are firmly grounded in the principles of learning theory and are the products of empirical research—a commodity which physicians and other professional disciplines value and respect. An alternative definition of behavioral medicine that accurately reflects this particular focus has been given by Pomerleau and Brady (1979):

> Behavioral medicine can be defined as (a) the clinical use of techniques derived from the experimental analysis of behavior—behavior therapy and behavior modification—for the evaluation, prevention, manage-

> ment, or treatment of physical disease or physiological dysfunction; and (b) the conduct of research contributing to the functional analysis and understanding of behavior associated with medical disorders and problems in health care. (p. xiii)

This definition clearly recognizes the historical antecedents from which behavioral medicine arose, namely, behavior therapy and behavior modification. Unlike the definition of behavioral medicine proposed by Schwartz and Weiss (1978), Pomerleau and Brady equate behavioral medicine with a specific school of thought. They also point out that the new technology of behavioral medicine is firmly grounded in an experimental analysis of behavior—in research.

It is apparent that both of these definitions have something important to offer the field of behavioral medicine. The first definition is quite broad and stresses the interdisciplinary approach. It has achieved substantial popularity, but it may lack the specificity needed to distinguish the field for the uninformed. The second definition is more specific and identifies behavioral medicine as an application of scientific experimentation, but uses language that may hinder popular acceptance. Of course, alternative definitions have been attempted. One that is similar to the second definition but succinctly focuses on the actual application of behavioral medicine has been given by Pinkerton, Hughes, and Wenrich (1982). This third definition proposes behavioral medicine to be:

> The clinical application of principles, techniques, and procedures of behavior therapy in the assessment, treatment, management, rehabilitation, and prevention of physical disease or concomitant behavioral reactions to physical dysfunction and the validation and refinement of such treatment techniques as applied to medical problems and health related issues through systematic investigations and research. (p. 3)

Just as behavior therapy has been conceptionalized to involve the application of the experimental method to the management of the individual case (Yates, 1970), in behavioral medicine the same experimental method is utilized, only its application is to medical problems rather than to problems more commonly reflective of behavioral dysfunction or psychopathology. The Pinkerton et al. definition clearly identifies what constitutes the clinical application of behavioral medicine, and, as the chapters in this and subsequent volumes will demonstrate, behavioral medicine involves the broad application of the experimental method to a host of problems not previously thought to be within the domain of psychology. In fact, a quite broad conceptualization of the scope of behavioral medicine appears progressively to be becoming the accepted norm. Thus, Surwit, Williams, and Shapiro (1982). propose that behavioral medicine be broadly defined to encompass the application of principles from all behavioral sciences to medical problems. And Neil Miller (1983) conceptualizes the field as involving the integration of relevant parts of epidemiology, anthropology, sociology, pharmacology, nutrition, neuroanatomy, endocrinology, immunology, and the various branches of medicine and public health.

ELEMENTS CONTRIBUTING TO GROWTH

Turning now from a discussion of the conceptual basis for and the domain of behavioral medicine to an analysis of the growth of the new speciality, it appears obvious that the shortcomings in the traditional biomedical model offer at least a partial explanation for the field's development. Krantz, Grunberg, and Baum (1985) address this point in the following terms:

> The role of behavior in today's most pressing health problems challenges the traditional medical model, which views disease as a purely biological phenomenon, that is, the product of specific agents or pathogens and bodily dysfunction. As a result, from both behavioral and biomedical communities there has been renewed interest in a broader model of health and illness encompassing psychological and social variables and their interaction with biological process. (p. 351)

Redd and Rusch (1985) cite several factors they see as responsible for the dramatic emergence of behavioral medicine. First, they feel there is a growing interest in a holistic approach to medicine that includes a consideration of psychological variables. This, in turn, has led to a concomitant awareness that behavior, or habits, play a major role in an individual's health. Further, Redd and Rusch cite the significance of the development of specific behavioral techniques capable of producing change in areas heretofore not thought to be under voluntary control. And, finally, they point to economic considerations and state that behavioral medicine is less expensive to the society than the "pharmacological alternatives" currently holding sway as largely the sole standard for intervention.

Basmajian (1985) points to several factors in accounting for what he terms "the next clinical revolution—behavioral medicine." He refers to the broad and behavioral approach to medical problems by Hippocrates, the failure of psychosomatic medicine to control symptomology, and the development of biofeedback as all being basic to setting the stage for the emergence of behavioral medicine. But Basmajian's most salient arguments in support of the recent growth of the field are as follows:

> What is new and particularly attractive about behavioral medicine is the emphasis on specific techniques derived from behavioral theories and research for the direct control or alleviation of physical symptoms of disease. Second is the reliance on objective definitions and measures of behavior and physiological response and the use of empirically based principles of intervention Third is its applicability to all medical disorders rather than only to disorders traditionally defined as psychological or psychophysiological in nature. (p. 593)

Basmajian also sees behavioral medicine as representing the incorporation of both physiological and behavioral knowledge to the management of the individual case.

Thoresen and Eagleston (1985) have pointed to historical conceptions of health, and they see a larger connection between mind and body and health and one's habits. They also pointed to "the growing evidence of links among behavior, health and disease as a rationale for the field's inception." These authors give an excellent overview of the field of what they refer to as "health psychology's" development.

Brownell (1984), highlighting the growth of the field, comments on the recent signs of the field's institutionalization, and considers whether the field is emerging or is already established. Brownell believes that the field is still emerging, and she appears to see behavioral medicine's major task as being an integrator of many disciplines from medicine and the behavioral sciences.

Upper et al. (1984), using a time frame of the last 15 years, offer two reasons for the growth of behavioral medicine during this period: first, introduction of innovative and effective treatment procedures; and second, the application of research method and findings of empirical psychology to the health field.

Inglis (1983) takes an approach somewhat different from the above authors' in describing the development of the field. Inglis considers that the roots of behavioral medicine lie in the behavioral sciences research and perspective of the early 1970s. He gives the following rationale for the events which set the stage for the emergence of behavioral medicine: (a) psychiatry's expanding role in medical education, (b) social change and innovation (this includes a shift in medical focus from treating the acutely ill to prevention), and (c) the involvement of the social sciences in health care. He also comments on the development in behavior therapy and its power to change abnormal behavior.

Neil Miller (1983), in his article "Behavioral medicine: Symbiosis between laboratory and clinic" for the *Annual Review of Psychology*, defines the field as follows:

> Behavioral medicine is an interdisciplinary field that integrates behavioral and biomedical knowledge relevant to health and disease. It involves the integration of relevant parts of epidemiology, anthropology, sociology, psychology, pharmacology, nutrition, neuroanatomy, endocrinology, immunology, and the various branches of medicine and public health, as well as related professions such as dentistry, nursing, social work, and health education. It is concerned with basic research, which at present is one of its greatest needs, and also with the application of its knowledge and techniques to prevention, diagnosis, therapy, and rehabilitation. (p. 3)

One can safely surmise from the title of Miller's article that he attributes the success of the field directly to success in the laboratory and the importance of the applied research which he surveys.

Weddington and Blindt (1983) discuss the development of behavioral medicine in terms of the movement away from the historical mind–body dualism. These authors see psychosomatic medicine as paving the way for a broader approach to disease. Rather than being antithetical to behavioral approaches, they feel psychosomatic medicine is a complementary field.

Blanchard (1982) attributes the success of the field to three factors; first, the success of behavior therapy, particularly when applied to more medically related problems; second, the development of a powerful technology, notably biofeedback; and third, the recognition of the role of risk factors or behaviors in health problems that represent the primary causes of mortality (i.e., heart disease and cancer). That the first two developments were able to impact the last development is particularly salient (see also Agras, 1982).

In summary, the most common themes reflecting the development of behavioral medicine in the literature include: (a) a movement towards a broader model of medicine that includes the role of behavioral variables, and is more holistic and less dualistic; (b) the development of effective behavioral techniques or a technology for behavior change; (c) the awareness of the role of personal habits, risk factors, or behaviors in health; and (d) the importance of applications or approaches based on research. These four themes, concerning the trend noted earlier in this chapter to define behavioral medicine in either a broad or narrow manner, now will be examined.

A BROADER MODEL OF MEDICINE

The broad approach to defining the field is often expressed in terms of a concern about the present model of medicine. The present biomedical model may well not be adequate to address the behavioral and social aspects of illness beyond a narrow biological approach. It is clear that, for some, behavioral medicine represents the modus operandi for a revolutionary approach to health and illness.

Many articles reviewed here, and particularly those which take the broad approach to defining the field (Krantz et al., 1985; Weddington & Blindt, 1983; Reading, 1982; Matarazzo, 1980; Schwartz & Weiss, 1977) make specific reference to an article by Engel (1977). In that article, "The need for a new medical model: A challenge for biomedicine," Engel summarizes the issue as follows:

> The dominant model for disease today is biomedical, and it leaves no room within its framework for the social, psychological, and behavioral dimensions of illness. A biopsychosocial model is proposed that provides a blueprint for research, a framework for teaching, and a design for action in the real world of health care. (p. 135)

That behavioral medicine is the broad representation of the biopsychosocial model is now clear. The quote given earlier in this chapter by Miller (1983), in which he lists all the areas that behavioral medicine envisions integrating, puts this idea into perspective. Brownell (1984) states that this enormous task of integration represents a major challenge presently for behavioral medicine. The accomplishment of this task would no doubt lend confirmation to statements by McDaniel (1984), who has called behavioral medicine "princely."

The trend of seeing behavioral medicine as the broadest category of health–behavior interactions has led to a host of new definitions for new corollary and subsumed disciplines under the behavioral medicine umbrella (Klippel & DeJoy, 1984). It was Matarazzo's (1980) opinion that the accepted broad definition of behavioral medicine given by Schwartz and Weiss (1978) did not emphasize enough the maintenance of health and the prevention of illness (other important themes in behavioral medicine). As such, Matarazzo (1980) proposed and defined a new domain in behavioral medicine, and called it *behavioral health.* Matarazzo (1980) defined this proposed new domain as follows:

> Behavioral health is an interdisciplinary field dedicated to promoting a philosophy of health that stresses individual responsibility in the application of behavioral and biomedical science knowledge and techniques to

> the maintenance of health and the prevention of illness and dysfunction by a variety of self-initiated and shared activities. (p. 813)

More simply, behavioral health might be called that domain which focuses on lifestyle modification. In the same article, Matarazzo (1980) clarifies the relationship between behavioral health and behavioral medicine and makes the following observation: "When the activities of these interfaces (medicine and psychology) are interdisciplinary, they fall under the heading of either behavioral health or behavioral medicine, depending on whether the activity is focused more on prevention or on remediation" (p. 815). Yet comprehensive behavioral medicine should include both prevention and health promotion. No doubt time will decide whether the identification of the specialty of behavioral health is necessary.

TECHNOLOGY FOR BEHAVIOR CHANGE

The narrower approach to defining behavioral medicine was given earlier in the quote by Pomerleau and Brady (1979). This approach defines the field, in part, by the use of techniques developed out of behavioral psychology. Effective technology in the service of behavior change is a central theme in the literature. A major technological advance associated with the early development of behavioral medicine is biofeedback. In fact the term behavioral medicine appears first to have been used in Birk's (1973), *Biofeedback: Behavioral Medicine.* Basmajian (1985), who calls behavioral medicine "a clinical revolution," considers that biofeedback was the catalyst for the start of this revolution. While such a perspective may be valid, Basmajian goes on to assert that, "along with other psychologic sources such as behavioral modification, biofeedback is today the very essence of behavioral medicine" (1985, p. 594).

Biofeedback is a technology that allows a patient to modify physiological responses not normally thought to be under voluntary control. Biofeedback involves using specialized equipment that directly monitors, analyzes, and displays physiological activity. The types of physiological activities that are commonly monitored include electromyographic (EMG), and electroencephalographic rhythms (EEG), heart rate (EKG), blood pressure (BP), blood flow, and skin temperature. Other responses that have been measured include stomach acid pH, sphincter activity, bowel sounds, respiration, sexual arousal, and blood alcohol level (Pinkerton et al., 1982). The basic concept of biofeedback, according to principles of learning, is that, when a patient is made aware of these responses, he or she will be able to develop some voluntary control over them to the extent that the response will be modified to occur in a desired direction. Disorders for which biofeedback has been utilized as a treatment method include the following: hypertension, cardiac arrhythmias, Raynaud's disease, fecal incontinence, ulcers, irritable bowel syndrome, spasmodic torticollis, cerebrovascular accidents, spinal cord injuries, asthma, chronic pain, migraine and tension headaches, and temporomandibular joint disorders. Biofeedback also has been used increasingly in neuromuscular reeducation, a procedure which is considered by some to be the most important present application of the technology.

Other techniques have been mentioned as important for behavioral medicine. These basic procedures include respondent conditioning with specific emphasis on systematic desensitization, flooding, and aversive conditioning, as well as operant conditioning procedures including contingency management, assertion, and social skills training. Self-management techniques also have been important to the emergence of the field. Self-management involves the therapist training the patient to modify aspects of his or her environment and perspective, which, in turn, serves to modify the problem behavior. Inevitably, however, beginning to offer perspective change soon opens the focus of the field to the cognitive domain—which then, of course, begins to call into question the scope of the so-called narrower definition of behavioral medicine. The direct application of behavior analysis and behavior modification are specified in the narrower definition of behavioral medicine (Pomerleau, 1979). Yet even within the narrow definition interventions are not confined solely to direct treatment, for behavioral medicine appears to include interventions involving: (a) prevention of medical disorders, (b) improvement of adherence to treatment regimens, (c) modification of patient's specific problem behavior, and (d) modification of health care providers behavior.

The narrower approach to defining the field appears less concerned with replacing the biomedical model with a broader conceptualization than with viewing behavioral medicine as a new medical specialty with its own effective techniques for addressing certain problems or types of problems. Of course, the development of behavioral medicine does not reflect the first attempt at a broad redefinition of medicine. The field of psychosomatic medicine historically has been concerned with the interplay between psychological and physiological variables, and it also has been very broad in its view of medicine, emphasizing a holistic rather than a dualistic approach (Weddington & Blindt, 1983). The field of psychosomatic medicine appears to have developed from a primarily psychoanalytic orientation based on the works of Freud and

Alexander. Initially, the field emphasized the etiology and pathogenesis of physical disease and focused on treating the hypothetical underlying causes of disease. Surwit et al. (1982) have offered the following comparison between a psychosomatic medicine approach and a behavioral approach to a problem:

> A patient presents with a disease or a set of isolated physical symptoms. According to the psychosomatic model, the physiologic disturbance is directly traceable to a neurotic conflict. The neurotic conflict in turn seems to be rooted in the disorder of the personality. Notice that both the neurotic conflict and the personality disorder are hypothetical constructs, the presence of which are based on inferred data. In contrast, the behavioral model dissects the patient's problem into changes in behavior and/or physiology. These changes can be determined from observable data that can be quantified. Whereas intervention in the psychosomatic approach is directed at a hypothetical problem, behavioral intervention is aimed at changing behavior and/or physiology directly. The effectiveness of this change is readily assessable through behavioral observation and conventional techniques of physiological monitoring. (p. 2)

From this, it is clear that the narrow definition of behavioral medicine would be fundamentally at odds with the approach of psychosomatic medicine; however, as mentioned previously, psychosomatic medicine has grown much broader and now includes contributions from general systems theory, learning theory, sociology, psychology, and behavior therapy (Lipowski, 1977; Weddington & Blindt, 1983). Following the broad biopsychosocial approach to medicine, some authors feel that behavioral medicine in the 1980s represents the psychosomatic medicine of the 1950s and 1960s (Schwartz & Weiss, 1977). Some authors consider behavioral medicine and psychosomatic medicine to be complementary approaches (Schwartz & Weiss, 1977; Schwartz, 1982; Weddington & Blindt, 1983), while other authors have been more critical of psychosomatic medicine and emphasize the view that psychosomatic medicine has not demonstrated effectiveness in the medical setting. Further, it is asserted that behavioral medicine represents a new and different approach altogether. Basmajian (1985) has quoted Shapiro (1977) on the demonstrated effectiveness of psychosomatic medicine as follows:

> The major inadequacies of psychosomatic medicine have been its excessive reliance on inadequately defined personality processes as a means of explaining why particular people develop particular diseases and, more importantly, its paucity of specific behavioral strategies for relieving or controlling symptoms. (p. 593)

In summary, it seems that a tension exists in defining the field of behavioral medicine. One trend is to define the field so broadly that it replaces the biomedical model with the biopsychosocial model and includes even the contributions of psychosomatic medicine. Yet the field then becomes so broad that the contributions of the themes of effective technology may tend to be lost. The prudence of the other trend, toward defining the field more narrowly, is in distinguishing behavioral medicine from psychosomatic medicine and aligning it with new advances from behavior therapy.

THE ROLE OF BEHAVIOR IN HEALTH

It has already been noted that the recognition of the role of personal behavior, habits, or risk factors was instrumental in creating this chapter's first theme of a broader model of medicine. A second theme, to which we now turn, is that health is habitual, consisting of persistent routines of action, for example, eating, exercising, relaxing, relating to others, etc. The expansion of the discipline of psychology from mental health to include behavioral factors affecting health and illness has been labeled specifically as *health psychology*, a term which refers to the psychologist's role in the broader definition of behavioral medicine. Krantz et al. (1985) reflect on this new field's growth as follows: "Since its inception in the late 1970's, health psychology has taken steps toward becoming a generic area of psychology by establishing its own division within the APA, its own journal, and a set of training guidelines. In addition, this problem-oriented field has brought together researchers and practitioners from a wide variety of psychological subspecialties" (p. 350).

The Division of Health Psychology was established in 1979 and already has over 2500 members. The first president of this division, Joseph Matarazzo, offered the following definition of health psychology:

> Health psychology is the aggregate of the specific educational, scientific, and professional contributions of the discipline of psychology to the promotion and maintenance of health, the prevention and treatment of illness, the identification of etiologic and diagnostic correlates of health, illness, and related dysfunction, and to the analysis and improvement of the health care system and health policy formation. (1982, p. 4)

An important further point made by Matarazzo (1982) is that health psychology not only involves clinical psychologists or applied psychologists but includes a much broader range of subspecialists throughout psychology. This cross-discipline focus is also illustrated by Krantz et al. (1985), who give a practical overview and some examples of the breadth of health psychology by discussing mechanisms linking behavior to physical disease, stress and its effects on health, psychoneuroimmunology, behavioral factors in cardiovascular disorders, cigarette smoking and tobacco use, and obesity and eating disorders.

A complete discussion of health psychology and definitions in behavioral medicine requires the consideration of one further term, *medical psychology*. Both medical psychology and health psychology have been used in connection with or synonymously with the term *behavioral medicine*. As behavioral medicine is a relatively new term, some authors have incorporated it into or assumed it to be a part of their preexisting field. Other authors, using the broad definition, have conceptualized behavioral medicine as the principle field subsuming other disciples and fields. Presently, some psychologists working in hospital settings label their work as health psychology and treat it as a subset of the broader discipline of behavioral medicine. Others use the terms synonymously, and still others see behavioral medicine as a subset of or techniques available to the preexisting field of medical psychology. All of these options are a possibility but not without obvious confusion, especially to those in other disciplines. Historically, medical psychologists have worked in departments of psychiatry. In the United Kingdom, Rachman (1980) has pointed out that the terms medical psychology and psychiatry are almost synonymous, and that the *British Journal of Medical Psychology* is predominately psychiatric in content. In the United States, medical psychologists have played an adjunctive role of relatively low status, applying broad psychological knowledge (usually from a psychodynamic orientation) to the diagnosis and assessment of the psychological bases or correlates of physical illness. Medical psychologists also have been involved as researchers in evaluating treatment outcome. Asken (1979) has pointed out that classical medical psychology consisted of health care studies, psychosomatics (psychodynamic understanding of physical illness), and somatopsychology (the study of body–brain relationships, including clinical neuropsychology). To this list Asken adds the new area of behavioral medicine.

Finally, in medical schools medical psychologists are likely to teach behavioral sciences courses, about human behavior and psychology, to medical students. It is the addition of behavioral medicine to the roles of the medical psychologist that represents a major change in the traditional conceptualization of this field. Rather than being concerned with simply assessing and understanding disorders, medical psychologists have come to take an active role in the prevention, assessment, management, and treatment of an increasing number of such disorders.

THE IMPORTANCE OF RESEARCH

The last and perhaps most crucial theme in the development of behavioral medicine concerns the importance of foundational research. Research is specifically mentioned in the narrow definition of behavioral medicine. Regardless of which approach to defining the field predominates, the importance of research continues to be primary as the field continues to grow. Matarazzo (1982) has made the following comments regarding the national and professional research priority in behavioral health:

> Yet, during the past several years, the National Institutes of Health, the National Science Foundation, and other federal funding agencies, responding to pressures from our citizens and their elected officials, almost monthly have asked graduate departments of psychology to submit proposals for basic and applied research in areas relating to physical health and behavior (Matarazzo, 1980). . . . It is up to those among us who are interested in behavioral health to take the initiatives that will allow us to participate in a new research and teaching enterprise. (p. 12)

Brownell (1984) reflects on the importance of more support for research in behavioral medicine, and considers that a lack of coherent research support will have direct negative effects on a broad behavioral medicine's attempt to integrate many disciplines.

Yet while there has been considerable research in the area of medical psychology, very little of that research has been done in conjunction with physicians. In the medical setting, psychology research remains too provincial and a little naive with regard to the multiplicity of variables affecting disease. So research should provide the impetus for integration of biomedical fields and psychology, yet this has not presently occurred.

Sanson-Fisher (1985) has analyzed the need for research in behavioral medicine in Australia and has proposed that such research be funded by that country's governmental agencies. He proposes that: "Without such research it will be impossible to develop cost-effective, valid and reliable mechanisms for measuring and monitoring health risk behaviors. Furthermore, without research in the field, mechanisms for modifying defined health risks on a group or individual basis will not be developed, with resulting costs to the health status of our community" (p. 279).

This chapter has presented the theoretical framework of and the general limits which encompass the present domain of Behavioral medicine. In the chapters to follow the field will be more specifically laid out through the perspectives of an internationally chosen set of contributors. It is the expectation of the present authors that from these perspectives the reader will appreciate both the scope and the potential of this relatively new yet rapidly developing domain of behavioral medicine.

REFERENCES

Agras, W. S. (1982). Behavioral medicine in the 1980's: Nonrandom connections. *Journal of Consulting and Clinical Psychology, 50*, 797–803.

Asken, M. J. (1979). Medical psychology: Toward definition, clarification, and organization. *Professional Psychology, 10*, 66–72.

Basmajian, J. V. (1985). Keynote address: The next clinical revolution-behavioral medicine. *Journal of American Osteopath Association, 85*, 592–594.

Birk, L. (Ed.). (1973). *Biofeedback: Behavioral medicine.* New York: Grune & Stratton.

Blanchard, E. B. (1982). Behavioral medicine: Past, present, future. *Journal of Consulting and Clinical Psychology, 50*, 595–596.

Brownell, K. D. (1984). Behavioral medicine. In G. T. Wilson, C. M. Franks, K. D. Brownell, & P. C. Kendall (Eds.), *Annual review of behavior therapy: Theory and practice, Vol. 9.* New York: The Guilford Press.

Engel, G. L. (1977). The need for a new medical model: A challenge for biomedicine. *Science, 196*, 129–136.

Gentry, W. D., & Matarazzo, J. D. (1981). Medical Psychology: Three decades of growth and development. In C. K. Prokop & L. A. Bradley (Eds.), *Medical psychology: Contributions to behavioral medicine.* New York: Academic Press.

Heslegrave, R. J. (1985). Behavioral medicine: Managing individual or corporate health? Comment on Cott & Pavloski. *Canadian Psychology, 26*, 168–173.

Inglis, M. (1983). Behavioral science and behavioral medicine revisited. *Canadian Journal of Behavioral Science, 15*, 305–317.

Klippel, J. A., & Dejoy, D. M. (1984). Counseling psychology in behavioral medicine and health psychology. *Journal of Counseling Psychology, 31*, 219–227.

Krantz, D. S., Grunberg, N. E., & Baum, A. (1985). Health psychology. *Annual Review of Psychology, 36*, 349–383.

Lipowski, Z. J. (1977). Psychosomatic medicine in the seventies: An overview. *American Journal of Psychiatry, 134*, 233–244.

Masur, F. T. (1979). An update on medical psychology and behavioral medicine. *Professional Psychology, 10*(2), 259–264.

Matarazzo, J. D. (1980). Behavioral health and behavioral medicine: Frontiers for a new health psychology. *American Psychologist, 35*, 807–817.

Matarazzo, J. D. (1982). Behavioral health's challenge to academic, scientific, and professional psychology. *American Psychologist, 37*, 1–14.

Matarazzo, J. D. (1984). Behavioral Health: A 1990 challenge for the health sciences professions. In J. D. Matarazzo, S. M. Weiss, J. A. Herd, N. E. Miller, & S. M. Weiss (Eds.), *Behavioral health*. New York: John Wiley & Sons.

McDaniel, C. (1984, November 10). Princely medicine. *The Medical Journal of Australia*, pp. 657–659.

Miller, N. E. (1981). An overview of behavioral medicine: Opportunities and dangers. In S. Weiss, A. Herd, & B. Fox (Eds.), *Perspectives on behavioral medicine*. New York: Academic Press.

Miller, N. E. (1983). Behavioral medicine: Symbiosis between laboratory and clinic. *Annual Review of Psychology, 34*, 1–31.

Owen, N. (1983). Commentary: Behavioral medicine. *Community Health Studies, 7*, 85–89.

Pinkerton, S. S., Hughes, H., & Wenrich, W. W. (1982). *Behavioral medicine: Clinical applications*. New York: John Wiley & Sons.

Pomerleau, O. F. (1979). Behavioral medicine: The contribution of the experimental analysis of behavior to medical care. *American Psychologist, 34*, 654–663.

Pomerleau, O. F. (1982). A discourse on behavioral medicine: Current status and future trends. *Journal of Consulting and Clinical Psychology, 50*, 1030–1039.

Pomerleau, O. F., & Brady, J. P. (1979). *Behavioral medicine, theory and practice*. Baltimore: Williams & Wilkins.

Rachman, S. (Ed.). (1980). *Contributions to medical psychology* (Vol. 2). New York: Pergamon Press.

Reading, A. E. (1982). Strategic and methodological aspects of behavioral medicine. *British Journal of Clinical Psychology, 21*, 79–84.

Redd, W. H., & Rusch, F. R. (1985). Behavioral analysis in behavioral medicine. *Behavior Modification, 9*, 131–154.

Sanson-Fisher, R. (1985). Commentary: Behavioral science and its relation to medicine—A need for positive action. *Community Health Studies, 3*, 275–283.

Schwartz, G. E. (1982). Testing the biopsychosocial model: The ultimate challenge facing behavioral medicine? *Journal of Consulting and Clinical Psychology, 50*, 1040–1053.

Schwartz, G., & Weiss, S. (1977). What is behavioral medicine? *Psychosomatic Medicine, 36*, 377–381.

Schwartz, G., & Weiss, S. (1978). Behavioral medicine revisited: An amended definition. *Journal of Behavioral Medicine, 1*, 249–251.

Surwit, R. S., Williams, R. B., & Shapiro, D. (1982). *Behavioral approaches to cardiovascular disease*. New York: Academic Press.

Tapp, J. T. (1985). Multisystems interventions in disease. In N. Schneiderman

& J. T. Tapp (Eds.), *Behavioral medicine: The biopsychosocial approach.* Hillsdale, NJ: Erlbaum.

Thoresen, C. E., & Eagleston, J. R. (1985). Counseling for health. *The Counseling Psychologist, 13,* 15–87.

Wedding, D., & Williams, J. (1983). Training options in behavioral medicine and clinical neuropsychology. *Clinical Neuropsychology, 5,* 100–102.

Weddington, W. W., & Blindt, K. (1983). Behavioral medicine: A new development. *Hospital and Community Psychiatry, 34,* 702–708.

Yates, A. J. (1970). *Behavior therapy.* New York: John Wiley & Sons.

2

Strategies of Assessment in Behavioral Medicine

D. G. Byrne

Department of Psychology
The Australian National University
Canberra

G. R. Caddy

Department of Psychology
Nova University
Fort Lauderdale, FL

ASSESSMENT AND CLINICAL PRACTICE

The comprehensive assessment of the individual patient is a necessary antecedent to any competent treatment. Without a background of systematic information which details both symptoms and the multitude of events preceding, accompanying, or following them, any attempt to intervene either with symptoms or their causes will, at best, amount to intuitive tamperings with human behavior and physiology. At worst, treatment without adequate assessment will lead to directionless excursions into clinical chaos. Just as buildings are not constructed without plans, nor electronic equipment without circuit diagrams, the modification of human behavior and physiology must also rely for its success on the guidance provided by the availability of clear-cut information regarding the nature of the problem and the individual within whom it occurs.

Medicine has had a long-standing tradition of assessment, typically taking the form of a clinical examination, accompanied perhaps by laboratory tests and culminating in the act of diagnosis. The pronouncement of a diagnosis commonly indicates by implication an understanding of those factors causing the symptoms and in the most ideal of situations points unfailingly to a strategy of treatment which, if applied according to a given set of rules, will lead to a reversal of the pathology and the removal of the symptoms. This rather idealized view of medical practice rests, of course, on a highly simplified model of illness. In such a model, tissue pathology which is readily observable and measurable is seen to arise from the operation of a single circumscribed cause. The formation of tissue pathology leads in turn to a situation in which the anatomical and/or physiological integrity of the organism is compromised. The individual will therefore experience this disruption to structure and/or functioning in the form of subjectively felt symptoms, often expressed as pain but frequently involving distress in all its many forms. The grouping together of individual symptoms into commonly held patterns of experience, either on the basis of accumulated clinical wisdom or, in latter times, using statistical procedures to establish categorizations, formed the visible part of the diagnosis and was taken to indicate both cause and treatment.

Such models as these sprang up in the days when simple, single causes were presumed to exist for all manner of illnesses. The historical context was that of classic bacteriological theory, in which momentous advances in the explanation of infectious diseases created the expectation, now known to be fallacious, that all illnesses might ultimately be explained in terms of single, potentially identifiable causes. Modern epidemiology has established that this is not so and that, with the possible exception of a handful of diseases of bacterial or viral origin, the present-day conception of illness is that of a complex and multifactorial process involving contributions, not just from physical pathogens, whether internally or externally encountered, but also from a broad range of individual, personal, behavioral, and social attributes of the individual.

This somewhat more contemporary conception of explanation in medicine comes close, of course, to the views encapsulated in the theme of this series, namely, that organic illness is, in many cases, as much a psychological phenomenon as it is a physical one. Moreover, while the conceptual steps from single cause explanations of illness to multifactorial views are enormous both intellectually and from a practical perspective, the implications for assessment are equally weighty.

Behavioral medicine has been variously described; however, for the purposes of the present chapter, we might take the following contribution as an appropriate basis for discussion:

> The interdisciplinary field concerned with the development and integration of behavioral and biomedical science, knowledge and techniques relevant to health and illness and the application of this knowledge and these techniques to prevention, diagnosis, treatment and rehabilitation. (Schwartz & Weiss, 1978)

Therefore, just as the detailed clinical assessment of the patient is an essential prerequisite to any medical procedure, so too is the clinical assessment of the patient unarguably necessary prior to the implementation of behavioral or psychological procedures designed to alleviate physical symptoms, eliminate behaviors constituting risk factors, or facilitate other behaviors concerned with health promotion. Of course, behavioral medicine itself derives from the science and practice of behavior therapy, which has a long and firmly held tradition of assessment and the evaluation of therapeutic outcomes (Yates, 1975). The most cursory scan of any recent textbook on behavior therapy will attest to the importance given to the role of assessment in the planning and design of behaviorally oriented intervention programmes. Insofar as behavioral medicine involves a unique combination of the scientific approaches espoused both by behavioral psychology and biomedical science, the tradition of systematic and comprehensive assessment prior to the implementation of clinical procedures aimed at intervention cannot be overemphasized.

OBJECTIVES OF ASSESSMENT

The assessment of the individual patient within the context of behavioral medicine has a number of objectives. These relate both to the behavioral and biomedical nature of the individual patient's condition as well as to the various stages which can be delineated in the processes of assessment, treatment, and follow-up. Such a process foreshadows the need for multimodal and sequential assessment covering multiple aspects of the individual's behavior and situation at several points in time. Once more, this is not an uncommon practice in behavior therapy and is to be seen in a number of standardized assessment formats, for example, that of Lazarus's BASIC ID (Lazarus, 1976).

A scan of the literature, both in behavioral medicine and behavior therapy, would indicate, however, that assessment in behavioral medicine should be designed to fulfill one or more of the following objectives.

The Specification of Target Behaviors, Symptoms, or Problems

While the practitioner in behavioral medicine must often face patient conditions which involve multiple foci, it is almost always necessary to limit the attention of behavioral intervention to one or at most a small number of related problems, at least in the first instance. This necessity is brought about, not only by limitations in the therapist's strategies of intervention and the need (possibly) to avoid the simultaneous implementation of potentially conflicting behavioral strategies, but also by the fact that patients themselves have limited capacities to cope with and comply with multiple therapeutic directions and practices. This does not mean that intervention in behavioral medicine must limit itself to simple problems or symptom manifestations. On the contrary, symptomatic patterns of individuals with psychological or behaviorally generated illness can be notoriously complex. It does mean, however, that the therapist, in association with the patient, must make sensible judgments about the degree to which particular components of the illness cause distress, and, of course, the potential complexity and demands of anticipated treatment strategies.

It is common in any behavior therapeutic exercise to establish hierarchies setting out the subjectively rated importance which individual patients attach to the various components of multifaceted problems. So, too, in behavioral medicine the patient and the clinician must typically work together in order to arrange the components of a complex problem into an order which is both amenable to systematic intervention and which suits the need of the individual patient for symptom relief. While this certainly implies that a series of problems rather than one single symptom may need to be worked through in a systematic fashion, it is a much more logical approach to therapy than a haphazard attack on the first symptom or problem which the patient may present in the opening minutes of a clinical interview. In essence, the therapist must structure assessment so as to ensure that the whole range of problems is open both to patient and therapist. Such a specification of target behaviors circumvents a difficulty, common in both medicine and clinical psychology, that the first symptom presented is not necessarily the one most distressing or important to be addressed. It is a commonly observed phenomenon in general practice, for example, that a relatively trivial or unimportant symptom or complaint will be presented as the means of establishing contact with the physician until the patient develops sufficient trust and confidence to reveal perhaps more distressing but more closely guarded difficulties.

The Establishment of Baselines

Both health-related behaviors and symptoms are notoriously variable phenomena. They vary over time in an apparently spontaneous way, and they also vary as a function of the conditions under which they are being observed, monitored, or measured. Importantly, however, both behaviors and symptoms should vary as a function of the implementation of treatment programs. In order to judge the value of a treatment program and the speed with which it is achieving its desired goals, appropriate baselines for target symptoms or behaviors must be measured as precisely as possible to provide the necessary reference point against which intervention strategies may be evaluated.

There are two potential pitfalls in the establishment of baselines which are particularly worthy of note. First, as was earlier pointed out, both behaviors and symptoms are intrinsically variable phenomena, and sufficient time must be devoted to treatment assessment to allow a representative sampling of periods and conditions which will allow the establishment of a realistic as opposed to a time-specific or situation-specific baseline. Relatively stable phenomena may require just a few days of monitoring or measurement, whereas less stable behaviors or symptoms may require a week or more of periodic assessment before the clinician can be confident that he or she has captured a representative sampling of the phenomenon and that the final baseline figure represents a realistic estimate. The time period for the establishment of a baseline will, of course, depend on the frequency of the symptom or behavior itself, so that for relatively infrequent phenomena a rather longer baseline measurement period may be necessary.

Secondly, many kinds of measurement procedures used to establish baselines are themselves *reactive*; that is, they exert a nonspecific but measurable therapeutic effect on the target behavior or symptom. Simple contact with a clinician during the course of a data collection interview may produce a series of nonspecific changes in the patient, all of which may result in therapeutic alterations of both the frequency and intensity of individual problems. The same may be said for patient self-monitoring of symptoms or behaviors. A number of studies have shown that the simple process of keeping a systematic record of behaviors or symptoms produces noticeable changes in the frequencies and amplitudes of those behaviors or symptoms in relation to self-reported baselines. Such a finding may reflect no more than that immediate self-reports of problems may be inaccurate and colored by a range of intervening variables which can neither be identified nor measured. It might also mean, however, that, by drawing a patient's attention to a particular symptom or behavior, there is some immediate behavior modification which works to influence the frequency and intensity of that symptom or behavior (Bellack & Hersen, 1977). The precise mechanism by which this reactivity works is not known; however, the cautious clinician must always note the potential discrepancy between self-reported baselines and those established over a period of systematic measurement, whether by the clinician or by patient self-monitoring.

The Establishment of Associations Between Health Risk Behaviors and the Presence of Symptoms or of Measurable Physical Pathology

Frequently, the relationship between behavior or other psychological attributes of the individual and the presence either of physical symptoms or of underlying organic pathology is no more than an implicit inference. Clinicians infer, often erroneously, from self-reported evidence that, because particular behaviors or psychological attributes exist coincidentally with the presence of symptoms, there is a proven causal association between such attributes and symptoms. In many instances the association may be totally fallacious, and indeed, in some circumstances, the direction of causality may be the reverse of that inferred by the busy clinician; that is, the presence of symptoms or the self-detection of pathology leading to the appearance of particular behaviors or other psychological attributes. There is no question, therefore, that, in competent assessment, the clinician must establish causal associations between aspects of behavioral or individual functioning and the presence of symptoms.

If intervention is to be successfully applied to any systematic manner, it must focus on antecedents of symptoms and not on consequences or on simultaneous events. An important focus of assessment, therefore, is to establish the real nature of associations between behaviors or psychological states and the experience of symptoms in such a way that it can be shown that the former predate the latter. This is not always an easy task, firstly, because of the fact that associations between behavioral or psychological states and physical symptoms are seldom linear or simple, and secondly, because the time course characterizing the influence of one on the other varies widely between individuals and between the nature of the symptoms in question. Moreover, a retrospective approach to this problem can never achieve a precise or in some cases even satisfactory solution. It is essential, therefore, at least to attempt the collection of serial data in an effort to provide an answer that is clinically useful.

Notwithstanding the potential difficulties of such an approach, there are many instances in which it can be successfully applied using brief prospective data collection procedures. Perhaps the best example of this has to do with the use of behavioral diaries in association with symptom check lists that are completed at discreet intervals over the course of a week or so. These intervals may be defined in units of time or by the experience of symptoms. Whichever way the clinician chooses to structure the exercise, it is possible to collect data which allow causal inferences to be drawn at a better than intuitive level.

The task is made simpler if the symptom in question is a simple one, for example, the experience of a headache or an episode of impotence. It is not impossible, however, to devise strategies in which the serial collection of data on more complex patterns of symptoms can provide equally useful results. These data, together with quite simple graphing procedures, are often sufficient to allow the clinician to devise therapeutic strategies with some certainty that these will focus on appropriate patterns of health risk behavior or other psychological states.

Determining Directions for Behavior Change and for Therapeutic Intervention

Where symptom complaints are simple and straightforward, the direction for behavior change, that is, the focus for therapeutic intervention, is typically clear-cut. However, where patients present with a multiple set of problems, some related and others distinct from each other, one of the initial therapeutic decisions must be the clinical domain in which the therapist will first focus. The determination of directions for therapeutic intervention will rest largely on two considerations. The first has to do with the patient's own view of the importance of the various problems being presented. Patients are typically asked in cases of multiple problem presentation to rank order the difficulties which they would like to deal with, from most to least difficult, and the therapeutic intervention is then focused on that problem which the patient sees as the one causing most concern. While this is a convenient way for the therapist to operate, it also presents a goal-oriented approach that many patients will find both comforting and least demanding of their own skills to participate in therapy. The second consideration concerns the clinician's own estimate of the relative importance of the various difficulties being presented. In many cases it is appropriate to allow the patient to make the decisions; however, where particular therapeutic interventions conflict with or contradict one another, it becomes the clinician's ethical responsibility to point this out to the patient in a clear and empathic manner. An example of this may be seen in the case of a patient presenting with the multiple problems of gastric pain, emotional tension, and disturbed marital relationships. While the patient's wish may be to remove pain and relieve tension, it may be the therapist's professional view that neither of these will happen until the marital problem is resolved. Thus, the therapist's responsibility to the client is to attempt to persuade by all necessary means that an alternative hierarchy will be most productive.

Clearly, the selection of a suitable and attainable direction for therapeutic change must be foremost in the therapist's mind at the beginning of any clinical venture. One might give many examples of the importance of this seemingly simple exercise, both in behavioral medicine and in other aspects of clinical psychology. It should be said, however, that the effectiveness of therapeutic intervention will rest to some extent on an eventual agreement between the patient and therapist about what directions behavioral and cognitive change should take, and any major disagreement in this respect is likely to provide an equally major obstacle to a successful therapeutic outcome.

Evaluating the Effectiveness of Therapeutic Intervention

While most clinicians will unreservedly agree on the need for assessment as an antecedent to therapeutic intervention, few will give more than tacit recognition to the need for systematic follow-up and evaluation. Courses in research methodology emphasize both the desirability of and the technology for achieving effective evaluation; however, clinical practice gives rather less attention to the application of this technology in a standard clinical exercise. Many patients are terminated for no other reason than that one or other of the parties (the therapist or the patient) has decided that some unspecified and unmeasured gains have been reached and that little more is likely to be accomplished through the course of structured encounters (Molloy & Sharpley, 1986).

What frequently goes unrecognized is that neither the parameters of therapeutic change nor the degree to which change has occurred have been identified and measured. Therefore, therapy may be prematurely terminated or, by contrast, may be allowed to proceed for a seemingly interminable period of time without demonstrable benefits, all because an appropriate evaluation strategy has not been built into the overall patient management plan.

Some clinicians may argue that the use of such evaluation strategies is not borne out in a cost–benefit analysis, and that therapeutic intuition or a cursory self-report by the patient of therapeutic progress is a sufficient metric to allow clinical judgments regarding termination or continuation of therapy to be made. Certainly, the establishment and implementation of an evaluation strategy within an overall management plan requires some additional effort and thought and certainly demands the undertaking of serial measures during the course of therapy and for a period thereafter. If the clinician is to take the trouble to establish baselines, however, he or she must surely proceed to the logical conclusion of testing therapeutic outcomes against those baselines in a systematic manner. The potential loss, both personally and economically to the patient, of having therapy extend fruitlessly beyond a reasonable period of time for no apparent further gain would seem to far outweigh the relatively small effort to evaluate therapy over the course of intervention.

A related benefit of systematic evaluation has to do with the phenomenon frequently observed in behavioral medicine, namely relapse. While many therapeutic interventions for symptoms of all kinds may well be successful to a greater or lesser degree in the short term, the continuation of success in the long term is a far less certain occurrence. Therapists may thus be persuaded that their initial therapeutic success will produce long-term benefits when in fact reversion to old risk behaviors or past patterns of symptoms is a common event. Without systematic evaluation of therapeutic outcome, therapists are frequently unaware of such reversions to baseline and a great deal of initial effort is then lost. While such evaluation may occur at an informal level by way of patients returning to therapists if symptoms or problem behaviors return, the use of even simple but systematic evaluation procedures over a time course of up to a year may result in very substantial therapeutic gains.

Estimating Compliance with Therapeutic Directions

Lack of compliance plays a notable part in the failure of any therapeutic intervention. It is prudent, therefore, at the outset of a therapeutic program to attempt to estimate the extent to which individual patients will choose to or be able to comply with instructions or directions given to them as part of their program.

Failure to comply with therapeutic instructions may be attributed to the operation of one or more of four general categories of influence—

these being a failure to adequately understand the instructions, a failure on the part of the therapist to recognize the degree of inconvenience which the therapeutic instructions might cause to the patient, a lack of motivation on the patient's part to achieve the degree or direction of change proposed by the therapist, and a failure of the program of therapy to meet the patient's expectations, either in terms of the direction of change or rapidity of change over the course of the therapeutic program (Masur, 1981).

There is a wide literature now indicating that failures of compliance may arise partly because patients are unable to fully understand and appreciate the nature of the instructions provided by the therapist. Where this is anticipated, it may well be important for the therapist to assess, at least at an informal level, both the patient's general ability to comprehend instructions and specific comprehension of the instructions given as part of the proposed program of therapy. Inconvenience too may present a measurable impediment to therapeutic progress. The therapist may therefore deem it wise to check very closely with the patient the extent to which therapeutic instructions will impinge on daily obligations, whether these be to occupational, family, or other concerns, and to attempt to structure a therapeutic program so that it produces the least general inconvenience for the patient. Of course, a balance must be struck between the necessary demands of therapy and the necessary obligations placed on the patient by factors external to the therapeutic situation; however, even brief questioning in this area should allow the therapist to gauge the extent to which a therapeutic program is likely to cause difficulties and therefore not be adhered to, or require specific motivation induction procedures to be implemented in order to maximize the prospects of compliance.

The motivation which individual subjects have to change health related behaviors or to lose symptoms is also a factor which needs to be assessed prior to the implementation of a therapeutic program. For the majority of patients the pain and discomfort of symptoms, or the potential health risk of behaviors, is sufficiently great to produce a substantial motivation for change. For others, however, the reasons for seeking help may be less clear-cut. Pressure to stop smoking, for example, may come more from relatives or physicians than from the individual himself or herself, and so the motivation to change this health related behavior may not be as great as if the patient had personally decided to stop smoking. Some patients may also gain particular advantages from the possession of pain or of symptoms. These advantages may come by way of abrogation of personal, occupational, or parental roles, as happens in the sociological concept of the sick role or in the elicitation of additional degrees of caring behavior from other people in response to the presence of symptoms, as may occur with abnormal illness behavior. In these and many other cases where the decision to seek help is not a personal one or where the value of symptoms may override the value of their removal, the potential reduction in motivation for change may have quite profound effects on the effectiveness of therapeutic outcome. The therapist must therefore attempt to ascertain the extent to which an individual patient is motivated to change behaviors or symptoms prior to the commencement of therapy.

Finally, ultimate compliance may be related to discrepancies between the actual rate of progress of a therapeutic program and expectations held by therapists and patients regarding rates of change. Where these expectations are aligned, dissatisfaction during the course of therapy is likely to be low and cooperation and compliance on the part of the patient will be correspondingly high. Where a major discrepancy occurs, however, patients may begin to wonder about the competence of the therapist, the extent to which symptom alleviation can be achieved, or the rapidity with which behavior change will take place. This resulting dissatisfaction may well produce corresponding decreases, or at least unfortunate fluctuations in compliance behaviors, which in turn may impair the progress and process of therapy. Simple questioning at the outset of any therapeutic programming regarding the client's expectations will serve to alert the therapist to any potential discrepancies which might occur and to allow the therapist to correct these before they impose on the patients and clients.

Establishing Contraindications and Fitting the Individual to the Program of Therapy

Clearly, not all patients will accept all kinds of therapeutic interventions, and in some cases there may be quite specific physiological or psychological reasons why a particular kind of therapy is not indicated for a certain patient. A patient, for example, with a long standing history of help-seeking behaviors may have attempted a large number of therapeutic interventions in order to overcome a particular problem, many of which may have been unsuccessful. The experience associated with this lack of success may create negative impressions of particular therapeutic styles of strategies, and, if the therapist is unaware of this, the potential outcome success of therapy may well be impaired. Assessment regarding past therapeutic experiences and the success or failure of these would, therefore, seem to be a necessary antecedent step to the implementation of any new program of therapy.

Some kinds of therapy demand particular activities which certain kinds of patients are unable to cope with. Difficulties such as inconvenience have been dealt with in previous sections. It is not uncommon, however, for patients to have particular aversions either to the ideology or the practice of certain kinds of therapeutic strategies. Patients sometimes, for example, express concerns regarding relaxation procedures which come too close to meditation with its spiritual connotations. Other patients may, for example, have great difficulty in externalizing cognitions or in achieving the process of visual imagery. These potential contraindications to particular kinds of therapies need to be assessed at the outset and the therapeutic strategy devised according to those parameters of therapy which the patient is likely to tolerate.

At a completely different level, there may be particular physiological contraindications to certain kinds of therapies which, if not assessed and avoided, may lead to potentially damaging physiological reactions. Active Jacobsonian relaxation procedures might, for example, produce transient but alarming increases in blood pressure in patients with reactive hypertension, and muscle relaxation procedures based on isometric techniques for muscle contraction have been known to produce episodes of chest pain in patients with unstable angina. Along similar lines, patients with specific bone disorders may experience considerable pain if relaxation exercises are too active or vigorous. Physiological and anatomical contraindications must, therefore, be checked quite scrupulously prior to the implementation of certain kinds of therapeutic strategies and particularly those based on psychophysiological methods. Some therapists go so far as to insist on a complete medical examination and a clearance from the physician prior to the implementation of therapy employing psychophysiological strategies.

THE FOCI OF ASSESSMENT

Clinical assessment is guided by a multitude of formats and styles, each of which directs the clinician's attention to the range of areas which require systematic scrutiny prior to the implementation of a therapeutic program. In clinical psychology, perhaps the most widespread and comprehensive of these is Arnold Lazarus's BASIC ID (Lazarus, 1976), which encourages the clinician, prior to the onset of active therapy, to inquire into the areas of behavior, affect, sensation, imagery, cognitions, interpersonal relationships, and drugs (biological influences). Such formats as these promote very comprehensive assessments and ensure that all areas of the individual are adequately, systematically, and appropriately assessed.

The demands of behavioral medicine do, however, differ somewhat from those of clinical psychology at large, and admirable as the BASIC ID or similar assessment formats are, the particular needs of behavioral medicine require the clinician to look again at the overall structure of assessment of individual functioning. Specifically, the model of illness usually seen in behavioral medicine is that of stress, where the occurrence of potentially unpleasant events in the individual's environment achieves, through a series of cognitive mechanisms, a set of affective and physiological responses which, if they are prolonged or if they impinge on vulnerable organ systems, may produce tissue damage and measurable pathology. The occurrence both of emotional and physiological responses to exposure to stressors, together with the pathology which may result, produce, in turn, a set of subjective experiences or symptoms which may themselves produce quite profound and incapacitating responses in the form of illness behaviors. This postulated sequence of events has been widely discussed in the literature and need not be gone into in further detail here. Those who are interested in reading further may be advised to consult a number of recent and authoritative review articles (Levi, 1977; Henderson, Byrne, & Duncan-Jones, 1981). This approach to conceptualizing the development of physical symptoms from behavioral and psychological antecedents does, however, point to a well-structured format for assessment in behavioral medicine which, if adhered to, will provide a systematic approach to the collection of clinical data prior to the implementation of a therapeutic intervention. While this approach is by no means the only one to provide useful data in behavioral medicine, its somewhat exhaustive coverage of the individual in his or her environmental context does provide the basis for the collection of very comprehensive data.

It is suggested, therefore, that, in collecting data on individual functioning within the environmental context prior to the implementation of an intervention program, the clinician should look systematically at the following areas in order to obtain the most complete overview of the patient and his or her environment.

The Environment

Individuals do not exist in isolation but within the confines of an environment which is defined in terms of its collective social, interpersonal, occupational, spiritual, and physical parameters. Interactions between the individual and the environment play a crucial role in the regulation of health and illness and are, therefore, of considerable importance in the study of behavioral medicine.

Perhaps the most prominent example of this relationship has emerged from the literature documenting the role of stressful life events in the onset of illness (Henderson et al., 1981). It is now widely accepted that those individuals who encounter a surfeit of events or occurrences in their environments which demand life change or which bring about feelings of distress or loss of control are more prone to the onset of illnesses of many kinds, including cardiovascular disease, gastrointestinal disease, minor infections, and respiratory diseases, than are those individuals whose lives are less punctuated by such events. While there has recently been some considerable debate, both on the measurement of life events or other environmental factors and on the extent to which life event occurrence contributes to the onset of illness (Byrne, 1986), there is now little question that such influences must be taken account of in epidemiological studies of human disease processes.

Just as such measurement is pertinent to epidemiology, it must also be seen as a prerequisite to individual clinical practice. One of the most common foci for assessment in behavioral medicine has been found to be that of environmental precursors to illness. It would, therefore, seem to be a necessary antecedent to clinical intervention in behavioral medicine that the individual's environment is assessed either for actual or potential stressors (Byrne, 1984). Even the most cursory scanning of this area frequently reveals the presence of major and easily remediable stressors which can be dealt with in the course of therapeutic intervention by means of quite modest life-style restructuring.

The Interpretive Process

While life events have been statistically linked with the onset of illness for some considerable time, more recent research has suggested that it is not simply the life event occurrence, but the way in which the individual interprets that life event occurrence, which determines the probability of illness. The work of Richard Lazarus (Lazarus, 1967) has demonstrated with great experimental sophistication that individuals interpret life events in different and highly idiosyncratic ways. Therefore, in addition to looking simply at the occurrence of life events or stressors, it is now considered to be important to assess the individual impact which these have on those to whom they occur.

Two sets of research studies from the area of cardiovascular disease serve to illustrate this point. The first has to do with the role of stressful life events in the onset of myocardial infarction. While a number of studies have indicated that the simple accumulation of life events predisposes to myocardial infarction, it has more recently been shown that it is the individual's interpretation of these life events which is the more important correlate of heart attack. A study by Byrne and Whyte (1980) showed that, while patients with documented myocardial infarction were not distinguished from noncardiovascular medical controls by the simple frequency of occurrence of life events, those patients who had sustained a major cardiovascular event had been, in the past, more likely to interpret those life events which had occurred to them as distressing than had the control subjects. This is very much in accord with the experimental work of Lazarus suggesting the interpolation of a cognitive filter or interpretive mechanism between the recognition of life event encounters and the organization of affective and physiological responses to these.

The second example concerns itself with responses to major illness. Once more, taking cardiovascular disease as the exemplar model, it has been shown that people with myocardial infarction vary widely in the magnitude of their responses to that event. Some respond in a fashion indicating acceptance of coping, while others are considerably traumatized by the experience of myocardial infarction. Investigation of this phenomenon would suggest once more that people interpret this life event in individually specific ways and in ways which are consistent with such factors as pain tolerance, past experience, societal expectation, and the like. Again, therefore, one must postulate the possibility of an interpretive mechanism which determines the extent to which an individual will respond to any major illness event in his or her life.

These findings do not necessarily attach only to cardiovascular disease. Similar conclusions may be drawn from evidence relating to other illnesses, both in terms of antecedents and consequences. Such evidence does, however, underscore the need to examine the tendency of each individual to respond adaptively or otherwise to major life events. There is some evidence that those individuals with the personality attribute of neuroticism will be more likely to respond in a maladaptive or catastrophic manner to major life events than those individuals free of this trait. There are, however, a wide range of additional factors which would seem to bear on the interpretation of life events, and this individual specific tendency should be investigated in conjunction with the clinical assessment of the patient's environmental load (Byrne, 1983).

Behavioral Predispositions to Health and Illness

A great deal of individual health risk is mediated through specific behaviors. Smoking, for example, is a discreet human behavior, as is eating to excess. Compliance with therapeutic regimes too, may be seen as a complex of individual behaviors. Thus, the process of development of many forms of illness, as well as the course which particular illnesses may take after onset, can be seen as having quite distinct behavioral contributions. It is important at the outset to recognize those behaviors which contribute to risk of illness or to prolongation or recurrence of illness after onset.

Some behaviors at odds with health may be quite simple both to conceptualize and to assess. Smoking behavior is a good example of this (though of course, the accuracy of recall and self-report of smoking behavior has occasionally been questioned). Others, such as compliance with therapeutic regimes, may be more complex and may, therefore, require a more detailed conceptualization and a multimodal approach to assessment. In either event, however, assessment prior to clinical intervention should include an evaluation of individual behaviors which might either promote ill health or prolong the course of recovery and rehabilitation following an episode of illness.

Affective State

Often the most immediate sign of the process of stress is that of affective distress. Individuals who have encountered a surfeit of life events and who have perceived these as distressing will frequently in the first stages show evidence of recognizable emotional upheaval. In the most immediate sense this usually takes the form of anxiety, though, if anxiety is prolonged, depression typically follows (Byrne, 1984).

Assessment of affective distress in behavioral medicine is important in a number of respects. Firstly, as we have just said, it is frequently the first sign of the onset of a stress reaction. Secondly, however, it is possible to trace biological pathways through which protracted affective distress may lead to transient physical symptomatology and eventually, in cases of severe distress over long periods of time, to actual physical pathology. Thus, emotional distress may provide the first psychological marker of deleterious, physiological affects which might follow.

Emotional distress may also impinge on the effectiveness of therapeutic intervention, since individuals who are highly anxious or deeply distressed may be less amenable to behavior change than those whose emotional state is more stable. The hopelessness surrounding depression, for example, may cloud an individual's ability to understand the necessity of modifying patterns of exercise after heart attack or of eating behavior in those who are pathologically obese. The presence of severe affective distress can, therefore, noticeably impair the success of behavior change in those requiring modification of physical symptomatology.

Assessment of individual behaviors, in so far as they relate to health risk or illness, is an important objective in the early assessment of the individual in behavioral medicine. Such assessment is usually a straightforward matter, however, in some instances health risk behaviors may be subtly hidden or guarded from the clinician and a degree of skill is often required in eliciting the necessary clinical data.

Physiological Responses

Psychophysiological reactivity in the fact of stressors or other environmental challenges is seen as the most likely mediator between psychological states and the development of physical pathology. Abundant evidence from a number of sources may be cited in support of this view, including evidence from studies of cardiovascular disease, gastrointestinal disease, and respiratory disease (Surwit, Williams, & Shapiro, 1981). The extent to which any individual demonstrates psychophysiological reactivity in the face of challenge must therefore constitute a potential focus for assessment in behavioral medicine.

There will, of course, be some contention surrounding this issue—firstly, in view of the evidence challenging the reliability of psychophysiological data, and, secondly, in view of the technical sophistication required in order to successfully achieve such an assessment. Determinants of psychophysiological reactivity are complex, and many factors apart from the underlying integrity of the individual's autonomic nervous system may contribute to variability in such measures. Simple environmental variables such as temperature and humidity, equipment variables such as electronic stability of preamplifiers, procedural factors such as the site and correctness of electrode placements, and psychological factors including fear of novel situations may all lead to widely varying results from psychophysiological testing in the same individual. Moreover, the technology of psychophysiological measurement has now reached such a level of sophistication that complex and expensive equipment and training in the use of that equipment is necessary before the clinician can be sure of stable and replicable measures. These considerations place some caution on the routine use of psychophysiological testing. There will, however, be instances in which simple psychophysiological assessment will contribute to the overall view of the patient. The use of brief electromyographical recording to demonstrate differential levels of muscle tension may, for example, establish the necessary focus for muscle relaxation in patients with diagnosed tension headache. Similarly, an examination of an electrocardiographic trace may provide useful information in determining the psychological treatment of psychogenic tachycardia. Therefore, while psychophysiological assessment should not be ruled out as too difficult, lengthy, or costly, it is perhaps not the area of assessment which will be seen as routine in behavioral medicine.

Symptoms of Illness

The primary emphasis in many aspects of behavioral medicine is the removal of symptoms of illness. It follows from this that a very detailed assessment of these symptoms must be undertaken prior to the initiation of therapeutic strategies. Symptoms may vary from simple reports of periodic pain through to complex patterns of experience and behavior which might be seen in such disorders as asthma. Moreover, the assessment of symptoms requires not only the self-report of subjectively perceived experiences but also information on the frequency and duration of these experiences, the intensity with which they are felt, the degree of distress and incapacity which they cause to all aspects of life, and the impact which these symptoms have on significant others. In this respect, it is also useful to have information on the perceptions of symptom frequency, duration, and intensity by significant other people in the patient's interpersonal environment.

Such information collection frequently requires the expenditure of some time and the serial accumulation of data. In certain cases it also requires that others, in addition to the patient, be interviewed with regard to the patient's symptoms. This is particularly important when the motivation for help seeking has come by way of pressure from another individual. In view of the central focus of symptomatology in the practice of behavioral medicine, however, it is essential that the most careful assessment of symptoms and their underlying pathology takes place prior to active treatment strategies.

Illness Behavior

In the field of behavioral medicine, psychological and behavioral factors should not only be considered in terms of their contribution to illness events. The experience of illness can bring with it a marked alteration in patterns of psychological and behavioral functioning that may be recognized as illness behavior. For some patients, the dominant response to illness is one of adaptation and coping, so that, while psychological and behavioral functioning may be impaired in direct result of the illness, this impairment is usually transient and consistent in degree with the nature of the illness.

Two aspects of this process should be borne in mind, however, in assessing the patient in a behavioral medicine context. Firstly, some patients may take on the sick role, which allows them to abrogate ordinary social, occupational, and interpersonal roles, and assume instead a role of dependency and reliance on others. If prolonged, this sick role may become, through reinforcement, an attractive alternative to ordinary social roles and a strong incentive to retain at least the external manifestations of illness. Not surprisingly, those patients who embrace the sick role may prove particularly resistant to treatment.

More recently, however, the concept of abnormal illness behavior has come into being. This has to do with emotional, behavioral, or cognitive responses to illness which are at odds with recovery, rehabilitation, and return to a preillness lifestyle (Pilowsky, 1969). Abnormal illness behaviors range from emotional responses to illness that are considerably in excess of those warranted by the nature of the symptoms or the seriousness of the pathology, to a complete denial of the importance of symptoms and of the need for their removal. Though the ramifications of these two extremes differ, they both have the end result of prolonging the experience of symptoms and, perhaps, of contributing to a deterioration in the underlying pathology. Individual responses to symptoms, and the responses of significant others in the interpersonal environment, should therefore be carefully assessed in order to elucidate those aspects of illness behavior which might prove to be deleterious to the expected course of recovery and rehabilitation following treatment.

Other Foci for Assessment

Specific individuals will inevitably require particular approaches to assessment, and these will also be determined by the nature of particular illnesses. In situations where substantial behavior change is required, for example, it may be necessary to undertake careful assessment of motivation for behavior change, and of the nature of social and interpersonal support systems which are available to assist this process.

It should always be remembered as well that, in behavioral medicine, we are dealing with disorders the pathology and appearance of which are essentially physiological and anatomical in nature, and it is incumbent on us as ethical practitioners to be aware of the underlying medical, genetic, and pathological states. In some cases, this may require the conduct of a thorough medical examination by a qualified physician prior to final decisions regarding the implementation of behavioral strategies. Some clinicians in behavioral medicine may even consider the medical examination to be a mandatory part of the overall assessment of the patient. It is certainly important if there are problems to do with medicolegal considerations, or if there are particular contrary indications to therapeutic strategies which must be taken into account. In any event, the patient's medical condition, and the knowledge of factors underlying this, should not be neglected in complete favor of a behavioral approach to the solution of clinical problems.

The area of personality is perhaps most contentious in the overlapping fields of behavioral and psychosomatic medicine (Bradley & Prokop, 1981). For some, personality is an historical irrelevance and need not be considered in any respect. For others, it is more theoretically palatable to give credence to underlying personality traits which may predispose either to particular kinds of stress reactions or to particular forms of illness. Assessment of personality will, therefore, depend very largely on the theoretical preconceptions held by individual clinicians. Some, however, will deem it necessary to undertake a comprehensive assessment of personality, particularly insofar as it relates to individual reactions to environmental stressors as a precursor to the treatment of the individual suffering from a stress reaction.

TECHNIQUES FOR ASSESSMENT

Assessment in behavioral medicine has no unique methodology of its own. As in many other areas of clinical practice, it draws on a variety of methods and techniques to produce an overall profile of the individual patient. These techniques are largely, but not exclusively, drawn from the area of clinical psychology, and a great deal has been written on the methodology of assessment from this perspective. Reference to any of a number of recent and widely respected texts will provide a very comprehensive overview of the process of clinical information gathering from the technical perspective (Bradley & Prokop, 1981; Ferguson & Taylor, 1980).

Assessment is typically, though somewhat simply, divided according to the three components of intake information, process, and evaluation of outcomes. Specific methodologies used in each of these three components will overlap to a very large extent, though some may be more suitable to specific components of the overall therapeutic strategy than others. Briefly, the principal techniques for clinical assessment may be categorized as follows.

The Clinical Interview

This is perhaps the most common form of data collection in clinical practice, and though it might vary from the totally structured and closed ended to the completely spontaneous and open ended, it relies on a dyadic interaction between the clinician and the patient for the purpose of data gathering. Such an interaction requires, at the very least, two things. The first is that the clinician has a relatively clear-cut view of the points of information which must be dealt with. That is, the clinician should decide beforehand on those areas of primary importance which are crucial to the presenting problem and about which information must be collected as a necessary prerequisite to the formation and implementation of a therapeutic intervention strategy. The second is that the clinician must necessarily build up a workable relationship or rapport with the patient prior to the inquiry regarding the detailed nature of the presenting problem. Such a relationship demands trust and mutual respect if it is to work in such a way that the patient is willing to disclose both painful and perhaps sensitive material regarding the problem for which help is being sought.

Interviews vary widely in duration. Some will, in the first instance, be very brief and may be seen as a mere preliminary to a more protracted data gathering exercise. Others will extend over one or more clinical sessions and will involve nothing more than data gathering for the first few days of patient contact. The choice of duration of a clinical interview is very much a matter for the particular clinician to decide. It is often decided, at least partly, on the basis of level of experience, so that some very experienced clinicians will choose to initiate the beginnings of therapeutic intervention after an apparently brief period of data gathering.

The degree of structure which an interview has as its basis is also a distinctly variable phenomenon. Some clinicians will use interviews, the structure of which is rigidly set and which may form the basis of a recognized assessment instrument, for example, the Present State Examination (Wing, Cooper, & Sartorius, 1974). Others will devise their own structures but stick more or less rigidly to the same pattern of questioning across all patients. Others will be entirely flexible regarding the data gathering and will use the interaction to collect information as it seems appropriate in the course of the interview.

Once more, these are matters essentially of a personal choice, and there are no absolute dictates. It is advisable, however, to remember the rule that the less experienced the interviewer, the more structured the interview should be, in order to insure that salient and subtle points of information regarding the patient, his or her symptoms, and the underlying biopsychosocial situation are not neglected.

Behavioral Self-Report

It is tacitly accepted that the most appropriate observer of individual behavior is that individual who is exhibiting the behavior in question. Thus, it is common in behavioral medicine to ask patients to observe their own behaviors as well as feelings and thoughts, and to record these over a period of time and in a variety of situations for later discussion with the clinician. The use of so-called behavioral diaries is a very common technique of data collection, both in clinical psychology and behavioral medicine.

Once more, the degree to which the data collection exercise is structured will vary from one individual to another and will reflect the degree of clinician's choice. Some clinicians allow a completely open-ended report of behaviors, thoughts, and feelings, while others will want to impose a degree of structure onto the manner in which patients make self-reports. In the latter case clinicians may want to specify the time period, the duration, the situation under which self-reports are being made, the format with which self-reports are made (direct narrative, the use of visual rating scales, or other formalized procedures), and the nature of the behaviors, thoughts, or feelings about which self-reports are required. While behavioral diaries can therefore take many forms, they are typically most useful when they contain a degree of structure, since structure implies at least that the clinician has a set of clinical hypotheses which are to be tested. The existence of such clinical hypotheses suggests, in turn, that the clinician has a degree of understanding of the nature of the problem.

Two cautions must be mentioned with regard to the use of behavioral self-report as a means of clinical data collection. The first is that individuals are not always the most reliable reporters of their own behaviors or experiences. A good example of this comes from the area of the self-reported collection of cigarette consumption rates, where it has been shown that self-reported rates do not always correlate highly with biological measures of the ingestion of cigarette smoke. For this reason it is always best to ensure that behavioral self-report is not the only means of the collection of clinical data. Secondly, it is now commonly accepted that behavioral self-report is a reactive measure. That is, the self-reporting of behaviors may result in a change in the frequency and intensity of those behaviors. Thus, the mere act of reporting and self-monitoring of one's own behaviors may exert a subtle therapeutic effect which might then contaminate or mask the effects of primary therapy. These two cautions should always be observed when employing behavioral self-report; however, this technique, in conjunction with appropriate techniques of simple statistical display, may provide a very powerful means of gathering clinical information over the course of time. Indeed, the sensible use of such data, appropriately displayed to patients, may play an important role in the process of therapy itself.

Direct Behavioral Observation

Perhaps the most comprehensive way of gaining clinical information, particularly where it regards specific behaviors, is that of direct behavioral observation. This involves the clinician or some other objective person spending time with the patient in specified situations, directly observing and recording the patient's behavior. When undertaken in a structured way, it provides a very detailed and comprehensive overview of the individual's activities.

There are, however, drawbacks to this technique. Firstly, it is exceptionally time consuming and requires the expenditure of a great deal of effort on the part of the therapist or technician. Thus, it is most likely to be useful only in cases where abnormal behaviors are relatively circumscribed and where these present with a reasonable frequency. Secondly, direct behavior observation is intrusive and may bring with it the disadvantages both that the behaviors in question will not be completed in the same way or to the same extent or with the same frequency as they might have been if unobserved. The observer may simply be unable to enter into some situations where the behaviors are most likely to be manifest. Therefore, while the direct observation of behavior has a distinct use in certain circumscribed situations, its use is limited to a large extent and most likely not to be seen as a routine form of assessment.

Questionnaires and Scales

Depending on the clinician's theoretical preconceptions of the nature of behavioral disorders, structured questionnaires and scales may be used to assess discrete aspects of the individual's experiences or psychological make-up. Mood scales are most frequently to be seen in this respect, since they provide convenient and relatively brief ways of assessing affective discomfort. The choice of scales will vary widely from one clinician to another. Some will prefer simple visual analogue scales with little semantic content, whereas others will require a more comprehensive approach to the assessment of mood, involving a number of questions each of which purportedly taps a different aspect of the emotion in question. One advantage of the brief and relatively unstructured visual analogue scale methods is that they may be used in a serial fashion to assess changes in mood over time and over the course of therapy and they may, therefore, be used as a means of evaluating both process and outcome.

More and more rarely, clinicians are using structured personality tests in order to guide therapeutic activities. The use of such tests requires an acceptance on the part of the clinician that personality is, firstly, a meaningful concept, and, secondly, that the trait scores which emerge from various tests provide useful information in attempting to modify behavior affect and thought.

Psychophysiological Measures

As we mentioned in the last section, the use of psychophysiological measures frequently requires some degree of technological sophistication together with access to a psychophysiological laboratory containing equipment of a kind necessary to make appropriate measures. For this reason, while psychophysiological measurement is certainly used and perhaps with greater and greater frequency in behavioral medicine, it is by no means a widespread technique of assessment. Nonetheless, with the progressive availability of psychophysiological equipment and with the continued emergence of research data indicating psychophysiological pathways between psychological and behavioral states and events of physical illness, it is anticipated that psychophysiological measurement will assume a greater importance in assessment in behavioral medicine in the future.

Enquiries to Significant Others

It has been previously mentioned that the individual patient may not be the most reliable or accurate observer of his or her own behaviors, thoughts, or feelings. For this reason, corroborative information is often sought from one or more significant other people. This approach provides useful cross-checks, and in situations involving family difficulties may itself be enlightening in terms of the disparities which emerge between patient and spouse reports. It does, however, raise two difficulties which must be attended to.

Firstly, the significant other may also not be an accurate or reliable reporter of information. It must not be assumed that, because an individual is close to the patient in question, the individual will necessarily provide an objective or accurate report of that person's behaviors or feelings that will be stable over time.

The second difficulty has to do with considerations of confidentiality and ethics. In many situations, patients will wish to discuss their particular problems only with the clinician and will not want the involvement of other people in any part of the clinical process. In these situations this request must be respected absolutely, and the use of significant others to collect clinical data without the express permission of the patient should be seen as a serious breach of professional ethics.

REFERENCES

Bellack, A. S., & Hersen, M. (1977). *Behavioral modification: An introduction.* Baltimore, MD: Williams and Wilkins.

Bradley, L. A., & Prokop, C. K. (1981). The relationship between medical psychology and behavioral medicine. In C. K. Prokop & L. A. Bradley (Eds.), *Medical psychology: Contributions to behavioral medicine.* New York: Academic Press.

Byrne, D. G. (1983). Personal determinants of life event stress and myocardial infarction. *Psychotherapy and Psychosomatics, 40,* 106–114.

Byrne, D. G. (1984). Personal assessments of life event stress and the near future onset of psychological symptoms. *British Journal of Medical Psychology, 57,* 241–248.

Byrne, D. G. (1986). Psychological factors and disease. In N. J. King & A. Remenyi (Eds.), *Health care: A behavioural approach.* Sydney, Australia: Grune & Stratton.

Byrne, D. G., & Whyte, H. M. (1980). Life events and myocardial infarction revisited: The role of measures of individual impact. *Psychosomatic Medicine, 42,* 1–10.

Ferguson, J. M., & Taylor, C. B. (Eds.). (1980). *The comprehensive handbook of behavioral medicine* (3 vols.). New York: Spectrum Publications.

Henderson, S., Byrne, D. G., & Duncan-Jones, P. (1981). *Neurosis and the social environment.* Sydney, Australia: Academic Press.

Lazarus, A. A. (1976). *Multimodal behavior therapy.* New York: Springer.

Lazarus, R. S. (1967). *Psychological stress and the coping process.* New York: McGraw-Hill.

Levi, L. (Ed.). (1977). *Emotions: Their parameters and measurement.* New York: Raven Press.

Masur, F. T. (1981). Adherence to health care regimens. In C. B. Prokop & L. A. Bradley (Eds.), *Medical psychology: Contributions to behavioral medicine.* New York: Academic Press.

Molloy, G. N., & Sharpley, C. F. (1986). Assessment strategies and experimental design. In N. J. King & A. Remenyi (Eds.), *Health care: A behavioural approach.* Sydney, Australia: Grune & Stratton.

Pilowsky, I. (1969). Abnormal illness behaviour. *British Journal of Medical Psychology, 42*, 347–351.

Schwartz, G. E., & Weiss, S. M. (1978). Behavioral medicine revisited: An amended definition. *Journal of Behavioral Medicine, 1*, 249–252.

Surwit, R. S., Williams, R. B., & Shapiro, D. (1981). *Behavioral approaches to cardiovascular disease.* New York: Academic Press.

Wing, J. K., Cooper, J. E., & Sartorius, N. (1974). *The measurement and classification of psychiatric symptoms.* Cambridge, England: Cambridge University Press.

Yates, A. J. (1975). *Theory and practice in behavior therapy.* New York: Wiley.

II

THE VASCULAR SYSTEM

3

The Pathophysiology of Vascular Disease

D. G. Byrne

Department of Psychology
The Australian National University
Canberra

THE ANATOMY OF THE HEART AND CIRCULATION

Gross Anatomy

The human heart is a four-chambered organ the sole purpose of which is to provide the pumping force necessary for the circulation of the blood to the body. It is fixed within the thoracic cavity by means of the pericardial sac. This sac is composed of layers of collagen tissue, fits closely around the epicardial surface of the heart, and is separated from the heart by pericardial fluid which serves a lubricating function, since the human heart is in constant motion. The pericardial sac is in turn attached at various points, both to the diaphragm and to the sternum, by a series of ligaments.

The tissue of the heart is composed of a series of muscle layers, which can be collectively termed the *myocardium*, and is divided into four precisely interconnected chambers. The atria, which are situated in the superior (upper) part of the heart, are separated from the ventricles, which are situated in the inferior (lower) part of the heart, by a fibrous ring of muscle bundles. Both the atria and ventricles are divided into right and left sections by septa. The flow of blood between the various chambers of the heart is, in the healthy individual, closely regulated by the presence of valves.

Venous blood enters the right atrium by means of the superior Vena Cava and descends through the tricuspid valve into the right ventricle. At a point where the myocardium is relaxed (diastole), this flow is unimpaired; however, when the myocardium is in a state of contraction (systole), the tricuspid valve closes to prevent the back-flow of blood into the right atrium. During systole, blood is pumped from the right ventricle through the pulmonary arteries to the lungs, where a process of gas exchange takes place and venous blood becomes reoxygenated by haemoglobin uptake of oxygen to form arterial blood. This blood is returned to the left atrium by means of the pulmonary veins. It descends through the mitral valve into the left ventricle, and, finally, during systole, it is ejected through the ascending aorta into the circulatory system to supply the organs of the body. Back-flow of blood from the left ventricle to the left atrium during systole is prevented by the closure of the mitral valve. Similarly, back-flow of blood from the large aortic vessel into the left ventricle during diastole is prevented by the closure of the aortic valve. Pressure within the ventricles is somewhat higher than that within the atria, and impairment of valve function allowing the back-flow of blood from ventricles to atria places considerable strain upon the heart. This is most often seen in mitral valve incompetence.

The rhythm of systole and diastole necessary for the maintenance of circulation is regulated by a series of motor fibers arising from the autonomic nervous system and embedded at various points in the myocardium. Both sympathetic and parasympathetic fibers are represented in this system, and neurophysiological disruptions may have serious consequences for the efficient functioning of the heart. Control is maintained by the presence of pressure receptors (baro-receptors) within the major arteries, which feed back information to the central nervous system related to blood pressure and can act to modify cardiac output.

Both the degree and efficiency of blood flow to the body are, however, a complex function of a number of attributes including heart rate, blood pressure, the ejection fraction (the volume of blood ejected from the left ventricle during systole), and the resistance of the circulatory system within the various body organs to the flow of blood (Surwit, Williams, & Shapiro, 1982). While a detailed consideration of the neurophysiological and haemodynamic factors regulating the circulation of blood is beyond the scope of this book, a number of recent accounts (Braunwald, Ross, & Sonenblick, 1976; Surwit et al., 1982) will provide a more than adequate grounding in this area. Any impairment to the integrity of the myocardium will have serious implications for the efficient delivery of blood through the circulatory system to the organs of the body.

The Coronary Arteries

The heart, together with arteries conveying blood from it and veins returning blood to it, forms a closed circulatory system. As Surwit et al. (1982) have remarked, the central purpose of this system is to meet the metabolic needs of the body by way of the delivery of oxygen and nutrient substances to body tissues and the removal of body wastes. As a functional organ in its own right, however, the heart has fundamental metabolic needs which must also be supplied by the circulation of blood within the myocardium. This circulation is undertaken by the coronary arteries.

The precise anatomy of the coronary circulation varies from one individual to another, though the basis for this is formed by two arteries, the right and left coronary arteries. Circulation to the myocardium surrounding the right ventricle is undertaken by the right coronary artery branches arising from it. The left common coronary artery branches into the left anterior descending artery and the left circumflex artery, which together circulate blood to the left side of the myocardium and, in particular, the tissue surrounding the left ventricle. As the coronary arteries branch into progressively smaller vessels, so as to serve broader areas of the myocardium, a detailed network of arterioles and capillaries can be seen ultimately to supply blood to individual muscle cells. Deoxygenated blood is taken up by the coronary veins, which form parallel though reverse networks to the arterial system. The bulk of the deoxygenated blood from the coronary circulation enters the right atrium.

The coronary arteries are elastic in make-up and are therefore suited to carry cardiac output at relatively high pressures during ventricular contraction. The physical properties of this elasticity in relation to the coronary circulation have been discussed in detail by Caulfield (1977). The internal lining of the coronary arteries consists of endothelial cells tightly bound to a basement membrane. This is in turn attached to the underlying stroma by filaments of collagen. The endothelial surface of the coronary arteries is normally smooth and allows the unhindered passage of blood. However, when damage occurs to the endothelial cell lining, there are several immediate pathological consequences. The first is that the flow of blood within the blood stream becomes disturbed. Secondly, the damaged lining of the vessel wall forms a focus for the deposit of dissolved foreign matter precipitating out of the blood stream. This in turn lays the foundation for the formation of atherosclerotic deposits which, if progressive, may finally result in the occlusion of the coronary arteries. Finally, since tissue containing collagen is thrombogenic, its exposure to blood increases the possibility of the formation of blood clots and thus also of blockage within the coronary arteries.

Disease of the coronary arteries, however this comes about, forms the substrate for clinical coronary heart disease. The maintenance of healthy coronary arteries is perhaps the single most important step in the prevention of coronary heart disease. A wide range of factors bear on the production of coronary artery disease, and an equally wide range of factors join with coronary artery disease to precipitate clinical episodes of coronary heart disease. Perhaps the most central issue relevant to the former, however, is that of atherosclerosis.

PATHOLOGICAL AND CLINICAL CONSIDERATIONS

Atherosclerosis

Weisfeldt and Flaherty (1977), in a recent discussion of coronary heart disease, stated that, in the overwhelming majority of cases, this is the "end result of the pathologic process designated as coronary atherosclerosis" (p. 346). While a number of other causes have been postulated and, in particular, subintimal haemorrhage and the sudden and largely unexplained spasm of coronary arteries, the bulk of opinion continues to indicate atherosclerotic damage to the coronary arteries as the most central precursor of coronary heart disease.

The basis of coronary atherosclerosis, in turn, is atheroma or atherosclerotic plaque. Pathological changes associated with this process involve the deposition of fatty substances, carried by blood, into the internal cellular structure of the coronary artery wall. It is possible that damage to the microstructure of the coronary artery wall provides a focus for this deposit, though the mechanisms leading to such damage are complex. This progressive pathology ultimately proliferates and destroys the internal surface of the elastic coronary arteries, the process being accompanied by fibrosis and calcification so that the end result is both thickening and hardening of the arterial walls. At the very least the consequences of the atherosclerotic process are a reduction in blood supply to parts of the myocardium distal to the arterial narrowing and local turbulence of the blood flow at points around the arterial lesion. However, in a significant proportion of persons with severe atherosclerotic damage, the aggregation of blood platelets, under the influence of a variety of thrombogenic factors, can lead to the formation of a thrombus or blood clot at one or other points in the coronary artery and, hence, to the complete occlusion of that vessel. The most obvious result of this is a cessation of blood supply to points in the myocardium further on from the blockage and the very rapid death or necrosis of myocardial tissue denied its regular complement of blood. Necrosis of the myocardium can occur within minutes of the cessation of blood flow.

Coronary Heart Disease

The clinical signs of coronary artery occlusion are clear-cut. A decrease in blood supply to the myocardium will eventually result in a myocardial demand for oxygen which cannot be met. The most immediate result of this is the condition of myocardial ischemia, whereby the myocardium, starved of an adequate blood supply, builds up lactic acid and other toxic waste products within muscle tissue. The clinical consequence of this disruption to myocardial metabolism is that of ischemic pain, which is clinically termed *angina pectoris*. This may occur either spontaneously or during physical exertion, when the demand by the myocardium for oxygen is markedly in excess of its normal requirements. However, in some patients with quite severe disease of the coronary arteries, angina pectoris can be experienced even during times of rest. Coincident with this clinical condition is a greater or lesser decrease in the efficiency of the heart to maintain bodily circulation and, therefore, a variety of clinical symptoms ranging from tiredness and breathlessness through to an almost complete incapacity to undertake physical work, these symptoms being in rough proportion to the extent of disease within the coronary arteries.

The increasing sophistication of medical investigatory techniques, and principally the use of coronary angiographic procedures, has allowed the early diagnosis of coronary artery disease before the patient experiences ischemic symptoms or discomfort of any severe kind. Increasingly often such patients are referred for coronary by-pass surgery, where a piece of healthy blood vessel, usually taken from the same individual, is grafted so as to shunt blood around a diseased portion of a coronary artery and restore circulation to the associated myocardial tissue. This process is sometimes aided by the natural growth of collateral vessels to compensate for the deficiencies of the diseased artery. However, a sizeable number of patients with symptoms of angina, usually secondary to quite severe disease of the coronary arteries, go on to experience one or more episodes of coronary heart disease.

Though the precise mechanisms underlying complete coronary occlusion are still to be totally understood, it is clear that severe narrowing of the coronary arteries, in conjunction with the presence of conditions which facilitate clotting of the blood (thrombogenic factors), may result in the aggregation of blood platelets and the formation of a blood clot which totally occludes the coronary artery. The subsequent cessation of blood supply results in very rapid death of myocardial tissue distal to the point of occlusion, and this loss of myocardial tissue is clinically termed *myocardial infarction*. Once lost, this tissue cannot be regenerated, and while other areas of the myocardium may be strengthened by physical exercise, and collateral circulation from other coronary arteries to surrounding areas of the myocardium established to maintain blood supply to intact muscle tissue, the total integrity of the myocardium and its subsequent efficiency in accomplishing an adequate systemic circulation has been decreased to an extent loosely related to the amount of tissue loss (though this depends on the site of the necrosis).

Another potential mechanism more recently implicated in the precipitation of coronary occlusion has been that of coronary artery vasospasm. While the processes underlying this are less clearly understood than those forming the basis of coronary thrombosis, the most likely determinant would appear to be an acute discharge of sympathetic neurons, both in and of the coronary artery wall, resulting in a total but transient constriction of the vessel and a cessation of blood flowing through it. Thus, while the vasospasm may subside and the coronary artery may reopen to reestablish blood supply to the myocardium, the result is nonetheless an area of myocardial necrosis and, therefore, of myocardial infarction. This mechanism has been linked particularly to the syndrome of sudden cardiac death, where postmortem examinations of patients who have died suddenly have revealed substantial areas of myocardial necrosis in the absence of significant coronary artery disease (Steptoe, 1981).

However, whatever the mechanisms underlying coronary artery occlusion, the clinical symptoms associated with acute myocardial infarction are usually quite characteristic. These consist of severe retro-sternal pain, usually described as constricting in nature and similar to anginal pain, together with nausea, faintness, loss of breath, and palpitations. In some cases the patient may lose consciousness. This pain may radiate to the left arm and, less commonly, to the throat and jaw. On clinical examination the patient is occasionally white and sweating, with an irregular pulse due to extra systolic beats. In a set of formal guidelines on the diagnosis of coronary heart disease for research purposes, the World Health Organization (1973) listed the following history of chest pain as that most typically signalling the onset of myocardial infarction. In the usual case, pain is (a) diffused through the chest either anteriorly or generally, though it may remain localized in the chest or radiate to the shoulder, arms, jaws, or abdomen on one or both sides; (b) resistant to nitroglycerine; (c) of a duration of more than 20 minutes; and (d) of severe or agonizing intensity. An atypical history is more likely to include symptoms such as dyspnoea, a feeling of suffocation, "indigestion," syncope, general malaise, sweating, or acute cardiac failure. Blood pressure is frequently elevated during the first few hours, though often decreases to normal levels after this. In some cases both coldness and cyanosis of the extremities may be seen, both of which indicate a disturbance in the efficiency of the circulatory system.

A number of clinical conditions, including infections of the pericardium, may mimic some symptoms of myocardial infarction, and particularly those of chest pain. Certain diagnosis of myocardial infarction is, therefore, dependent on a series of electrophysiological and laboratory investigations in the first days following the onset of symptoms. Characteristic electrocardiographic (EKG) changes are found in over 95% of patients shortly after the onset of chest pain. In order to attract an unequivocal diagnosis of myocardial infarction, the World Health Organization (1973) has suggested that these should involve (a) the development of a pathological Q wave, and (b) the evolution of an injury current lasting for more than 1 day (this necessitates the collection of serial EKG traces in order to confirm these changes over a period of time). The World Health Organization's guidelines go on to indicate a series of EKG changes providing more equivocal evidence of myocardial infarction, including (a) the presence of an injury current which later disappears, (b) the presence of a stationary injury current, (c) symmetrical inversions of the T wave, (d) bundle-branch block with additional Q wave, and (e) presence of a pathological Q wave in a single EKG record.

In addition to clinical history of chest pain and the detection of EKG changes, it is also necessary to establish the presence in the blood of certain enzymes indicating the process of myocardial tissue necrosis. Typically, this process results in the presence of serum glutamic oxaloacetic transaminase (SGOT) and lactic dehydrogenase (LDH), the former appearing in elevated levels between 8 and 36 hours after myocardial infarction, and the latter peaking at between 3 and 6 days after the clinical event (Willerson, Hillis, & Buja, 1982). The presence of all three of these signs provides almost certain evidence of myocardial infarction.

RISK FACTORS FOR CORONARY HEART DISEASE

Willerson et al. (1982) provide a comprehensive list of risk factors for the development of coronary heart disease. These are conveniently divided into the categories of risk factors related to fundamental biology (e.g., age, sex, and inherited characteristics), those related to endogenous regulatory mechanisms (e.g., hypertension, hyperlipidemia, and the relative ratios of blood fat fractions), those concerned with environmental factors (e.g., cigarette smoking, physical activity, and psychological and behavioral characteristics), and those to do with organ system pathology (e.g., chronic renal disease or hypothyroidism). The bulk of epidemiological evidence, however, indicates that four risk factors, namely high serum lipids, high blood pressure, cigarette smoking, and presence of a characteristic pattern of time-pressured, hard-driven, and hostile behaviors (the Type A behavior pattern), contribute most strongly and most consistently to risk of coronary heart disease.

The evidence documenting associations between elevated levels of serum lipids and the incidence of coronary heart disease is both large and variable. Keys (1970) showed that population rates of coronary heart disease were positively correlated with population levels of serum cholesterol. The National Cooperative Pooling Project in the USA (Doyle & Kannel, 1970) demonstrated that, while rates of first major coronary events were 45 per 1,000 in men with serum cholesterol levels of 175 mg %, these rose to 162 per 1,000 in men with serum cholesterol rates greater than 300 mg %. Data in general agreement with this trend have been reported by Stamler (1974), Kannel, McGee, and Gordon (1976), and Rosenman, Brand, Jenkins, Friedman, Straus, and Wurm (1975). Based on data such as these, it would seem that approximately one-third of survivors of acute myocardial infarction aged 60 years or less are characterized by an elevation of lipids in the blood (Willerson et al., 1982).

While this evidence is persuasive, a number of questions remain to be answered. The first concerns the mechanisms responsible for the regulation of serum lipid levels. Biosynthesis of cholesterol, which appears to be the lipid substance most implicated in the pathology of coronary artery disease (the role of triglycerides as an independent risk factor is much more contentious), occurs primarily in the liver (Willerson et al., 1982). Cholesterol attaches to protein molecules of varying densities and is thereby transported to peripheral tissues. The biochemistry of this process has been extensively investigated (Gotto, Miller, & Oliver, 1978; Schaefer, Eisenberg, & Levy, 1978), and while the issue is indeed a complex one, it is not by and large controversial.

Cholesterol attached to low density lipoprotein (LDL) is strongly associated with the risk of coronary heart disease, while levels of high density lipopritein (HDL) appear to have a consistently negative association with coronary heart disease risk.

What is controversial is the role of diet in the regulation of serum lipids. While Keys' (1970) study popularized the notion that diet, insofar as it influences serum lipids, can be a coronary risk factor, and while this has more recently attracted epidemiological support (Shekelle, Shryock, Paul, Lepper, Stamler, Liu, & Raynor, 1981), there is now evidence at odds with this opinion (Byrne, Rosenman, & Schiller, 1985). Questioning of the evidence linking diet, serum cholesterol, and coronary heart disease has arisen both from methodological concerns (Armstrong, Mann, Adelstein, & Eskin, 1975; Mann, 1977) and because of conflicting epidemiological data (Nichols, Ravenscroft, Lamphiear, & Ostrander, 1976; Byrne, Rosenman, & Schiller, 1985). Findings failing to relate diet to serum cholesterol have cast doubt on the area, and, while the association between serum cholesterol and risk of coronary heart disease must continue to be given credence, the regulation of this risk factor by means of patterns of dietary intake is contentious. The role of behavior in the regulation of serum lipids has recently attracted attention (Dimsdale & Heid, 1982) and the environment–person interaction presents itself as a fertile area for future epidemiological study of the risk of coronary heart disease endowed by serum lipids.

Data from the National Cooperative Pooling Project (1978) can also be used to demonstrate the importance of blood pressure as a coronary risk factor. These data show that men with a diastolic pressure of less than 75 mm Hg have an age-adjusted rate of first major coronary events of 48 per 1,000, whereas men with diastolic pressure of 105 mm Hg or greater, have an age-adjusted risk rate for major coronary events of 188 per 1,000. The World Health Organization considers the area of risk to include diastolic pressures of 95 mm Hg and greater, and, for the range of 95–104 mm Hg, the age-adjusted rate for first major coronary events was 99 per 1,000. It is therefore clear from these data that increases in diastolic pressure constitute a noticeable risk for coronary heart disease.

A similar picture is evident for systolic blood pressure. Data from the National Cooperative Pooling Project (1970, 1978) show a steady rise in the incidence of both sudden cardiac death and first major survived coronary events in middle-aged men in parallel with increases in systolic blood pressure. While the physiological mechanisms underlying the determination of blood pressure are complex and continue to be subject to intensive investigation (Steptoe, 1981; Surwit et al., 1982), high blood pressure is a risk factor for coronary heart disease which must continue to be accepted.

Data from a variety of sources confirm the association between cigarette smoking and risk of coronary heart disease. The National Cooperative Pooling Project (1978) reported the death rate from coronary heart disease to be 20 per 1,000 from men who have never smoked in contrast to a death rate of 60 per 1,000 among men who had smoked greater than one packet of cigarettes per week. This death rate fell in proportion to decreases in the number of cigarettes smoked per day. Moreover, it was shown that, while pipe and cigar smoking introduced a modest increase in risk of death from coronary heart disease, it was not substantially above that for nonsmokers and was certainly considerably below that for cigarette smokers. This may have to do with differential rates of absorption of toxic substances from cigarette smoking in the lungs and in the mouth; cigarette smokers tend to inhale into the lungs, whereas cigar and pipe smokers are more likely to keep the smoke within the mouth. The evidence here, however, is somewhat tenuous. Most interesting, the rate of coronary heart disease deaths among those who had smoked in the past but had subsequently given up was marginally below the coronary heart disease death rate for those who had never smoked.

Reported risk attributed to cigarette smoking was rather greater when the first major survived coronary event and not coronary heart disease death constituted the epidemiological end point. In this case the risk associated with past smoking was greater than that associated with those who had never smoked cigarettes. In all other respects, however, the pattern of risk for survived coronary heart disease among smokers paralleled that found for coronary heart disease deaths.

More recently, a succession of reports from the United States Surgeon General (see, for example, United States Surgeon General's report on smoking and health, 1983) have consistently reported strong epidemiological associations between cigarette smoking and risk of coronary heart disease. The Surgeon General's report for 1979 cited 26 major epidemiological studies in which it was shown that smokers had a higher incidence of heart attacks, both fatal and nonfatal, than did nonsmokers.

While the mechanisms linking cigarette smoking with damage to coronary arteries and to initiation of coronary heart disease are somewhat poorly understood, there is evidence that these links might act both through the exacerbation of existing coronary artery atherosclerosis and also by the production of regional cardiac ischaemia which in turn may promote electrical instability, fibrillation, and ultimate destabilization of electrical conduction within the myocardium. Cigarette smoking is, of course, a human behavior, and any risk of coronary heart disease endowed by this factor can be viewed as much as a behavioral risk as a physiological one.

Among all risk factors for coronary heart disease the Type A behavior pattern is perhaps the most controversial. This behavior pattern is characterized by a sense of time urgency, a high need for achievement and excessive ambition, impatience and intolerance of frustration, an unusual degree of job involvement, and overt hostility and aggression (Byrne, 1981). While Type A behavior has been linked with the incidence of coronary heart disease in a number of retrospective and prospective studies, three of these stand out for their magnitude and methodological care.

The Western Collaborative Group Study (Rosenman et al., 1975) assessed Type A behavior in 3,154 male subjects who were healthy at the time of initial examination. These subjects were followed through for 8.5 years, during which serial medical and other investigations provided close to complete data on coronary events, whether survived or otherwise. Simultaneous adjustment for all other risk factors at termination of the study revealed that Type A men had had between 1.87 and 1.98 times more risk of coronary heart disease over 8.5 years than did men in whom Type A behavior was not evident.

Similar results emerged from an 8-year follow-up of subjects in the Framingham Study (Haynes, Feinleib, & Kannel, 1980). Taking all other risk factors into account, male subjects between 45 and 54 years of age who had Type A behavior showed a risk of coronary heart disease around 50% greater than men in the same age group who were not Type A. When men between 55 and 64 years were considered, the risk of coronary heart disease attributable to Type A behavior increased to twice that among men without the behavior pattern.

In a major retrospective study involving more than 6,000 employees in Belgian industrial organizations, the presence of Type A behavior was also found to be strongly related to the prevalence of identified coronary heart disease, and this was independent of other coronary risk factors (Kornitzer, Kittel, De Backer, & Dramaix, 1981).

A number of issues remain to be resolved with regard to Type A behavior as a coronary risk. A great deal of work remains to be done both on the definition and on the measurement of Type A behavior (Byrne, Rosenman, Schiller, & Chesney, 1985). Moreover, the pathophysiological links between the Type A behavior pattern and coronary artery pathology are yet to be established with any certainty. Still, the weight of evidence from well-conducted epidemiological studies clearly indicates the Type A behavior pattern as an independent and causal risk factor for coronary heart disease.

The discussion to this point has concerned the potency of single risk factors considered independently of all other risk factors. While it is, of course, possible for an individual to have only one of a number of coronary risk factors, it is more likely the case that a single individual will possess several risk factors in combination. The rules by which these risk factors add together are not well understood and are almost certainly a function of the relative level of risk factors in any individual. Nonetheless, there is some data from major epidemiological studies dealing with the additivity at least of the three risk factors of serum cholesterol, high blood pressure, and cigarette smoking.

This situation, too, can be represented by data from the National Cooperative Pooling Project (1970). The age-adjusted rate for a first major coronary event (myocardial infarction) among cigarette smokers with normal blood pressure and serum cholesterol levels is somewhat more than twice that for persons with no risk factors. The presence of high blood pressure or serum cholesterol, again in the absence of other risk factors, raises the rate of first major coronary events marginally higher, even, than this. A combination of any two risk factors raises the rate of illness events to between three and four times that where no risk factors are in evidence, while the presence of all three risk factors (high blood pressure, elevated serum cholesterol and cigarette smoking) almost doubles the rate of first major coronary events relative to the effects of two risk factors only.

There is no precise formula which can explain the ways in which coronary risk factors combine to increase the observed rates of myocardial infarction. It is unlikely to involve a simple process of addition, since each risk factor would not appear to carry equal weight in the determination of risk. On the other hand, the data from the National Cooperative Pooling Project (1970, 1978), as well as evidence from a persuasive body of independent, epidemiological studies accumulating over the past two decades, indicates quite conclusively that high blood pressure, elevated levels of cholesterol (and perhaps other lipid substances) in the blood, and cigarette smoking, either singly or in combination, endow substantially increased risks of sustaining coronary heart disease.

REFERENCES

Armstrong, B. K., Mann, J. I., Adelstein, A. M., & Eskin, F. (1975). Commodity consumption and ischaemic heart disease mortality with special reference to dietary practices. *Journal of Chronic Diseases, 28*, 455–463.

Braunwald, E., Ross, J., & Sonenblick, E. H. (1976). *Mechanisms of contraction of the normal failing heart.* Boston, MA: Little, Brown.

Byrne, D. G. (1981). Type A behaviour, life events and myocardial infarction: Independent or related risk factors? *British Journal of Medical Psychology, 54*, 371–377.

Byrne, D. G., Rosenman, R. H., & Schiller, E. (1985). *Patterns of dietary intake and serum lipids in a sample of employed, Australian males*. Unpublished manuscript, Department of Psychology, Australian National University, Canberra.

Byrne, D. G., Rosenman, R. H., Schiller, E., & Chesney, M. A. (1985). Consistency and variation among instruments purporting to measure the Type A behavior pattern. *Psychosomatic Medicine, 47*, 242–261.

Caulfield, J. B. (1977). Anatomy of the cardiovascular system. In J. T. Willerson & C. A. Sanders (Eds.), *Clinical cardiology*. New York: Grune & Stratton.

Dimsdale, J. E., & Heid, J. A. (1982). Variability of plasma lipids in response to emotional arousal. *Psychosomatic Medicine, 44*, 413–430.

Doyle, J. T., & Kannel, W. B. (1970). *Coronary risk factors: 10 year findings in 7446 Americans*. Paper presented to VI World Congress of Cardiology, London.

Gotto, A. M., Miller, N. E., & Oliver, M. F. (Eds.). (1978). *High density lipoproteins and atherosclerosis*. Amsterdam: Elsevier.

Haynes, S. G., Feinleib, M., & Kannel, W. B. (1980). The relationship of psychosocial factors to coronary heart disease in the Framingham Study: III. Eight year incidence of coronary heart disease. *American Journal of Epidemiology, 111*, 37–58.

Kannel, W. B., McGee, D., & Gordon, T. (1976). A general cardiovascular profile: The Framingham Study. *American Journal of Cardiology, 38*, 46–51.

Keys, A. (1970). Coronary heart disease in seven countries. *Circulation, 41*, 1–211.

Kornitzer, M., Kittel, F., De Backer, G., & Dramaix, M. (1981). The Belgian heart disease prevention project: Type A behavior pattern and the prevalence of coronary heart disease. *Psychosomatic Medicine, 43*, 133–145.

Mann, G. V. (1977). Diet-heart: End of an era. *New England Journal of Medicine, 297*, 644–650.

Nichols, A. B., Ravenscroft, C., Lamphiear, D. E., & Ostrander, L. D. (1976). Independence of serum lipid levels and dietary habits. *Journal of the American Medical Association, 236*, 1948–1953.

Rosenman, R. H., Brand, R. J., Jenkins, C. D., Friedman, M., Straus, R., & Wurm, M. (1975). Coronary heart disease in the Western Collaborative Group Study. *Journal of the American Medical Association, 233*, 872–877.

Schaefer, E. J., Eisenberg, S., & Levy, R. I. (1978). Lipoprotein, apoprotein metabolism. *Journal of Lipid Research, 19*, 667–687.

Shekelle, R. B., Shryock, A. M., Paul, O., Lepper, M., Stamler, J., Liu, S., & Raynor, W. J. (1981). Diet, serum cholesterol and death from coronary heart disease. *New England Journal of Medicine, 304*, 65–70.

Stamler, J. (1974). The prevention of coronary heart disease. In E. Braunwald

(Ed.), *The myocardium: Failure and infarction.* New York: H. B. Publishing.

Steptoe, A. (1981). *Psychological factors in cardiovascular disorders.* London: Academic Press.

Surwit, R. S., Williams, R. B., & Shapiro, D. (1982). *Behavioral approaches to cardiovascular disease.* New York: Academic Press.

U.S. Surgeon General's Report. (1983). *The health consequences of smoking: Cardiovascular disease.* Bethesda, MD: U.S. Department of Health and Human Services.

Weisfeldt, M. L., & Flaherty, J. T. (1977). Myocardial infarction. In J. T. Willerson & C. A. Sanders (Eds.), *Clinical cardiology.* New York: Grune & Stratton.

Willerson, J. D., Hillis, L. D., & Buja, L. M. (1982). *Ischaemic heart disease: Clinical and pathophysiological aspects.* New York: Raven Press.

World Health Organization. (1973). *Evaluation of comprehensive rehabilitative and preventive programmes for patients after acute myocardial infarction.* Copenhagen, Denmark: Regional Office for Europe.

4

The Type A Behavior Pattern and Coronary Heart Disease

D. G. Byrne

Department of Psychology
The Australian National University
Canberra

The introduction by Friedman and Rosenman (1974) of the concept of Type A or coronary-prone behavior began a debate which has perhaps been the most prominent and controversial in the behavioral study of coronary heart disease (CHD) in the past decade. *Type A behavior* was the term coined to refer to a loosely related constellation of attributes, typically time urgency and impatience, competitiveness and ambitiousness, need for achievement and poor frustration tolerance, high occupational involvement, hostility, and aggression, which might be observed in the activities of any given individual (Rosenman & Chesney, 1982). Early observations (Friedman & Rosenman, 1959; Friedman, St. George, & Byers, 1960) suggested these attributes to be associated both with overt coronary disease and with elevations in coronary risk factors and cardiovascular arousal which might be expected to precede CHD. More recent studies based on systematic assessments of the TABP and in relation to CHD both as an existent disease (retrospective studies) and as a developing phenomenon (prospective studies) have lent support to these initial findings, though the literature has not reported entirely unequivocal results.

Retrospective studies using both interview assessments of the TABP (Keegan, Sinha, Merriman, & Shipley, 1979; Orth-Gomer & Ahlbom, 1980) and assessments based on individual self-report by questionnaire (Jenkins, Zyzanski, & Rosenman, 1971; Kenigsberg et al., 1974; Shekelle, Schoenberger, & Stamler, 1976; Cohen, Syme, Jenkins, Kagan, & Zyzanski, 1979; Kornitzer, Kittel, De Backer, & Dramaix, 1981) have lent uniform support to an association between the TABP and CHD. Broadly, patients with diagnosed CHD appear to have higher levels of the TABP, either self-reported or independently observed, than healthy control groups or groups of patients hospitalized for illness other than CHD. The interpretation of retrospective evidence does, however, pose difficulties. Thus, some criticism has been attached to these studies along the lines that self-reports, at least, of the TABP might be influenced by the patients' need to justify the presence of CHD in terms of imagined attributes of a hard-driven lifestyle. Nonetheless, the overall consistency of the evidence, together with the observation that the finding holds across interview as well as self-report measures of the TABP, suggests that retrospective studies do indicate a real link between the TABP and CHD.

Any postulated association in epidemiology is, of course, strengthened by prospective evidence, and this has been forthcoming from at least two major studies. The first of these, the Western Collaborative Group Study (WCGS), initiated by Rosenman and his colleagues (Rosenman et al., 1964), involved around 3000 healthy male subjects at commencement for whom extensive data were available, not just on the TABP, but also on standard physical risk factors for CHD. Careful follow-up of these subjects (Rosenman, Friedman, Straus, Jenkins, Zyzanski, & Wurm, 1970; Rosenman, Brand, Jenkins, Friedman, Straus, & Wurm, 1975), terminating at 8.5 years after commencement, showed that, when all other risk factors were accounted for, males with TABP were around twice as much at risk of CHD as those in whom the TABP was absent. This finding has been confirmed by independent analyses of the data (Matthews, Glass, Rosenman, & Bortner, 1977; Brand, Rosenman, Jenkins, Sholtz, & Zyzanski, 1978).

While the Framingham Study of Coronary Risk (Haynes, Feinleib, Levine, Scotch, & Kannel, 1978) was not intended to examine the role of the TABP, a re-analysis of its data has been used to confirm this role. Haynes, Feinleib, and Kannel (1980) used items from a psychosocial questionnaire originally administered in the Framingham Study to construct a scale reflecting attributes of the TABP. This measure of the TABP was found to be unrelated to premorbid levels of CHD risk based on weighted combinations of physical risk factors and derived from the Framingham logistic equations (Haynes et al., 1978). The scale was, however, significantly related to the incidence of a variety of manifestations of CHD occurring up to 8 years after the initial administration of the questionnaire to a cohort of initially healthy subjects (Haynes et al., 1980). By contrast to the WCGS, the Framingham study included female subjects as well as males. Men identified as Type A on the Framingham scale had around a twofold risk of developing angina pectoris, MI, and other forms of CHD over 8 years, when compared with subjects not showing the behavior pattern. These findings were evident in men up to 64 years of age and moreso in white- than in blue-collar occupations, but were not evident among subjects 65 years and older. Importantly, the findings were independent of the influence of all other measured risk factors.

Patterns of association were similar for female subjects, with women 45 to 64 years who developed CHD also scoring significantly higher on the Type A scale than those remaining healthy over the 8-year incidence period. Type A women experienced twice the rate of MI and three times the rate of angina pectoris as those without the behavior pattern, and, once more, these associations were independent of the influence of other risk factors.

As an investigation of coronary risk, the methodological credibility of the Framingham Study is accepted without question. If these findings have a weakness, therefore, it is in the retrospective nature of the scale construction. The Framingham Type A scale has been validated against more usual measures of the TABP (Byrne, Rosenman, Schiller, & Chesney, 1985) and has been found to correlate well both with interview and self-report measures of the behavior pattern. These data then, add substantially to the evidence indicating a causal link between the TABP and the incidence of CHD.

Analyses arising from the WCGS data have shown that the TABP is also a strong predictor of recurrent CHD following an initial clinical event. Jenkins, Zyzanski, and Rosenman (1971, 1976) compared men who had experienced a single clinical episode of CHD over the 8.5 years of the study with those who had sustained recurrent CHD in the same period. Multivariate analyses showed the TABP to be the strongest single predictor of recurrent CHD (independent of other measured risk factor levels), followed by cigarette smoking and serum cholesterol levels.

While psychophysiological mechanisms which might link the TABP to pathological levels of cardiovascular arousal and hence to risk of CHD have been widely investigated (Myrtek & Greenlee, 1984), a discussion of these is beyond the scope of the present chapter. More apposite to the issue of clinical CHD, however, are the findings that TABP relates positively to the degree of coronary atherosclerosis as determined by angiography (Zyzanski, Jenkins, Ryan, Flessas, & Everist, 1976; Blumenthal, Williams, Kong, Schanberg, & Thompson, 1978; Frank, Heller, Kornfeld, Sporn, & Weiss, 1978).

Still, not all evidence has provided unequivocal support for a link between the TABP and CHD. Firstly, several recent prospective studies have been unable to demonstrate associations between the TABP and either first episode of CHD (Shekelle, Gale, & Norusis, 1985) or its recurrence (Case, Heller, Case, & Moss, 1985). Some criticism may be attached to these contradictory studies, and particularly those failing to relate the TABP to incidence of primary or recurrent CHD, on the grounds that they were general studies of coronary risk and the measurement of the TABP was dictated more by convenience than by primary interest. Thus, the epidemiological association between the TABP and risk of CHD, while sometimes challenged, maintains its credibility as an explanatory concept in behavioral medicine.

DEFINITIONS OF TYPE A BEHAVIOR

Definitions of *Type A behavior* are both broad and variable, though a number of existing definitions and descriptions do set a useful context within which to discuss the overall notion. While the introduction of both the term and the idea of Type A behavior are undeniably attributed to Friedman and Rosenman (1974), the essence of this idea was eloquently stated as early as 1892 by Sir William Osler in his textbook *The Principles and Practice of Medicine.*

Contemporary definitions are best represented by that of Friedman (1978), who defined Type A behavior as:

> A relatively specific type of continuous emotional disquiet that is initiated and sustained in an individual by (1) his abnormally intense, chronic struggle to achieve more and more objectives or to participate in more and more events in less and less time, or (2) his exaggerated hostile reactions to various activities of other human beings. (p. 137)

A number of descriptions of Type A behavior may serve to extend these definitions into recognizable aspects of human activity. Byrne (1981) said of this phenomenon:

> The literature collectively suggests that persons manifesting this behaviour pattern are characterised by a sense of time urgency, are ambitious with a high need for achievement, are impatient and intolerant of frustration and exhibit an unusual degree of job involvement. (p. 371)

Herman, Blumenthal, Black, and Chesney (1981), with encouraging similarity, describe the Type A individual as:

> typically aggressive, competitive, ambitious and hostile with a pervasive quality of time urgency and impatience. (p. 405)

There are, of course, many such descriptions. Each paper on Type A behavior seems to contain its own. However, the differences between these are subtle at most, and one can assume a fair amount of agreement as to the various components of behavior which have been observed to make up the overall pattern.

Factorial descriptions of Type A behavior tend to confirm those based on observation. Zyzanski and Jenkins (1970) use data from the Western Collaborative Group Study to examine the factor structure of responses to the Jenkins Activity Survey (Jenkins, Rosenman, & Friedman, 1967). This was a self-completed questionnaire designed specifically for use in the study as one of several methods for assessing the Type A behavior pattern. A factor analysis of these data which can be described as statistically meticulous yielded three independent factors. The first of these was termed *Hard Driving and Competitiveness.* Items significantly loading on this factor identified a pattern of behavior concerned with task commitment, expenditure of effort, and the perception of activities and interactions as challenges to be accepted and dominated. While such behaviors might be most prominently observed within the work situation, there are many other environments, such as those involved in competitive sport or other activities, which might allow this pattern to become manifest. The second factor was labeled *Job Involvement.* Items significantly loading on this factor were identified specifically with the workplace and describe behaviors involving the acceptance or establishment of difficult and challenging deadlines, the tendency to extend work past normal hours, the acceptance and, indeed, soliciting of work in excess of personal capacity, and the conviction that job demands should take precedence over all other considerations. The final factor attracted the label *Speed and Impatience.* This was identified by items portraying undue haste and rapidity in both motor and cognitive activities, a self-imposed time pressure, an intolerance of slowness in others, and an inordinate degree of irritability and distractibility.

Reference to this study serves several purposes. Firstly, it provides empirical confirmation of the more impressionistic descriptions arising from earlier work. Secondly, it begins the process of delineating the several elements of the Type A behavior pattern, so establishing it as a complex and nonunitary set of behaviors. The idea that the Type A behavior pattern is in fact composed of a number of independent elements has recently been discussed by Jenkins and Zyzanski (1982). Finally, the statistical work arising from this study lays the ground for a more detailed measurement of Type A behavior, and so for the establishment of more specific associations between Type A behavior and clinically manifest cardiovascular disease.

One facet of Type A behavior understated in earlier studies but recently assuming prominence is that of hostility. While the attribute of aggression appears in most descriptions of Type A behavior, its emergence either as a predictor of myocardial infarction or as an element in factorial descriptions of the behavior pattern is only now attracting interest. Both Francis (1981) and Smith (1984) have reported modest but consistent correlations between measures of Type A behavior and self-reported expressions of anger and hostility. In addition, more recent factorial examinations of common methods of assessing the Type A behavior pattern have indicated hostility to be a notable component of the pattern (Anderson & Waldron, 1983; Matthews, Krantz, Dembroski, & McDougall, 1982). Prospective studies (Barefoot, Dahlstrom, & Williams, 1983; Shekelle, Gale, Ostfeld, & Paul, 1983; Williams, Haney, Lee, Kong, Blumenthal, & Whalen, 1980) have significantly related both to risk of coronary heart disease and mortality from it. Moreover, a more modest study of the experience of angina in patients with diagnosed coronary artery disease (Smith, Follick, & Korr, 1984) showed that the frequency of angina attacks was quite strongly related to the possession of self-reported anger. Data such as these would indicate that future work on the relationship between Type A behavior and coronary heart disease should not ignore the potentially important role of anger and hostility as components of the former.

STRESS AND TYPE A BEHAVIOR

Traditional views of the TABP have sought to dissociate it from any notion of stress, neuroticism, or psychiatric impairment (Jenkins, 1978). However, while standard definitions of the TABP emphasize its essentially behavioral character (Rosenman & Chesney, 1982), an early and perhaps broad overview portrays it, inter alia, as an action–emotion complex, so recognizing, at least in principle, the role of an affective element in the overall construct. More recent conceptualizations of the TABP are more explicit in their acceptance that, insofar as Type A behaviors confer coronary risk, both behavior and emotion (and particularly emotional distress) must bear conjoint responsibility (Price, 1983).

Support for this can be drawn from two interrelated sources. Firstly, despite the opinion that those with the TABP are largely unaware of the character of their behaviors (Herman, Blumenthal, Black, & Chesney, 1981), there is mounting evidence that Type A behaviors are accompanied by significant emotional discomfort. Dimsdale, Hackett, Block, and Hutter, (1978) reported associations between measures of the TABP and indices of subjective tension, depressive mood, and anger in a sample of patients awaiting cardiac catheterization, while Bass (1984) and Smith (1984) found significant relationships between the TABP and both neuroticism and psychiatric symptomatology in similar groups of patients. In order to counter the very real argument that data obtained by self-report from patient samples may be too prone to contamination, significant relationships between the TABP and a range of measures of emotional distress (but not conspicuous psychiatric impairment) have also been found in several samples of healthy subjects free of coronary disease (Chesney, Black, Chadwick, & Rosenman, 1981; Francis, 1981; Wadden, Anderson, Foster, & Love, 1983; Byrne & Rosenman, 1987). The most extreme interpretation of these data, based largely on correlations between measures of the TABP and those of both trait and state anxiety, holds that the TABP and neuroticism are conceptually equivalent (Eysenck & Fulker, 1982; Irvine, Lyle, & Allon, 1982). The TABP is, however, strongly typified by overtly time-pressured behaviors (Friedman, 1969) and, under some conditions, induces a state of heightened autonomic arousal (Myrtek & Greenlee, 1984). In view of this, Byrne and Rosenman (1987) have argued that the subjective experience of these phenomena, either singly or in combination, can reasonably explain the emotional discomfort which many Type A individuals admit to.

Secondly, a little recent evidence has suggested that possession of the TABP facilitates the accumulation of stressful life events. Following a close examination of the thematic character of the TABP, Byrne (1981) made the claim that individuals with Type A behaviors may act, albeit unwittingly, to place themselves in personal, social, and occupational circumstances which increase the likelihood of their encountering stressful life events. Data from both patient samples (Dimsdale et al., 1978; Falger, Bressors, & Dijkstra, 1980; Byrne, 1981) and a sample of individuals free from CHD (Byrne & Rosenman, 1986) have all shown consistent significant correlations between measures of the TABP and self-reported frequency of stressful life event encounters. Moreover, it has been shown that Type A patients, at least, tend to interpret those life events which have occurred to them as being of greater emotional impact than control subjects free of coronary disease (Byrne, 1981). Interestingly, associations between the TABP and measures of life events have been strongest for those categories of life events independently judged to be under greatest personal control. This has led to the view that some part of the noxious character of the TABP has to do with the need, by those with Type A behaviors, to impose control, not only on the environment, but on their responses to it (Vickers, Hervig, Rahe, & Rosenman, 1981; Vingerhoets & Flohr, 1984).

The definition of stress given by Tennant et al. (1985) encompasses both external events and individual responses, whether emotional or physiological. Within the meaning of this definition, the TABP is clearly interconnected with the notion of stress though the relationship might be situation-specific (Scherwitz, McKelvain, & Laman, 1983). A distinction must be made, however, between conceptual and empirical relationships, and while it may be argued that the nature of the TABP could create circumstances both within and outside of the individual which might facilitate the stress response, some care must be taken lest the evidence presently to hand is extrapolated too far.

MEASUREMENT OF TYPE A BEHAVIOR

The measurement of Type A behavior assumes several important roles. Firstly, the presence and extent of Type A behavior needs to be established in some systematic way. Secondly, if the object of the exercise is to modify this behavior, then the effectiveness of that modification strategy needs to be evaluated, and this involves systematic measurement both before and after the application of any intervention strategy. Finally, since Type A behavior is not a unitary concept but is made up of several distinct elements (Zyzanski & Jenkins, 1970; Jenkins & Zyzanski, 1982), and since these elements are neither uniformly related to the risk of coronary heart disease (Jenkins, 1978) nor evenly distributed among all those exhibiting Type A behavior (Chesney et al., 1981), it would seem useful to know, for any single individual, the relative presence of the components of Type A behavior, so that appropriate foci for intervention could be adopted. Useful reviews of this field may be obtained from several sources (Byrne et al., 1985; Chesney et al., 1981), and the psychometric properties of the various Type A measuring instruments have been particularly well covered by Byrne et al. (1985).

Two measures of Type A behavior are most commonly used. These are the structured interview (Rosenman et al., 1964; Rosenman, 1978) and the Jenkins Activity Survey (Jenkins, Zyzanski, & Rosenman, 1979). Considerable debate exists as to the relative efficacy of these two.

The Structured Interview

This was first developed for use in the Western Collaborative Group Study, and reports of associations between Type A behavior and myocardial infarction have arisen largely from its use (Rosenman et al., 1975). In view of strong and consistent associations between categorizations of Type A behavior based on the Structured Interview and the onset of various manifestations of cardiovascular disease, this technique has achieved a useful reputation as a Type A measure. The qualitative and thematic structure of the interview arose from a series of clinical observations which were cast into the form of questions or other forms of information gathering interactions. These set out to address (a) the degree of drive and ambition, (b) the degree of past and present aggressive competitive hostile feelings, and (c) the degree of time urgency (Chesney et al., 1981) exhibited by an individual. The items making up the Structured Interview are presented in detail by these authors. These items are administered as part of an interview in such a way that the interviewer is not only able to note the verbal content of subjects' responses, but to encourage the person with Type A predispositions to display these in response to challenges during the interview. This is achieved, for example, by the interviewer omitting to complete the ends of sentences, so that the Type A person, in order to rush through, will go on ahead of the interviewer. The interviewer is, therefore, able to note actual instances of Type A behavior when they occur throughout the interview.

On the basis both of verbal responses to questions and of judgments of actual instances of Type A behavior manifested throughout the interview, the interviewer makes ratings concerning the presence of Type A behavior or its absence (Type B behavior), and also of the degree to which Type A or Type B behaviors are apparent. A five-point scale is used to give the following distinctions:

A1: Fully developed Type A pattern;
A2: Many Type A characteristics, but not the complete pattern;
X: An even mix of Type A and Type B characteristics;
B3: Many Type B characteristics but some Type A characteristics as well;
B4: A relative absence of Type A characteristics.

Since the Structured Interview acts as a situational challenge for Type A behaviors, the conditions surrounding the interview are crucially important. Interviewers must be consistent with respect to vocal style (speed, volume, intonation, and inflection), length of the interview, question content, and interviewer behavior.

Reliability between several interviewers has been found quite acceptable. Caffrey (1968) reported interrater reliability coefficients as varying between 0.64 and 0.84, with the more modest correlations occurring for relatively newly trained interviewers. Test–retest reliability, too, has been examined (Jenkins, Rosenman, & Friedman, 1968), with reliability coefficients of around evident 0.82 over periods of between 12 and 20 months.

THE JENKINS ACTIVITY SURVEY

The Jenkins Activity Survey (Jenkins, Zyzanski, & Rosenman, 1979) is the major rival to the Structured Interview in the measurement of Type A behavior. This is a self-completed questionnaire the content of which arose from the item content of the interview instrument. The present version (there have been several developments over the past years) contains 52 items (Jenkins et al., 1979). Factor analytic work on earlier versions of this scale (Zyzanski & Jenkins, 1970) revealed the three dimensions of hard driving and competitiveness, job involvement, and speed and impatience. Use of the Jenkins Activity Survey produces a global Type A score and three subscores representing the three factors just listed. The value of this lies with the finer dissection of the substructure of the Type A behavior pattern.

Internal reliability for the four Jenkins Activity Survey scales (the Global Scale and three subscales) ranges between 0.73 and 0.85, while test–retest reliability over a 4- to 6-month interval ranges between 0.65 and 0.82 (Jenkins et al., 1979).

Chesney et al. (1981) questioned the advantages of the Jenkins Activity Survey over the Structured Interview in at least three respects. Firstly, the prospective evidence linking Type A behavior with myocardial infarction is weaker for Jenkins Activity Survey scores than for structured Interview classifications (Brand et al., 1978). Secondly, the relation between Jenkins Activity Survey scores and coronary angiographic findings has been brought into question (Blumenthal et al., 1978). Finally, Structured Interview ratings are more strongly related to cardiovascular reactivity during experimentally induced stress than are Jenkins Activity Survey scores (Dembroski et al., 1978). The Jenkins Activity Survey does, however, have the advantages both of convenience (it is self-completed) and of dividing up the Type A behavior pattern into its relative components.

OTHER MEASURES OF TYPE A BEHAVIOR

Vickers (1973) developed a brief nine-item self-completed questionnaire for use in epidemiological surveys. This scale was found to correlate around 0.80 with the Jenkins Activity Survey and to be associated with the presence of a number of coronary risk factors. It did not, however, distinguish between patients with myocardial infarction and those with the less serious illnesses (Byrne, 1981), and has been criticized for failing to assess the entire universe of Type A behaviors (Caffrey, 1978). Therefore, while this short instrument has the advantage of being convenient and simple to use, it is unlikely to provide an adequate measure of a complex behavior pattern and cannot, therefore, be recommended for use in the clinical setting.

A scale which is almost as brief was reported by Bortner (1969), though this instrument failed to correlate at all with Jenkins Activity Survey scores. It provided a 66% agreement with classifications of Type A behavior arising from the Structured Interview, and patients with myocardial infarction were found to have higher scores on the Bortner scale than healthy control subjects (Heller, 1979). There is, however, little epidemiological evidence to link scores on this scale to prospective risk for myocardial infarction.

Rather more epidemiological evidence has accumulated from the Framingham Study (Haynes et al., 1980), where, in its latest stages, a short, self-completed instrument was developed for the assessment of Type A behavior. Items contained in this instrument were chosen on the grounds that they were "typical of the Type A behavior pattern." This scale was found to be a significant predictor of myocardial infarction at 8-year follow-up. The evidence linking this measure of Type A behavior with risk of myocardial infarction is rather stronger than that attached to the two previously discussed, short measures of the Type A behavior pattern. This immediately makes it a potential prospect as a clinical measure of Type A behavior. More work is still to be done, however, on its use within the clinical context, and, as yet, it is unlikely to supplant the more established means for assessing Type A behavior.

Both Chesney et al. (1981) and Byrne et al. (1985) have reported modest correlations between standard measures of Type A behavior and scales arising from established, psychometric measures of personality. These have included the California Psychological Inventory, the activity scale of the Thurstone Temperament Schedule, the dominance scale of the Adjective Checklist, the Nemoticism Scale of the Eysenck Personality Inventory and the State-Trait Anxiety Inventory. There is no evidence, however, either clinical or epidemiological, that scores on these scales relate to risk of myocardial infarction. Therefore, they do not present useful alternatives for the clinical assessment of Type A behavior.

THE MODIFICATION OF TYPE A BEHAVIOR

In an area where the epidemiological association between a behavior pattern and a disease category is so persuasive, the amount of systematic research on the modification of Type A behavior is remarkably sparse. Several recent reviews of this are (Gentry, 1978; Suinn, 1978, 1980; Chesney et al., 1981) reveal only a small number of studies which have postulated intervention strategies based on adequate conceptualizations of Type A behavior and which have then gone on to implement and evaluate these strategies.

Perhaps the only study which has directed its attention specifically to survivors of myocardial infarction has been that of Friedman (1978). This is not in itself a problem, since there is no evidence to suggest that the principles, or those with identification of Type A behavior in healthy subjects, or those with identified coronary risk should not generalize adequately to persons who have experienced and survived myocardial infarction. One might even speculate that the survivor of myocardial infarction would more readily accept a program aimed at modifying Type A behavior, since the presence of serious illness should act as a motivator for behavior change.

Advice and Clinical Anecdote

Friedman and Rosenman (1974) suggested a series of simple, self-directed strategies directed at the alteration of Type A behavior. The focus of their program was twofold. The first related to personal awareness of Type A behaviors. This arose from the notion that, while many people may exhibit Type A behaviors in a variety of situations, it is commonly reported that these behaviors are neither perceived as being Type A in character nor associated with feelings of undue stress or tension (Rosenman, 1978). In order to make people aware that they may be responding in a Type A fashion without recognizing it, Friedman and Rosenman (1974) produced an illustrative list of typical Type A behaviors extending across a variety of circumstances.

The second phase of this program related to a set of exercises designed to eliminate Type A behaviors whenever and wherever these were seen to occur. These strategies involved the deliberate imposition of alternative behaviors immediately a Type A behavior was identified, and emphasized self-management. This is of course, closely akin to the long-standing behavioral strategy of response substitution (Rimm & Masters, 1979).

Useful as such a program might be, however, there is no empirical data which attests to its effectiveness. It is simply presented as exercises based on clinical observation and practice, and on the conceptualization of the Type A behavior pattern which Friedman and Rosenman (1974) held. Rosenman and Friedman (1977) presented data from a small pilot study involving twelve Type A men in a group program lasting 18 months. Groups were conducted by a therapist with a psychoanalytic background, and intervention strategies were based on the notions espoused by Friedman and Rosenman (1974). There is little evidence to indicate the outcome of this program, though Chesney (1978) reported that anecdotal results arising from it were encouraging.

Systematic Studies of Type A Behavior Modification

The seminal work in this area has come from the studies of Suinn and his colleagues. This work, to which they have given the collective title Cardiac Stress Management Program (CSMP), was based on five premises (Suinn, 1980) considered essential in conceptualizing the process of Type A behavior modification. Firstly, they argued that stress management must be an early focus of intervention, since initial attempts to modify and reverse very ingrained patterns of Type A behavior may themselves lead to situational tension, and patients require the skills to combat this. Secondly, since time urgency and impatience were prominent components of Type A behavior, patients should experience relatively rapid changes in their behavior patterns so as to allay frustration which might arise from protracted intervention strategies. In order to achieve this, they adopted a form of accelerated anxiety management training previously developed by Suinn (1975, 1976). Thirdly, since persons with Type A behaviors frequently see these as equating with productivity and efficiency (Rosenman, 1978), any alternative behaviors or life styles put forward should be seen as carrying the same advantages. Fourthly, behavioral retraining should emphasize a self-control of patients' own activities to others. Finally, it seemed most productive to give Type A persons the actual experience of producing alternative behaviors rather than simply instructing in these. For this reason they devised a program of visuomotor behavior rehearsal (VMBR) (Suinn, 1972, 1976), where subjects rehearsed alternative behaviors under controlled conditions so that resulting stress could be effectively and rapidly alleviated.

In some respects, Suinn's conceptualization of the modification of

Type A behavior seems similar to that originally advanced by Friedman and Rosenman (1974), with the emphasis on both awareness of Type A responses and the deliberate practice of alternative behaviors to these. The advance is, of course, that Suinn has refined this model and proposed concrete intervention strategies based on the principles of behavior modification.

Two studies have been undertaken to evaluate these strategies. In the first of these, Suinn (1975) investigated type A behavior modification in patients who had survived myocardial infarction. Ten patients were given five group sessions composed of both anxiety management training and VMBR, and their progress was compared with a similar group of 10 subjects undergoing standard medical rehabilitation procedures. Outcome measures centered on indices of coronary risk, and in particular on serum lipid measures. Substantial decreases in both cholesterol and triglyceride level were found for intervention subjects, both within the group (pre- vs. posttest levels), and when the intervention group was compared with the control group. These findings were replicated in a further sample of 17 survivors of myocardial infarction who later undertook the intervention program (Suinn, 1980). However, while the intent of the program was to modify Type A behavior, no specific measures of this were used, and there is no way of telling whether changes in the behavior pattern were in fact achieved. Certainly, it is encouraging that intervention produced changes in coronary risk as indexed by cholesterol levels. Changes in Type A behavior, whether they were simultaneous or casual, cannot, however, be inferred from these results.

In a subsequent study based on a similar conceptualization of Type A behavior modification, Suinn and Bloom (1978) used subjects drawn from a population of healthy volunteers. Behavioral intervention strategies closely similar to those employed in the previous study were offered to one group of these subjects, and outcome measures were compared with a control group to which no intervention program was offered. Each group consisted of seven subjects. This, perhaps, says something of the differential effects of intervention between myocardial infarction patients and ostensibly healthy subjects.

More importantly, however, measures of both Type A behavior and anxiety were employed in the study. Using these as outcome measures, it was found that intervention subjects showed significant decreases both in state and trait anxiety measures, and also in the Speed and Impatience and Hard Driving scales of the Jenkins Activity Survey, when compared with control subjects. This evidence is more pertinent to the issue, and provides some support for the contention that at least some aspects of Type A behavior are open to effective modification. The results, however, must be viewed cautiously, for at least two reasons. Firstly, the sample sizes were small and there were discrepancies between serum lipid results emerging from the first study (Suinn, 1975) and this subsequent study. Secondly, as Chesney et al. (1981) have pointed out, the Jenkins Activity Survey total Type A scores were not significantly lower in the intervention group than in the control group, and it is only this total score which has been found in epidemiological studies to be reliably predictive of myocardial infarction.

The other systematically evaluated approach to the modification of Type A behavior has arisen from the work of Roskies and her colleagues (1978, 1979), though the conceptual basis of this work differs markedly from that adopted by Suinn. The propositions upon which this work is based appear to be psychoanalytic in nature and involve the notion that Type A behavior arises from continued striving for maternal love, and guilt over competition with the father. All other considerations aside, this appears to be something of a sexist notion of Type A behavior in view of Waldron et al.'s (1977) evidence that women as well as men may manifest Type A attributes.

To examine this approach, Roskies, Spevack, Surkis, Cohen, and Gilman (1978) offered a program of 14 group sessions of psychotherapy run along psychoanalytic lines to a group of 13 healthy subjects with identified Type A behavior. The focus of these group sessions was to sensitize Type A persons to their apparent need to exert control over the environments within which they lived, and to facilitate recognition of the maladaptive aspects of this situation. A second group of 12 healthy subjects, also with identified Type A behaviors, were taught in 14 group sessions to modify their Type A responses by means of standard stress management procedures. These procedures involved the continual monitoring of tensions during daily life and the use of deep muscle relaxation exercises to counteract this tension. The group was identified as a behavior therapy group. A final and rather small group of six subjects consisted of patients with identified cardiovascular disease and was treated in the same way as the behavior therapy group.

Reductions in both cholesterol levels and systolic blood pressure were evident over the course of treatment for all groups; however, there were no significant differences between groups. A measure of psychological well-being, the General Health Questionnaire, which can be seen as a measure of state anxiety (Henderson, Byrne, & Duncan-Jones, 1981), also showed decreases over time for all groups. Once more, however, no standard measure of Type A behavior was consistently used. Subjects were asked for subjective self-reports of competitiveness and time urgency, and it was found that these self-reported attributes decreased over the course of treatment for all groups. Decreases were significantly greater for the behavioral group than for the psychotherapy group. In the absence of specific and recognized measures of Type A behavior, however, the results must be viewed tentatively.

Roskies et al. (1979) published a 6-month follow-up to their 1978 study, in which it was found that changes in risk factor levels for the behaviorally treated group with identified cardiovascular disease were significantly more enduring than changes in risk factor levels for the group of healthy subjects treated with psychotherapy. Outcome measures for healthy subjects who were also treated behaviorally lay somewhere between these two groups.

Jenni and Wollersheim (1979) used volunteer subjects both with and without a history of cardiovascular disease, but with identified Type A behavior. These were assigned either to a behavioral intervention group emphasizing the restructuring of cognitions associated with Type A behavior, a stress management group involving the monitoring of tension and the use of procedures to counteract this, and a waiting list control group. Each of the intervention groups involved six sessions. The cognitive therapy group showed decreases in serum cholesterol levels over the course of treatment relative to a minor increase in cholesterol in the waiting list control group. There was, however, a substantial increase in cholesterol during the course of stress management, and this result, which clearly indicates an elevation in cardiovascular risk, is unexplained. Indices of both state and trait anxiety decreased over time in both intervention groups relative to the control group; however, these changes were not enduring.

While the Structured Interview was used to assess subjects for Type A behavior at the beginning of the study, it was not readministered either after intervention or at follow up. The Bortner scale (Bortner, 1969) was administered as a postintervention measure, and Type A behaviors were not evident in the sample to any excessive degree. Direct comparisons between pretest and posttest measures cannot, however, be made, since the scales differed appreciably between these two points of data collection.

Suinn (1980) quoted two unpublished studies which give some more support for the notion that Type A behavior is amenable to modification. Curtis (1974) used a collection of behavioral techniques, including stress management and autogenic training, as the basis for behavior modification in a group of healthy Type A subjects. Comparison of intervention subjects with a control group also possessing Type A attributes revealed reductions among the former, in both cholesterol and triglyceride levels over the course of intervention, relative to the latter. Yarian (1976) used electromyographic biofeedback as a Type A intervention strategy and was able to demonstrate reductions in levels of frontalis muscle activity among Type A intervention subjects relative to Type A control subjects. In neither case, however, were explicit measures of Type A behavior used, and so once more it is not possible to attribute changes either in risk factor levels (serum lipids) or tension levels (muscle activity) to preceding changes in Type A behavior.

The focus of a systematic study reported by Levenkron, Cohen, Mueller, and Fisher (1983) was a comparison of three methods (comprehensive behavior therapy emphasizing self-control procedures, group support but without specific behavioral procedures, and the provision of basic health information) for the modification of Type A behavior among healthy male volunteers. Pretreatment assessment included measures of self-reported Type A behavior together with scales of affective distress and measures of coronary risk factors. Both behavior therapy and group support conditions involved weekly meetings of 90 minutes spread over 8 consecutive weeks, while the final condition (information giving) involved a single 2-hour session. At follow-up 1 week after termination of each treatment condition, subjects involved in both behavior therapy and group support exhibited significantly lower scores on the Jenkins Activity Survey than did subjects in the information-only groups. This pattern was evident also in self-reported reactions to a stress challenge test. Neither temporal changes nor differences between groups were, however, apparent for standard coronary risk factors (heart rate, blood pressure, or blood fats). This study singled out anger and impatience, in particular, as useful targets for treatment.

Certainly, the most ambitious program of research yet to be undertaken in this area is that initiated under the direction of Friedman (1978). In this study, a cohort of 862 Type A males who had recently survived myocardial infarction were offered a variety of intervention strategies aimed at modifying their Type A behaviors. Of these, 592 were randomly assigned to groups using broad spectrum approaches, including self-observation and monitoring to increase awareness of Type A behavior, self-management of the environment, behavioral contracting, deep muscle relation, anxiety management training, and cognitive restructuring directed towards modifying Type A behavior. The remaining 270 were allocated to groups which emphasized traditional procedures of rehabilitation and included a "conventional education regarding the need to reduce traditional risk factors and group psychotherapy to deal with problems of anxiety and depression" (Surwit et al., 1982, p. 210).

Results of this large study have been encouraging, due in large part to a more than adequate sample size, the use of multiple measures of Type A behavior, and the prospective design of the investigation. A

2-year follow-up of patients taking part in the study has shown quite persuasively that Type A behavior is amenable to modification (Powell, Friedman, Thoresen, Gill, & Ulmer, 1984). Patients taking part in programs designed specifically to modify the behavior pattern were, after 2 years, significantly lower on Type A behavior as measured by self-support, the report of a spouse, and the report of a co-worker than were patients whose cardiac rehabilitation program was aimed at general issues. Type A behavior was judged by independent raters viewing a videotape of the Structured Interview method of assessment. Of those involved in the Type A modification program, 17.9% showed reductions in multiple measures of Type A behavior, and a further 29.4% on a single measure of the behavior pattern; only 21.5% failed to demonstrate any reduction, while 26.5% dropped out of the study.

The clinical importance of this program is evident, however, in a further report of the same cohort (Friedman et al., 1984) in which it can be seen that decreases in the rate of coronary events follow from reductions in the level of Type A behavior. The 3-year cumulative recurrence rate for myocardial infarction among those receiving Type A behavior modification was, at 7.2%, significantly lower than the 13% found in those receiving a more medically oriented rehabilitation program. The implications of this finding are of considerable importance in the secondary prevention of myocardial infarction; however, the full realization of this benefit must await the demonstration that modification of the Type A behavior pattern, when applied to those free of cardiac symptoms, results in significant reductions in the primary incidence of heart attack.

With the exception, then, of the work of Suinn and his colleagues (Suinn, 1975, 1980; Suinn & Bloom, 1978), and the extensive study of Friedman and his group, there has been little attempt either to spell out the conceptual basis for intervention strategies or to describe in sufficient detail the nature and course of the intervention processes undertaken. This is a critical deficit, since it allows neither the systematic replication of these studies nor translation of the intervention techniques into feasible strategies for routine clinical management of cardiac patients. This makes the adequate description of the intervention foci a crucial consideration in any future study of Type A behavior modification, whether it be experimental or clinical.

General Principles in the Modification of Type A Behavior

While the studies quoted above may be criticized both on conceptual and methodological grounds, the results are encouraging when viewed collectively. The evidence points to the conclusion that deliberate strategies of behavior modification designed to counteract one or more of the elements of Type A behavior can achieve measurable reductions in primary or secondary coronary risk. Two basic questions remain unanswered, however. The first concerns the specific aspects of Type A behavior which, if successfully modified, are likely to provide the greatest benefit in terms of reduced coronary morbidity and mortality. The second concerns the most appropriate strategies of intervention to modify these aspects of behavior.

It will be clear from the earlier sections of this chapter that Type A behavior is not a unitary phenomenon but is composed of a number of components (Jenkins & Zyzanski, 1982). With this is mind, one can see sense in the argument of Chesney et al. (1981) that the first step in any program of Type A behavior modification, whether it be experimental or clinical, is the specification of target behaviors. Two things need to be borne in mind in this respect. The first of these is that Type A behaviors take several forms and that those aspects which are present in one individual need not necessarily be present in another. The second is that, while Type A behavior contributes to coronary risk, it is rather less clear which components of Type A behavior are most damaging. All of this points to the need for individually tailored programs of Type A behavior modification designed to fit the specific demands of each individual patient. This assumes that the components of Type A behavior can and will be accurately measured as a precondition to modification. The notion of individual programs also conflicts, to an extent, with the potential benefits arising from intervention with groups of patients. Assuming, then, that we are at least able to specify for any individual, those aspects of Type A behavior which are most prominent, it should be possible to list the available intervention strategies which might be brought to bear on the modification, whether these strategies have been examined specifically in relation to Type A subjects or arise more generally from the literature in behavior modification.

Cognitive strategies. It seems clear that Type A behaviors, as manifest responses, arise from some predisposing set of cognitions or personal constructions of the environment. The most fundamental of the intervention strategies would, therefore, appear to be those based on the restructuring of these cognitions. Jenni and Wollersheim (1979) reported their most promising results from the cognitive therapy group, and elements of cognitive restructuring can be discerned within the therapeutic strategies of Suinn (1980) and of Roskies et al. (1978), though, in the latter study, much of this is phrased within a psychoanalytic context. An examination of the range of strategies proposed by Friedman and his group also indicates a considerable reliance on those to do with cognitive restructuring. Clearly, the effective utilization of cognitive strategies will depend on the effective externalization and specification of what the offending cognitions may be. This is standard practice in any form of cognitive therapy. Having disclosed the internal dialogue hypothesized to cause people to respond to their environments in Type A ways, there is every reason to believe that those cognitive restructuring strategies may be used effectively to modify cognitions which initiate and promote Type A behaviors.

Environmental management. A prominent aspect of the literature in this area has related to the ways in which social and cultural contexts might reinforce and maintain Type A behaviors once these are established (Rosenman, 1978). This presents a potential difficulty, since it might be surmounted only by social change on a large scale, and while this may be a desirable objective, it is infrequently a practical proposition. Environments can, of course, be changed in more modest ways. Chesney et al. (1981) point to the possibility of modifying home and work environments at an individual level without the need to consider social change on a grander scale. Modification of the social and occupational environments at this level may involve both monitoring, to discern those elements of the environment that are likely to reinforce Type A behaviors, and the use of deliberate strategies such as those suggested by Friedman and Rosenman (1974) to change these situations. This may be particularly useful in the work environment (Chesney & Rosenman, 1980), where the individual may be encouraged to exercise a degree of control over the amount of work undertaken, the amount of effort and time put into work, and the extent to which occupational considerations should override other activities such as those involving leisure and recreation. However, in societies where the level of employment relates strongly to social and economic status, this should be undertaken with the patient's explicit acceptance that previously valued aspects of life style may incur change. This may prove difficult, given the common tendency to equate the time urgency and excess activity associated with Type A behavior with efficiency and productivity in one's work life.

Direct behavior change. Type A behaviors take a wide variety of forms, and though they come about as the result of situational determinants, their common characteristic is that they are overt and observable aspects of activity and lifestyle. Such behaviors, therefore, form a very apparent focus for intervention strategies. Indeed, the thrust of Friedman and Rosenman's (1974) suggestions to Type A individuals to alter their behaviors was that they should quite deliberately adopt patterns of activity which were diametrically opposed to Type A behaviors. This area does, however, bear on the very mainstream of behavior therapy, and a wide range of well-established and evaluated techniques are available for the modification of unwanted behaviors, Type A or other. Much of the emphasis of Suinn's (1980) work had to do with the immediate alteration of behaviors which were identified as Type A. This was based on the rationale that Type A subjects are most likely to respond favorably to procedures in which they can become experientially involved, and where relatively rapid changes, at least during the course of therapy, are likely to be evident. Two well-accepted procedures in behavior therapy, those of behavior rehearsal and response substitution, both using role play methods, are important in this respect. Within the context of Type A behavior modification, the patient would be encouraged to continually monitor personal behaviors for Type A responses. When these were likely to occur, the selection of an alternative non-Type A response, perhaps from a prearranged list, and the deliberate initiation of this behavior, would be practiced. When coupled with the technique of role play, where the patient is able to practice these response substitution procedures in the absence of threat from the real environment, the process may form the basis for a useful strategy for the direct modification of Type A behaviors.

Time management. The prominence of time urgency within the Type A behavior pattern points to the potential effectiveness of time management in intervention. Individuals with this component of Type A behavior are typically poor managers of time, and this is perhaps most evident in their struggle to obtain an unlimited number of poorly defined things from their environment in a short period of time (Friedman, 1969). Procedures for the training of effective time management are, however, now available and have been evaluated (Lakein, 1973; Ferner, 1980). These procedures involve the monitoring and definition of areas where time management is ineffective, and the more rational allocation of available times to necessary tasks. Given the prominence of time urgency and its variety of manifestations within the overall Type A behavior pattern, it is likely that procedures for the retraining of time management will receive greater attention in future strategies of Type A intervention.

Hostility management. Overt hostility as a manifestation of Type A behavior is perhaps less prominent than one might expect, given its repeated appearance in descriptions of the Type A behavior pattern (Herman et al., 1981) though these same authors reported that 62% of

Type A subjects rated themselves as "aggressive," while Francis (1981) found that Type A subjects reported significantly higher levels of "state hostility" as evidenced on the Multiple Affective Adjective Check List than did their non-Type A colleagues. The procedures developed by Novaco (1975) for the management of anger and hostility, which emphasize self-monitoring the restructuring of hostile cognitions and the substitution of passive or neutral responses, would be well suited where hostility was found to be a prominent component of the presenting Type A pattern for any individual.

Stimulus control. Consideration of the direct modification of behaviors within the Type A pattern does raise one rather general issue in behavior therapy. The prevailing conceptions of the Type A pattern (Rosenman & Chesney, 1980) suggest that the overt and manifest behaviors are directly initiated by situational and environmental circumstances which may themselves be transient. That is, Type A behaviors seem, to an extent, to be under stimulus control. The area of stimulus control has been well documented in behavior therapy (Goldfried & Merbaum, 1973), and several of the intervention strategies alluded to above may well have been discussed within the ambit of stimulus control. While no work has yet been done in this area, formalizations of intervention strategies based on the identification of situational determinants of Type A behavior, and the gradual dissociation of behaviors from their determinants, would seem to hold some conceptual promise.

Stress management. As will be evident from earlier discussions, the appearance of distress or other affective disturbances as a consequence of Type A behaviors is still in debate (Byrne, 1981). Nonetheless, there is growing evidence that persons manifesting the Type A behavior pattern will also experience and report signs of affective distress (Suinn, 1980). Indeed, as Suinn pointed out, the very process of attempting to modify Type A behaviors may lead to frustration and distress if the subject is unable to experience early success with behavior modification. The need to incorporate procedures for stress management into a comprehensive strategy of Type A behavior modification would, therefore, seem to be indicated.

There is much to recommend Suinn's programs of anxiety management (Suinn, 1975; Suinn & Richardson, 1971; Suinn & Bloom, 1978), to the extent that these are based both on well-researched processes of anxiety management and have been evaluated with cardiac patients. Progressive muscle relaxation clearly has an important role to play both in these programs and in others (Jenni & Wollersheim, 1978; Roskies et al., 1978). However, three cautions are advised in its use.

The first is that, in isolation, relaxation is unlikely to be particularly effective, since it focuses on the consequences of Type A behaviors while doing little to modify the behaviors themselves. The second is that people with extreme degrees of Type A behavior may be unwilling to engage in the somewhat rigorous time demands of relaxation training, in the absence of relatively immediate effects. Thus progressive muscle relaxation in the management of affective distress associated with Type A behavior is to be seen more as a component of intervention than as its central focus.

The final caution concerns the potentially damaging physiological effects of isometric procedures of muscle relaxation on the vulnerable myocardium in recent survivors of myocardial infarction. While the evidence suggests that ordinary procedures of muscle relaxation are unlikely to severely challenge the myocardial integrity of cardiac patients (Davidson, Winchester, Taylor, Alderman, & Ingels, 1979) the use of more passive strategies for muscle relaxation must be advocated, at least in the early stages of recovery from myocardial infarction.

It should be borne in mind that, where intervention is undertaken with the recent survivor of myocardial infarction, the affective picture may be confounded by the patient's immediate emotional responses to illness (Byrne, 1979; Byrne & Whyte, 1978). Thus, the pattern of affective distress evident in this period may not necessarily characterize the individual's state either before illness onset or in the long term after. This does not detract from the potential value of the management of affective distress at this point, though the therapist should be aware that it is not necessarily Type A behavior which is being treated.

Psychophysiological management. There is little doubt that, at least under some circumstances, Type A behavior has definite psychophysiological consequences. A range of behavioral techniques, including deep muscle relaxation (Blanchard & Miller, 1977) and biofeedback of various kinds (Schwartz & Beatty, 1977) have been advocated for the control of this activity. It is worth bearing in mind, however, that, if the cognitive and behavioral aspects of Type A behavior have been adequately addressed in any program of intervention, the need to consider treatment at the physiological stage should have diminished. Indeed, this may even be seen as an instance of "putting the cart before the horse," and there would be some who would argue that, if the psychophysiological consequences of Type A behavior are so pronounced as to pose a future threat, then they should be treated pharmacologically with the use of a beta blocking agent (Rosenman, 1983), while psychological management should simultaneously focus on the modification of events earlier in the process. This perhaps goes too far and denies the potential usefulness of behavioral techniques which might help to control physiological arousal, but it does underscore the primary importance of behavior modification at the level of cognitions and of Type A behaviors themselves.

REFERENCES

Anderson, J. R., & Waldron, I. (1983). Behavioral and content components of the structured interview assessment of the Type A behavior pattern in women. *Journal of Behavioral Medicine*, *6*, 123–135.

Barefoot, J. C., Dahlstrom, W. G., & Williams, R. B. (1983). Hostility, CHD incidence and total mortality: A 25 year follow-up of 255 physicians. *Psychosomatic Medicine*, *45*, 59–63.

Bass, C. (1984). Type A behavior in patients with chest pain: Test-retest reliability and psychometric correlates of Bortner scale. *Journal of Psychosomatic Research*, *28*, 289–300.

Blanchard, E. B., & Miller, S. T. (1977). Psychological treatment of cardiovascular disease. *Archives of General Psychiatry*, *34*, 1402–1413.

Blumenthal, J. A., Williams, R., Kong, Y., Schanberg, S. M., & Thompson, L. W. (1978). Type A behavior pattern and coronary atherosclerosis. *Circulation*, *58*, 634–639.

Bortner, R. W. (1969). A short rating scale as a potential measure of Pattern A behavior. *Journal of Chronic Diseases*, *22*, 87–91.

Brand, R. J., Rosenman, R. H., Jenkins, C. D., Sholtz, R. I., & Zyzanski, S. J. (1978). Comparison of coronary heart disease prediction in the Western Collaborative Group Study using the structured interview and the Jenkins Activity Survey Assessments of the coronary-prone Type A behavior pattern. In R. M. Dembroski, S. M. Weiss, J. L. Shields, S. G. Haynes, & M. Feinleib (Eds.), *Coronary-prone behavior*. New York: Springer-Verlag.

Byrne, D. G. (1979). Anxiety as state and trait following survived myocardial infarction. *British Journal of Social and Clinical Psychology*, *18*, 417–423.

Byrne, D. G. (1981). Type A behaviour, life events and myocardial infarction: Independent or related risk factors? *British Journal of Medical Psychology*, *54*, 371–377.

Byrne, D. G., & Rosenman, R. H. (1986). The Type A behaviour pattern as a precursor to stressful life-events: A confluence of coronary risks. *British Journal of Medical Psychology*, *59*, 75–82.

Byrne, D. G., & Rosenman, R. H. (1987). Type A behaviour and the experience of affective discomfort. *Journal of Psychosomatic Research*, *30*, 663–672.

Byrne, D. G., Rosenman, R. H., Schiller, E., & Chesney, M. A. (1985). Consistency and variation among instruments purporting to measure the Type A behavior pattern. *Psychosomatic Medicine*, *47*, 242–261.

Byrne, D. G., & Whyte, H. M. (1978). Dimensions of illness behaviour in survivors of myocardial infarction. *Journal of Psychosomatic Research, 22*, 485–491.

Caffrey, B. (1968). Reliability and validity of behavioral measures in a study of coronary heart disease. *Journal of Chronic Diseases, 21*, 191–204.

Caffrey, B. (1978). Psychometric procedures applied to the assessment of the coronary-prone behavior pattern. In T. M. Dembroski, S. M. Weiss, J. L. Shields, S. G. Haynes, M. Feinleib (Eds.), *Coronary-prone behavior*. New York: Springer-Verlag.

Case, R. B., Heller, S. S., Case, N. B., Moss, A. J., & the Multicenter Post-Infarction Research Group. (1985). Type A behavior and survival after acute myocardial infarction. *New England Journal of Medicine, 312*, 737–741.

Chesney, M. A. (1978). *Coronary-prone behavior and coronary heart disease: Intervention strategies*. Unpublished manuscript.

Chesney, M. A., & Rosenman, R. H. (1980). Type A behavior in the work setting. In C. L. Cooper & R. Payne (Eds.), *Current concerns in occupational stress*. New York: John Wiley & Sons Ltd.

Chesney, M. A., Black, G. W., Chadwick, J. H., & Rosenman, R. H. (1981). Psychological correlates of the Type A behavior pattern. *Journal of Behavioral Medicine, 4*, 217–229.

Cohen, J. B., Syme, S. L., Jenkins, C. D., Kagan, A., & Zyzanski, S. J. (1979). Cultural context of Type A behavior and risk for CHD: A study of Japanese American males. *Journal of Behavioral Medicine, 2*, 375–384.

Curtis, J. (1974). *The effects of educational intervention on the Type A behavior pattern*. Unpublished manuscript, University of Utah.

Davidson, D. M., Winchester, M. A., Taylor, C. B., Alderman, E. A., & Ingels, N. B. (1979). Effects of relaxation therapy on cardiac performance and sympathetic activity in patients with organic heart disease. *Psychosomatic Medicine, 41*, 303–309.

Dembroski, T. M., Macdougall, J. M., Shields, J. L., Petitto, J., & Lushene, R. (1978). Components of the Type A coronary-prone behavior pattern and cardiovascular responses to psychomotor performance challenge. *Journal of Behavioral Medicine, 1*, 159–176.

Dimsdale, J. E., Hackett, T. P., Block, P. C., & Hutter, A. M. (1978). Emotional correlates of Type A behavior pattern. *Psychosomatic Medicine, 40*, 580–583.

Eysenck, H. J., & Fulker, D. (1982). The components of Type A behaviour and its genetic determinants. *Activitas Nervosa Superieur (Prague), Supplement 3*, 111–125.

Falger, P., Bressors, I., & Dijkstra, P. (1980). Levensloop patronen van hartinfarct patienten en van controlegroegen: Enkele overeenkomsten en verschillen. *Gerontologie, 11*, 240–257.

Ferner, J. D. (1980). *Successful time management*. New York: Wiley.

Francis, K. T. (1981). Perceptions of anxiety, hostility and depression in subjects exhibiting the coronary-prone behavior pattern. *Journal of Psychiatric Research, 16*, 183–190.

Frank, K. A., Heller, S. S., Kornfeld, D. S., Sporn, A. A., & Weiss, M. (1978). Behavior pattern and coronary angiographic findings. *Journal of the American Medical Association, 240*, 761–763.

Friedman, M. (1978a). Type A behavior: Its possible relationship to pathogenic processes responsible for coronary heart disease. In T. M. Dembroski, S. M. Weiss, J. L. Shields, S. G. Haynes, & M. Feinleib (Eds.), *Coronary prone behavior*. New York: Springer-Verlag.

Friedman, M. (1978b). Modifying "Type A" behavior in heart attack patients. *Primary Cardiology*, pp. 9–13.

Friedman, M., & Rosenman, R. H. (1959). Association of a specific overt behavior pattern with increases in blood cholesterol, blood clotting time, incidence of arcus senilis, and clinical coronary artery disease. *Journal of the American Medical Association, 169*, 1286–1296.

Friedman, M., & Rosenman, R. H. (1974). *Type A behavior and your heart*. New York: Knopf.

Friedman, M., St. George, S., & Byers, S. O. (1960). Excretion of catecholamines, 17-ketosteroids, 17-hydroxycorticoids and 6-hydroxy-indole in men exhibiting a particular behavior pattern (A) associated with high incidence of clinical coronary artery disease. *Journal of Clinical Investigation, 39*, 758–764.

Friedman, M., Thoresen, C. E., Gill, J. J., Powell, L. H., Ulmer, D., Thompson, L., Price, V., Rabin, D., Breal, W. S., Dixon, T., Levy, R., & Bourg, E. (1984). Alteration of Type A behavior and reduction in cardiac recurrences in post myocardial infarction patients. *American Heart Journal, 108*, 237–248.

Gentry, W. D. (1978). Behavior modification of the coronary-prone behavior pattern. In T. M. Dembroski, S. M. Weiss, J. L. Shields, S. G. Haynes, & M. Feinlab (Eds.), *Coronary-prone behavior*. New York: Springer-Verlag.

Goldfried, M. R., & Merbaum, M. (1973). *Behavior change through self-control*. New York: Holt, Rinehart & Winston.

Haynes, S. G., Feinleib, M., & Kannel, W. B. (1980). The relationship of psychosocial factors to coronary heart disease in the Framingham Study: III. Eight year incidence of coronary heart disease. *American Journal of Epidemiology, 111*, 37–58.

Haynes, S. G., Feinleib, M., Levine, S., Scotch, N., & Kannel, W. B. (1978). The relationship of psychosocial factors to coronary heart disease in the Framingham Study: II. Prevalence of coronary heart disease. *American Journal of Epidemiology, 107*, 384.

Heller, R. F. (1979). Type A behavior and coronary heart disease. *British Medical Journal, 2*, 368.

Henderson, A. S., Byrne, D. G., & Duncan Jones, P. (1981). *Neurosis and the social environment*. Sydney, Australia: Academic Press.

Herman, S., Blumenthal, J. A., Black, G. M., & Chesney, M. A. (1981). Self-ratings of Type A (coronary prone) adults: Do Type A's know they are Type A's. *Psychosomatic Medicine, 43*, 405–413.

Irvine, J., Lyle, R. C., & Allon, R. (1982). Type A personality as psychopathology: Personality correlates and an abbreviated scoring system. *Journal of Psychosomatic Research, 26*, 183–189.

Jenkins, C. D. (1978). A comparative review of the interview and questionnaire methods in the assessment of the coronary-prone behavior pattern. In T. M. Dembroski, S. M. Weiss, J. L. Shields, S. G. Haynes, & M. Feinleib (Eds.), *Coronary-prone behavior*. New York: Springer-Verlag.

Jenkins, C. D., & Zyzanski, S. J. (1982). The Type A behaviour pattern is alive and well—when not dissected: A reply. *British Journal of Medical Psychology, 55*, 219–223.

Jenkins, C. D., Rosenman, R. H., & Friedman, M. (1967). Development of an objective psychological test for the determination of the coronary-prone behavior pattern in employed men. *Journal of Chronic Diseases, 20*, 371–379.

Jenkins, C. D., Rosenman, R. H., & Friedman, M. (1968). Replicability of rating the coronary-prone behavior pattern. *British Journal of Preventive and Sociological Medicine, 22*, 16–22.

Jenkins, C. D., Zyzanski, S. J., & Rosenman, R. H. (1971). Progress toward validation of a computer-scored test for the Type A coronary-prone behavior pattern. *Psychosomatic Medicine, 33*, 193–201.

Jenkins, C. D., Zyzanski, S. H., & Rosenman, R. H. (1976). Risk of new myocardial infarction in middle-aged men with manifest coronary heart disease. *Circulation, 53*, 342–347.

Jenkins, C. D., Zyzanski, S. J., & Rosenman, R. H. (1979). *Jenkins activity survey manual (Form C)*. New York: The Psychological Corp.

Jenkins, C. D., Zyzanski, S. J., Rosenman, R. H., & Cleveland, G. L. (1971). Association of coronary-prone behavior scores with recurrence of coronary heart disease. *Journal of Chronic Diseases, 24*, 601–611.

Jenni, M., & Wollersheim, J. (1979). Cognitive therapy, stress management training, and the Type A behavior pattern. *Cognitive Therapy and Research, 3*, 61–73.

Keegan, D. L., Sinha, B. N., Merriman, J. E., & Shipley, C. (1979). Type A behavior pattern: Relationship to coronary heart disease, personality and life adjustment. *Canadian Journal of Psychiatry, 24*, 724–730.

Kenigsberg, D., Zyzanski, S. J., Jenkins, C. D., Wardwell, W. I., & Licciardello, T. (1974). The coronary-prone behavior pattern in hospitalized patients with and without coronary heart disease. *Psychosomatic Medicine, 36*, 344–51.

Kornitzer, M., Kittel, F., De Backer, G., & Dramaix, M. (1981). The Belgian heart disease prevention project: Type A behavior pattern and the prevalence of coronary heart disease. *Psychosomatic Medicine, 43*, 133–145.

Lakein, A. (1973). *How to get control of your time and your life*. New York: Signet.

Levenkron, J. C., Cohen, J. D., Mueller, H. S., & Fisher, E. B. (1983). Modifying the Type A coronary-prone behavior pattern. *Journal of Consulting and Clinical Psychology, 51*, 192–204.

Matthews, K. A., Glass, D. C., Rosenman, R. H., & Bortner, R. W. (1977). Competitive drive, pattern A and coronary heart disease: A further analysis of some data from the Western Collaborative Group Study. *Journal of Chronic Diseases, 30*, 489–498.

Matthews, K. A., Krantz, D. S., Dembroski, T. M., & McDougall, J. M. (1982).

Unique and common variance in structured interview and Jenkins Activity Survey measures of the Type A behavior pattern. *Journal of Personality and Social Psychology, 42*, 303–313.

Myrtek, M., & Greenlee, M. W. (1984). Psychophysiology of Type A behavior pattern: A critical analysis. *Journal of Psychosomatic Research, 28*, 455–466.

Novaco, R. W. (1975). *Anger control.* Lexington, MA: Heath.

Orth-Gomer, K., & Ahlbom, A. (1980). Impact of psychological stress on ischaemic heart disease when controlling for conventional risk indicators. *Journal of Human Stress, 61*, 7–15.

Powell, L. H., Friedman, M., Thoresen, C. E., Gill, J. J., & Ulmer, D. K. (1984). Can the Type A behavior pattern be altered after myocardial infarction? A second year report from the recurrent coronary prevention project. *Psychosomatic Medicine, 26*, 293–313.

Price, V. A. (1983). *Type A behavior pattern: A model for research and practice.* New York: Academic Press.

Rimm, D. C., & Masters, J. C. (1979). *Behavior therapy: Techniques and empirical findings* (2nd ed.). New York: Academic Press.

Rosenman, R. H. (1978). The interview method of assessment of the coronary-prone behavior pattern. In T. M. Dembroski, S. M. Weiss, J. L. Shields, S. G. Haynes, & M. Fernleib (Eds.), *Coronary-prone behavior.* New York: Springer-Verlag.

Rosenman, R. H. (1983). *Psychosomatic risk factors and coronary heart disease: Indications for specific preventive therapy.* Bern, Stuttgart, and Vienna: Hans Huber Publishers.

Rosenman, R. H., & Chesney, M. A. (1980). The relationship of Type A behavior pattern to coronary heart disease. *Activitas Nervosa Superieur, 22*, 1–45.

Rosenman, R., & Chesney, M. (1982). Stress, Type A behavior and coronary disease. In L. Goldberger & S. Bresnitz (Eds.), *The handbook of stress.* New York: MacMillan.

Rosenman, R. H., & Friedman, M. (1977). Modifying Type A behavior pattern. *Journal of Psychosomatic Research, 21*, 323–331.

Rosenman, R. H., Brand, R. J., Jenkins, C. D., Friedman, M., Straus, R., & Wurm, M. (1975). Coronary heart disease in the Western Collaborative Group Study: Final follow-up experience of 8½ years. *Journal of the American Medical Association, 233*, 872–877.

Rosenman, R. H., Friedman, M., Straus, R., Jenkins, C. D., Zyzanski, S. J., & Wurm, M. (1970). Coronary heart disease in the Western Collaborative Group Study: A follow-up experience of 4½ years. *Journal of Chronic Diseases, 23*, 173–90.

Rosenman, R. H., Friedman, M., Straus, R., Wurm, M., Kositchek, P., Hahn, W., & Werthessen, N. T. (1964). A predictive study of coronary heart disease: the Western Collaborative Group Study. *Journal of the American Medical Association, 189*, 15–22.

Roskies, E., Kearney, H., Spevack, M., Surkis, A., Cohen, C., & Gilman, S. (1979). Generalizability and durability of treatment effects in an intervention program for coronary-prone (Type A) managers. *Journal of Behavioral Medicine, 2*, 195–207.

Roskies, F., Spevack, M., Surkis, A., Cohen, C., & Gilman, S. (1978). Changing the coronary-prone (Type A) behavior pattern in a non-clinical population. *Journal of Behavioral Medicine, 1*, 201–216.

Scherwitz, L., McKelvain, R., & Laman, C. (1983). Type A behavior, self-involvement, and coronary atherosclerosis. *Psychosomatic Medicine, 45*, 47–57.

Schwartz, G. E., & Beatty, J. (1977). *Biofeedback: Theory and research.* New York: Academic Press.

Shekelle, R. B., Gale, M., & Norusis, M. (1985). Type A score (Jenkins Activity Survey) and risk of recurrent coronary heart disease in the Aspirin Myocardial Infarction Study. *American Journal of Cardiology, 56*, 221–225.

Shekelle, R. B., Gale, M., Ostfeld, A. M., & Paul, O. (1983). Hostility, risk of coronary heart disease and mortality. *Psychosomatic Medicine, 45*, 109–114.

Shekelle, R. B., Schoenberger, J. A., & Stamler, J. A. (1976). Correlates of the JAS Type A behavior pattern score. *Journal of Chronic Diseases, 29*, 381–94.

Smith, T. W. (1984). Type A behavior, anger and neuroticism: The discriminant validity of self-reports in a patient sample. *British Journal of Clinical Psychology, 23*, 147–148.

Smith, T. W., Follick, M. J., & Korr, K. S. (1984). Anger, neuroticism, Type A behaviour and the experience of angina. *British Journal of Medical Psychology, 57*, 249–252.

Suinn, R. M. (1972). Behavior rehearsal training for ski racers. Brief report. *Behavior Therapy, 3*, 519.

Suinn, R. M. (1975). The cardiac stress management program for Type A patients. *Cardiac Rehabilitation, 5*(4).

Suinn, R. M. (1976). Anxiety management training to control general anxiety. In J. Krumboltz & C. Thoresen (Eds.), *Counseling methods.* New York: Holt.

Suinn, R. M. (1978). The coronary-prone behavior pattern: A behavioral approach to intervention. In T. M. Dembroski, S. W. Weiss, J. L. Shields, S. G. Haynes, & M. Feinleib (Eds.), *Coronary-prone behavior.* New York: Springer-Verlag.

Suinn, R. M. (1980). Pattern A behaviors and heart disease: Intervention approaches. In J. M. Ferguson & C. B. Taylor (Eds.), *Behavioral medicine.* Lancaster, England: MTP Press.

Suinn, R. M., & Bloom, L. J. (1978). Anxiety management training for Type A persons. *Journal of Behavioral Medicine, 1*, 25–35.

Suinn, R. M., & Richardson, F. (1971). Anxiety management training: A nonspecific behavior therapy program for anxiety control. *Behavior Therapy, 4*, 498.

Surwit, R. S., Williams, R. B., & Shapiro, D. (1982). *Behavioral approaches to cardiovascular disease.* New York: Academic Press.

Tennant, C., Langeluddecke, P., & Byrne, D. G. (1985). The concept of stress. *Australian New Zealand Journal of Psychiatry*, *19*, 113–118.

Vickers, R. (1973). *A short measure of Type A personality*. Unpublished manuscript, University of Michigan, Institute for Social Research.

Vickers, R. R., Hervig, L. K., Rahe, R. H., & Rosenman, R. H. (1981). Type A behavior pattern, coping and defense. *Psychosomatic Medicine*, *43*, 381–396.

Vingerhoets, A. J. J. M., & Flohr, P. J. M. (1984). Type A behaviour and self-reports of coping preferences. *British Journal of Medical Psychology*, *47*, 15–21.

Wadden, T. A., Anderson, C. H., Foster, G. D., & Love, W. (1983). The Jenkins Activity Survey: Does it measure psychopathology? *Journal of Psychosomatic Research*, *27*, 321–325.

Waldron, I., Zyzanski, S., Shekelle, R. B., Jenkins, C. D., & Tannenbaum, S. (1977). The coronary-prone behavior pattern in employed men and women. *Journal of Human Stress*, *3*, 2–18.

Williams, R. B., Haney, T. L., Lee, K. L., Kong, Y., Blumenthal, J. A., & Whalen, R. E. (1980). Type A behavior, hostility and coronary atherosclerosis. *Psychosomatic Medicine*, *42*, 539–549.

Yarian, R. (1976). *The efficacy of electromyographic biofeedback training as a method of deep muscle relaxation for college students displaying either coronary or non-coronary prone behavior patterns*. Unpublished manuscript, University of Maryland.

Zyzanski, S. J., & Jenkins, C. D. (1970). Basic dimensions within the coronary-prone behavior pattern. *Journal of Chronic Diseases*, *22*, 781–792.

Zyzanski, S. J., Jenkins, C. D., Ryan, T. J., Flessas, A., & Everist, M. (1976). Psychological correlates of coronary angiographic findings. *Archives of Internal Medicine*, *136*, 1234–1237.

5

Psychophysiological Mechanisms in the Etiology and Treatment of Essential Hypertension

Sarah S. Knox

Associate Professor of Psychiatry
Wayne State University School of Medicine
Detroit, MI
and
The Karolinska Institute of Environmental Medicine
Stockholm, Sweden

INTRODUCTION

Primary hypertension is widespread in Western industrial societies, and approximately 90% of all diagnosed cases are essential, that is, of unknown origin (Guyton, Cowley, Coleman, DeClue, Norman, & Manning 1974). In addition, only about 34% of those on medication gain control over their blood pressure (Rowland & Roberts, 1982). These facts have generated a great deal of scientific inquiry into the causality and treatment of essential hypertension. But the profusion of research has both facilitated and complicated understanding of the underlying etiological mechanisms. There seems to be a general consensus only in that the disease is multifactorial and heterogeneous (Weiner, 1979; Folkow, 1982). A number of studies, both animal (Okamato, 1972) and human (Heiberg, Magnus, Berg, & Nance, 1981; Iselius, 1983) have led to agreement among many authors that some combination of genetic predisposition is usually involved in the initial stages. But the heterogeneity of disease manifestations, even in same age populations, renders differentiation of causal mechanisms and the interplay of genetic and environmental variables extremely difficult. To complicate matters still further, the factors involved in initial elevations of blood pressure are not necessarily those which maintain them.

A comprehensive review of the literature would take several volumes and is beyond the scope of this chapter. What will be done here is to examine some of the psychophysiological processes involved in hypertension as well as some of the methodological problems which have led to contradictory results.

METHODOLOGICAL ASPECTS

One of the major confounding factors in many of even the most systematic studies of psychosocial variables and hypertension is the way in which the hypotheses are formulated. Large numbers of these studies are designed with systolic and diastolic blood pressure as dependent variables and a variety of personality, socioeconomic, and/or environmental variables as the independent variables postulated to influence blood pressure. The underlying assumption of simple cause/effect relationships neglects the obvious fact that permanent or often-recurring blood pressure elevation is the resulting symptom of a complicated disease process involving many physiological changes. The fact that there is still a great deal of discussion and uncertainty concerning the physiological parameters involved in the development and maintenance of hypertension causes complications in the design and interpretation of studies concerning psychosocial influences on its etiology.

The problems involved with hypertension research are well illustrated by the parable of the blind men and the elephant. Three blind men who did not know anything about elephants were shown an elephant and asked to describe their impressions. The first blind man felt the tusks and described the elephant as thin, smooth, and hard. The second felt the elephant's leg and described elephants as being very rough and shaped like a tree. The third began to feel around in the elephant's mouth and described him as warm and rather slimy. Each man described a partial truth—the result of his own interactions with the elephant. Yet these descriptions did not coincide.

The most glaring problem facing anyone trying to interpret or synthesize results from hypertension research is the number of studies ostensibly investigating the same variables, but yielding contradictory results. These contradictions have two principal sources: (a) measurement error, and (b) the focusing of attention on only one or a few hypothetically relevant variables, to the exclusion of others which covary or interact with those being investigated.

Both of these problems can be exemplified by the large amount of research dealing with aggression, where a potpourri of methods for measuring aggression and inhibition of aggression has been used. These include questionnaires which measure frequency, type, and inhibition of anger (e.g., *HDHQ*—Cochrane, 1973; *FPI*—Mayer, 1972; Weyer, 1977; *Edwards Personality Inventory*—Siegel, Matthews, & Leitch, 1981; *KSP*—Schalling & Svensson, 1983; and the *Harburg Scale*—Harburg, Blakelock, & Roeper, 1979; Gentry, Chesney, Gary, Hall, & Harburg, 1982; *Forced Choice Inventory*—Schill, 1972), as well as recall of aggressive stimuli (Lee, Carstairs, & Pickersgill, 1971), individual questions about being angry (Baer, Collins, Bourianoff, & Ketchel, 1979; Goldberg, Comstock, & Graves, 1980), and projective techniques (McClelland, 1979). Needless to say, these studies measure different aspects of the dimension anger/hostility with quite varying degrees of accuracy.

Though a majority of the studies dealing with this dimension do yield significant results with respect to some aspect of systolic or diastolic blood pressure, by far not all of them do. And before any attempt at interpretation can be made, a large number of other factors must be taken into consideration: reliability and validity of the instruments used; definition of blood pressure groupings and of hypertension; other physiological parameters measured; whether or not the study was performed post hoc (i.e., after the diagnosis of hypertension), longitudinally, or prognostically; and in what type of situation the measurements were made. It is also important to look at the number and constellation of postulated influencing factors which were included in a particular study to see whether important covarying factors were controlled for.

The importance of these methodological aspects becomes clearer when we look more closely at some of the factors whose influence on hypertension has been investigated. The number of variables postulated to affect blood pressure are many, but, for the purposes of this chapter, they will be grouped generally into: socioeconomic factors, working environment, social support, life events, personality, and genetic–biological influences (e.g., sympathetic reactivity, salt sensitivity, etc.). The literature in each of these areas is copious, but an overview is a necessary first step in understanding the complicated interactions involved in hypertension development.

It is the thesis of this chapter that individual and environmental factors crucial for the development of essential hypertension can only be defined relevantly in terms of each other. The presence or absence of particular individual or environmental components are only critical in the development of hypertension when they occur in certain combinations which are maladaptive in the individual's interactions with his environment. *Maladaptive* in this sense means the generation or perpetuation of a state of unpleasantness and discomfort. What will be discussed here are some of the nonconstructive interactions specific to the development of hypertension.

PSYCHOSOCIAL FACTORS

Socioeconomic Factors

The label *socioeconomic* applies to a large range of variables, including marital status, race, income level, geographic factors, educational level, and so on.

There are a number of studies which have reported blood pressure differences between different geographical areas. However, these differences (e.g., rural/urban) are not consistent but seem to covary with other factors. A study of 74,000 18-year-olds in the greater Stockholm area (Theorell, Svensson, Knox, & Ahlborg, 1982) showed a higher average systolic BP in rural as opposed to urban areas. The rural areas were characterized by recessive economies with low median income and a high number of subjects on welfare. Gentry et al. (1982) reported a higher frequency of hypertension in high stress areas of Detroit. High- and low-stress areas (both urban) were defined by differences in median income, median level of education, percentage of unemployment, and social instability (crime and divorce rate). These results were adjusted for age and body weight. But the relative risk for hypertension in this study was best defined by an equation combining race, sex, socioecological stress area, and anger expression—the highest risk being for black males characterized by suppression of anger expression and living in high-stress areas. Here, the importance of the individual/situation interaction begins to emerge.

Many studies have found higher blood pressures among blacks than whites, and these differences have been postulated to be genetic. However, Marmot and Khaw (1982) point out that, though blacks in the United States have higher BP and higher mortality from hypertension than whites, blacks in some parts of rural Africa have low pressures. Results from a number of studies indicate that high pressures in blacks may be at least partially due to environmental factors.

Harburg, Erfurt, Hauenstein, Chape, Schall, and Schork (1973) examined race in connection with high- and low-stress areas. Areas with high stress were defined as those having low socioeconomic status, high crime rates, high density, high resident mobility, and high rates of marital break-up. This study showed the highest BP levels among black males living in high stress areas, but no difference between black low-stress and white living areas. However, these results were complicated by the dimensions of anger suppression and guilt. Suppressed anger was associated with high BP levels and percentage of hypertension for black high-stress and white low-stress males. Black men in low-stress areas with high pressures showed associations with anger suppression accompanied by denial of guilt. Again, the results point clearly to an interaction between individual coping strategies and socioeconomic factors.

Fulton (1980) reported that blacks and whites of middle-class socioeconomic status do not differ significantly in blood pressure levels, but that there are racial differences in the proportion of BP variance explained by personality.

Also a prospective study of demographic data in Massachusetts (Jenkins, Tuthill, Tannenbaum, & Kirby, 1979) showed that racial composition of areas did not correlate with death rate in hypertension, but that low education and low occupational status did. It would seem that the importance of race for hypertension development covaries with the presence of such factors as socioeconomic status, environmental stress, and personal coping strategies.

A population study in Norway (Eide, 1982) supports the data showing that level of education and occupation are important factors with respect to hypertension, but this study reported that these influences were not the same for males and females. Male skilled workers had higher systolic blood pressure than professional and unskilled workers. Semiskilled workers had higher diastolic blood pressure than professionals. But among females, professionals had higher diastolic pressure than semiskilled workers. This may reflect the conflicts attached with changing roles. Females with mainly physical labor had higher systolic and diastolic BP levels than those with partially physical and partially mental work. This is undoubtedly due to physical biological factors.

These studies are only a selection of many dealing with socioeconomic variables. But they are representative of the intimate interaction between biological, environmental, and individual variables and demonstrate the confusion to which the interpretation of isolated factors can lead.

Working Environment

A large part of each day for most men, and an increasing number of women, is spent traveling to and from or being at work. As a result, a number of epidemiological studies of hypertension have included work related factors. However, there are relatively few in-depth studies investigating working environment in relation to blood pressure elevations. One of these, Karasek, Schwartz, and Theorell (1982) investigated the effects of high-strain occupations on BP levels from the U.S. Health and Nutrition Examination Survey (HANES) between 1971 and 1974, and came to the conclusion that psychological work load contributed significantly to variations in diastolic blood pressure, and that low job decision latitude contributed significantly to variations in systolic blood pressure. These variables were significant even after control for age and relevant socioeconomic variables.

Results of a study of 100 employees in industrial firms (Novaco, Stokols, Campbell, & Stokols, 1979) showed that distance and speed of the commute to work accounted for significant proportions of variance in both systolic and diastolic blood pressures measured upon arrival at work. Locus of control (internality) also showed significant regression effects on systolic blood pressure when entered with these variables.

These results coincide with those from the population study in Norway (Eide, 1982) that was cited earlier as showing significant effects of types of employment on blood pressure. Here also, a significant regression effect of travel distance for both systolic and diastolic blood pressures was found in females, as well as a significant effect of "travel stress" (a combined measure of distance, time, and way of travel to work) on diastolic blood pressure in males. Resting blood pressure measures were used in this study.

In another study, men from the greater Stockholm area were followed up 10 years after their draft examinations, at age 28 (Knox, Theorell, Svensson, & Waller, 1984). Participants were selected on the basis of their blood pressure at age 18: 56 hypertensives, 27 normotensives, and 23 hypotensives. The main purpose of this study was to investigate the effect of working environment on blood pressure. However, its results demonstrated the necessity of including individual variables even in studies whose main interest is the effect of situational factors.

When the regression of resting systolic and diastolic blood pressures on comprehensive self-report measures of the working environment, plus job strain classifications (Alfredsson, Karasek, & Theorell, 1982) were calculated, none of them were significant at the .05 level. However, work satisfaction was significant at the .10 level in both analyses—in the opposite direction from that expected; that is, blood pressure increased with increasing work satisfaction. These results were at first difficult to understand but became more logical after analysis of the personality inventories which had been administered. These revealed that a high degree of socialization and a low degree of self-perceived aggression, in relation to the environment, were both associated with high blood pressure at rest. This may indicate that these hypertensives have more willingness to function socially and to describe their environment in a positively skewed way. Had personality factors not been included in this study, the results concerning working environment would have been very difficult to interpret.

They would also have been underestimated if the authors had looked only at blood pressure levels and not at blood pressure variations or at the underlying physiological mechanisms involved in these elevations.

This can be illustrated by differences in blood pressure during and outside of work. No simple association between kind of occupation and resting BP level could be observed. However, each subject was also given portable apparatus for self-measurement of blood pressure and asked to measure his BP every waking hour of a normal working day. Results showed that only those persons who had been hypertensive at age 18, and who had high-strain (hectic, not controllable) occupations at the time of the study, showed significant increases in systolic BP at work. The tendency for diastolic pressure increases was the same, though not significant. There were no indications of self-selection to these kinds of jobs, either with regard to personality or with regard to BP level at age 18.

When no direct relationship between working environment and BP levels at rest were found, it was decided to examine the association between working environment variables and the physiological variables, which explained a significant amount of the variance in resting BP levels. In addition to BP, relative weight and heart rate; blood samples were taken and analyzed for plasma adrenaline and noradrenaline, plasma renin activity, blood hemoglobin, hematocrit, and serum cholesterol. Thirty-three percent of the variance in resting diastolic BP could be explained by hemoglobin (positive), renin (negative), and heart rate (positive). And 38% of the variance in systolic pressure could be explained by hemoglobin, relative weight, adrenaline, and renin. All of these except for renin, correlated positively with systolic BP.

Multiple regression analyses were then performed to evaluate the linear regression of these BP, relevant physiological variables on self-reported working environment and strain occupation. None of the working environment variables accounted for a significant amount of the variance in hemoglobin, but high decision latitude was significantly associated with low renin (which in turn was associated with high resting systolic and diastolic BP). Analyses performed on adrenaline revealed no significant effects of self-reported working environment but positive association between job classifications "influence over working tempo" and "heavy lifting." Relative weight, on the other hand, was not influenced by any of the job classification variables, but by several aspects of self-reported working environment. Employment security, and an inclination to react to a feeling of being unjustly treated at work by showing anger, were both negatively correlated to relative weight. Also, degree of congruence between actual and desired amounts of work satisfaction was positively correlated with relative weight. With regard to heart rate, there was one significant work related variable—reacting with anger to a feeling of being unjustly treated at work. The less this type of coping, the higher the heart rate.

As will be revealed in the next section, these results were further altered when buffer variables involving social network were added to the equations. However, this study demonstrates several important methodological points: (a) reliance on self-report measures alone can give rise to erroneous interpretations, (b) both individual and situational variables must be investigated if reliable results concerning etiological mechanisms in hypertension are to be achieved, and (c) drawing inferences from simple analyses between psychosocial factors and blood pressure (in itself the symptom of a complicated disease process) can lead to a gross underestimation of effects, especially in younger populations.

Social Support

The dimension of social support is comparatively new in hypertension research and has been investigated as a protective *buffer factor*. Amount and quality of social support are due partly to such environmental factors as type of residence area, family structure, and atmosphere at work, as well as such individually determined factors as ability to express feelings, awareness of needs, and capacity for giving. However, even here the results vary. Insel, Fraser, Phillips, and Williams (1981) reported a significant positive correlation between support as measured by the Family Clinical Inventory and systolic blood pressure in male children between 10 and 16 years of age. But due to the fact that this sample was composed of children, the authors hypothesized that what they had referred to as support may have been looked upon by the children as parental pressure.

Dressler (1983) found that persons with lower psychosocial resources—a combination of social support (a three-item measure) and coping strategy (active vs. passive) had higher blood pressure, as did persons who were overweight. But the effects of relative weight were negligible when psychosocial resources were high. When social support and coping strategy were examined separately, there was no significant effect of either on systolic pressure, but a significant interaction for coping × weight on systolic pressure. Persons with a nonactive coping style who were overweight had higher systolic BP. For diastolic pressure there was a significant effect of social support and a significant effect of coping × weight. Again, the main difference was between those who had a nonactive coping style, low social support, and were overweight as opposed to those who used nonactive coping, had high social support, and normal weight.

The Scandinavian research already mentioned has examined the effects of social support network more extensively in relation to blood pressure.

In the Norwegian study (Eide, 1982) a significant effect of social network (an index based on quality of relationships to spouse, relatives, neighbors, and a feeling of acceptance in the environment) was seen in multiple regressions of both systolic and diastolic BP in men and women. The moderator effects of social support were exemplified in the interactions between diastolic BP, support, and travel stress. Women with more support tolerated longer travel without harm.

In the Stockholm study (Knox et al., 1985) a modified version of the Interview Schedule for Social Interaction (Henderson, Duncan-Jones, Byrne, & Scott, 1980) was employed. This instrument measures two main dimensions, attachment and social interaction, and consists of a number of subscales. These are: acquaintance, friendship, attachment, reassurance of worth, and reliable alliance. All of these scales except "reassurance of worth" were used. This scale contained missing data due to a restructuring of the interview (based on new information concerning these scales) halfway through the study. An additional scale measuring amount of physical contact (ranging from a casual pat on the back to the intimacy of sexual intercourse) was also included.

Multiple regression analyses were performed with the physiological variables accounting for a significant amount of variance in resting systolic and diastolic BP as the dependent variables (Knox, Theorell, Svensson, & Waller, 1985). First, self-report measures of working environment were entered into the equations. In the next step only those self-report measures with significant regression effects were entered, together with job classifications ("strain occupations"). In a third set of analyses, social support variables were entered together with those variables which had achieved significance in the second set of analyses. There were no effects of social support on blood hemoglobin, plasma renin, or relative weight.

However, the picture for adrenaline changed with the addition of social support in stage 3 of the analyses. In the first two stages, only the job classifications "influence over work tempo" and "heavy lifting" were significant. When social support was added to the equation, "contacts with acquaintances" and "attachment" were entered in steps 1 and 2 of the equation. The fewer contacts with acquaintances and the poorer amount of attachment, the higher the adrenaline. In step 3 of this equation, the job classification "jobs offering possibilities for learning new things" was significant, indicating that the less this possibility exists, the higher the level of adrenaline. Work tempo was entered first in step 4 of the equation, then, in step 5, the support variable "reliable alliance." Together, these variables accounted for 44% of the variance in adrenaline.

A similar picture can be seen for heart rate. In the first two equations, the only significant variable was reacting with anger to a feeling of being unjustly treated at work. But when social support was added to the equation, number of contacts with acquaintances came first in order of importance, "anger coping" second, and physical contact third.

On the basis of these analyses, it was decided to test a structural model which would explain these relationships. This was done to clarify some of the problems involved with interpreting multiple regression analyses employing large numbers of variables, where there exists an interdependence or simultaneous causation among the observed response variables. The results of these Lisrel path analyses are presented in Figures 5.1 and 5.2.

Life Events

Recent life change is a variable first defined in a questionnaire by Holmes and Rahe (1967), which has been used in several studies investigating hypertension related factors. It consists of 43 common life occurances such as marriage, death of people to whom one is close,

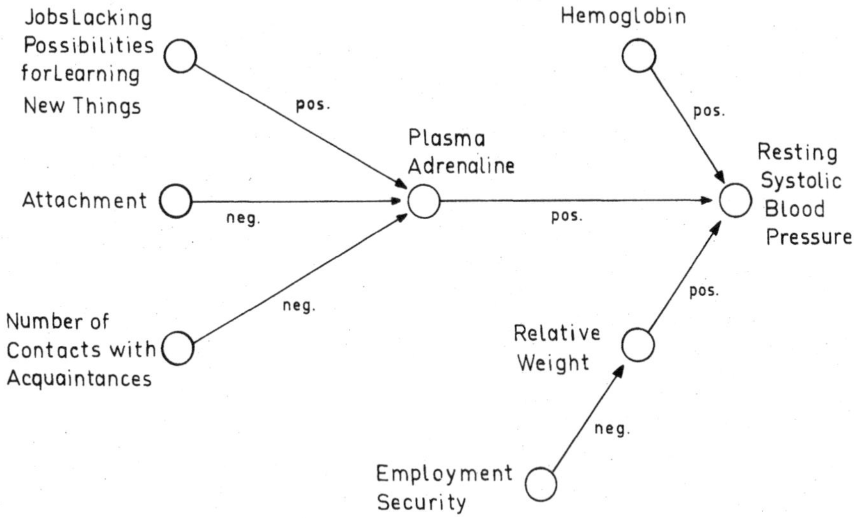

FIGURE 5.1. Lisrel analysis of psychosocial and physiological factors in relation to systolic blood pressure at rest

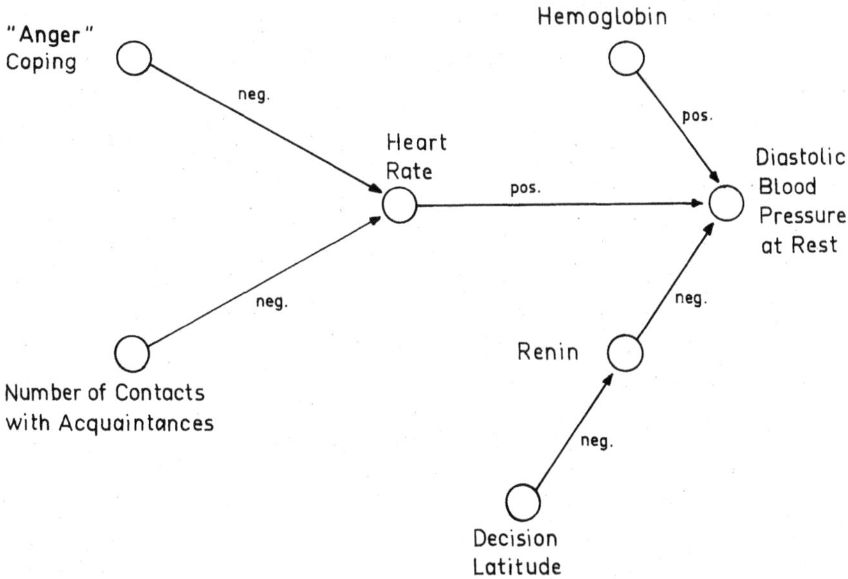

FIGURE 5.2. Lisrel analysis of psychosocial and physiological factors in relation to diastolic blood pressure at rest

birth of children, divorce, etc. The subject states whether he has experienced these and rates them according to relative amount of stress. A study by Beard (1982) found significant differences between number of life events in two age groups (20–35 and 50–65 years). The blood pressure of these groups differed significantly in the expected direction, namely, that the pressure of the older group was higher. However, neither of the groups were hypertensive. In general, the older group had fewer life events, but among older people with high life events, an electrolyte imbalance was found.

In another study (Osti, Trombini, & Magnani, 1980) comparing 20 hypertensive patients with 20 nonhypertensive cardiovascular patients matched for age, sex, social status, years of schooling, social class, and duration of illness, the 20 hypertensive patients had significantly more undesirable life events. These data are supported by another study (Myers & Miles, 1981), which compared normotensives (mean age 26 years) and hypertensives (mean age 46 years). After the effects of age were controlled for, the hypertensive group showed more anxiety and tension, a greater amount of subjective stress, and a greater number of total negative life change units, as well as a greater proportion of negative to total life stress events.

However, two other studies have reported different results. In a study of 166 individuals, LaPensee (1981), found that hypertension could not be predicted by life events. Theorell, Svensson, Knox, Waller, and Alvarez (1986) found fewer life events in a nonclinical population of 28-year-old hypertensives than in other men. It is possible that discrepancies between this latter study and earlier studies reporting a greater number of events might reflect an artifact. Seeking a doctor for help may be preceded by an accumulation of life events. In such cases an excess prevalence of reported recent life events may reflect help-seeking in an acute situation rather than primary hypertension as such. There are also indications that the lower value reported here may be a "true" value. Interviews with the patients in this study revealed that they had a smaller social network than other men (Knox et al., 1985). This could mean that their "world is smaller" and diminish the likelihood that events would occur.

COPING PROCESSES: INDIVIDUAL–SITUATION INTERACTION

It was stated as the thesis of this chapter that individual and environmental factors crucial for the development of primary hypertension can only be defined in terms of each other. The foregoing section on psychosocial factors has demonstrated the problems which arise when attempts are made at interpreting situational factors separately. It was shown, for example, that effects of race interact with such diverse variables as socioeconomic status, personality, and place of habituation, that the effects of work stress are modulated by social support outside of work, and that social support in turn interacts with coping strategies.

In the following section, we will see how theories of personality in relation to hypertension have been modified to account for the dynamics of the continuous interaction between the individual and his environment.

Personality Characteristics

Research concerning personality and hypertension is profuse and contradictory. Early investigations in this area relied greatly upon questionnaires designed to measure trait characteristics such as anxiety, hostility, depression, extraversion, neuroticism, and so on. Numerous different instruments were used in these studies, and the problems of interpretation began with defining what exactly was measured. An example pertaining to hostility was discussed in the methods section.

But complexities of measurement error are only one aspect of the difficulties involved in these studies. Another problem is that their underlying assumptions were basically naive. The theory behind emphasis on traits assumes a generalized and static way of reacting to environmental stimuli. It ignores the dynamics of an individual's interactions with his or her surroundings. A simple example may illustrate this. A teenager with a fairly harmonious background, low "anxiety" and low "hostility" as defined by a number of these tests, finishes his obligatory schooling and goes out to look for a job. Unfortunately, there is a recession, and unemployment is high. He realizes that finding work will be difficult but is full of self-confidence and enthusiasm. However, at the end of a year he is still without work. His self-confidence has been diminished by many rejections and by his parents' growing irritation at his not contributing economically to the household. His level of "anxiety" has clearly increased, and he is beginning to feel hostility. To reduce his anxiety, he begins avoiding job interviews; during the few he accepts, he is prepared for defeat and has difficulty hiding the resentment he feels at the way life has treated him. This in turn reduces his chances of finding a job even further and provides further fuel for his increasingly negative attitude.

According to a WHO report (Warr, 1985), an "aspect considered to be important in determining a person's mental health is a position within a social structure which carries some esteem from others. In practice, a person may be a member of several social structures (for instance, a family, a manufacturing company, a local community, and society as a whole). . . . Esteem within a social structure is generated primarily through the value attached to activities inherent in a role and the contribution these make." Obviously, there is continuous feedback between the individual and his environment, which influences future interactions.

The previous section on psychosocial factors demonstrates quite clearly that there are factors outside of the individual which can influence his blood pressure. The simple application of one or several personality questionnaires to a group of hypertensives and a matched group of normotensives does not provide a great deal of insight into the complicated interreactions between an individual and his surroundings. And it is therefore not surprising that the results of such studies are confusing and contradictory.

More recent research has therefore focused its attention on the interaction between individual and environmental factors. This interaction is to a great extent influenced by the way a person perceives the actual situation (Magnusson, 1982). His perception is in turn influenced, not only by the objective characteristics of the situation, but also by his personality and previous experience.

A study concerning self-disclosure (Handkins & Munz, 1978) may illustrate this. In this study, hypertensives disclosed less personal information on high intimacy topics than normotensives but perceived themselves as revealing equally as much. In contrast to normotensives, they also reported no change in stress level in anticipation of the interpersonal interview, and no reduction of stress afterwards. The fact that the interview situation involved discussing details about oneself with a stranger made it potentially quite stressing—as is shown by the unwillingness on the part of hypertensives to disclose intimate information. Yet, overtly, this potential threat was denied. Unfortunately, blood pressure measurements were not made during the interview, so we know nothing about the actual reactivity in this situation.

However, the results reported by Knox et al. (1984) that work satisfaction and aggression inhibition were positively associated with higher blood pressure at work than outside of work seem to show a connection between how an individual perceives his situation and how his blood pressure reacts. Hypertensives in this study also reported more psychological motives than other men when asked, 'Why do you work?' (Theorell, Alfredsson, Knox, Perski, Svensson, & Waller, 1984). Together, these facts lead to the conclusion that the hypertensives in this study perceived their work in a positively skewed way.

In still another study (Meyer, Derogatis, Miller, & Reading, 1978), it was reported that patients (blacks) who reported to a hospital with the complaint of hypertension reported significantly less distress than a control group.

Manuck et al. (1984) have referred to "a defensive style that may promote submissive, differential and inhibited behavior in hypertensives by permitting a more benign appraisal of situations typically calling for assertive responding."

This group demonstrated greater heart rate and diastolic blood pressure reactivity to mental arithmetic among men with parental history of hypertension than in men who had no parental history. However, a closer look revealed that only those hypertensives who experienced anxiety or anger during the task actually showed increases in heart rate and blood pressure.

Manuck formulated a theory that hypertensives might have problems with assertiveness and performed an investigation involving role playing with both normotensives and hypertensives. The normotensives showed no reliable relationship between blood pressure and behavior. But hypertensives could be divided into two groups psychophysiologically. Group 1 had the greatest increases in pulse pressure while role playing, and these were due mostly to systolic reactions. Group 2 had low pulse pressure responses. Systolic reactions were mostly attenuated, but diastolic reactions were substantial. Though there is no direct evidence, one interpretation of this is that group 1 reacted with cardiac output and group 2 with peripheral resistance. Group 1 hypertensives were significantly more assertive than group 2 and as assertive as normotensives. They were, however, significantly more hostile than normotensives in verbal contact. Group 2 was so inassertive as to fall well below the scale point of appropriate assertiveness.

Perini et al. (1982) also found subgroups of hypertensives by using a projective technique—the Rosenzweig picture-frustration test. Hypertensive patients with high adrenaline were somewhat more assertive, externalized their aggression, and had a stronger need to solve problems immediately, than patients with low adrenaline. Hypertensive patients with high noradrenaline were less assertive, had less externalized and more internalized aggression, showed more initiative to please others, and were more willing to submit in a passive way, than either hypertensives with low noradrenaline or a control group. But they had a stronger need to solve conflicts immediately. Thus, these latter hypertensives had two incompatible tendencies: the avoidance of conflicts coupled with a strong need to solve them. Perini et al. have also found this profile of suppressed aggression and reduced assertiveness in hypertensive patients with high renin.

This section will close with a discussion of inhibited power motivation (McClelland, 1979). Three different samples of subjects ($N = 27$, $N = 235$, and $N = 78$, all males) were given projective tests where they were asked to write stories to pictures. These were then rated according to need for power, need for affiliation, and activity inhibition. In all three samples, those with high power and high inhibition—"the inhibited power motive syndrome" had higher mean blood pressure. In addition, it was found in a longitudinal study that the inhibited power motive syndrome measured in men in their mid-30s significantly predicted elevated blood pressure 20 years later.

McClelland points out similarities between inhibited power motivation and suppressed hostility. He also says that executives are usually characterized by high power and activity inhibition, but that they do not have elevated rates of cardiovascular problems. One reason for this could be that, in their positions, they meet few challenges to their assertiveness. Thus, inhibited power motivation, together with strong situational challenges to one's power needs, would contribute to blood pressure elevation. It is also interesting to note that high power needs, together with high affiliation, did not increase risk. In this case, people are more important than position, which would coincide with the "buffer" theory of social support.

These are but limited examples of studies involving coping strategies. However, they suffice in illustrating the importance of individual/situation interaction in hypertension development.

Reactivity

Obrist (1976) was one of the first to apply the terms *active* and *passive* coping to describe cardiovascular reactivity to environmental stimuli. According to this report, the heart is more under vagal control and blood pressure dominated by vascular processes during passive situations, such as classical conditioning, where the subject cannot himself influence the outcome. But during active coping, such as shock avoidance, the heart is more under sympathetic control, which is directionally independent of somatic activity.

In a continuation of this work, Light (1981) interpreted their findings of effortful active coping, together with sympathetically mediated heart rate and blood pressure increases, as reflecting an inappropriate mobilization of mechanisms. The sympathetic nervous system, whose main function is to mobilize the body for action, is called into action in situations which mainly require mental (but not physical) response.

Fredrikson (1985, 1986) has summarized the major research in the area of reactivity and come to several conclusions, among them the following:

1. Both sustained hypertension and borderline hypertension subjects with a family history of hypertension show hyperreactivity to situations requiring behavioral activity.
2. Reactivity differences between hypertension and normotension may be more readily observed with tasks including behavioral demands than those that are nondemanding.
3. Hyperreactivity in hypertension seems specific to the cardiovascular system and is not part of generalized sympathetic activation.

MULTIFACTOR MODEL

The preceding has been an overview of how psychosocial factors and interactions between the individual and his environment influence blood pressure. The most important information emerging from this research is the multifactorial nature of influences on hypertension. What remains to be seen is how these behaviorial factors interact on a physiological level.

We will begin with a brief summary of individual genetic–biological influences on subsequent development of primary hypertension.

Genetic–Biological Influences

Space does not allow an in-depth discussion of genetic influences. However, as stated earlier, their importance has been established in both animal and human research. Folkow (1982) estimates their influence, on the basis of population studies, to be over 10%. The consensus seems to be that these influences are triggered by the presence of certain environmental factors. These interactions are illustrated by the studies of family history and cardiovascular reactivity and are important because of the generally held assumption that it is the amount and strength of reactivity which eventually brings about long term changes in blood pressure elevation.

Another biologically important factor for hypertension is age. The BP levels clinically defined as normal increase with age ("Why does blood pressure," 1981), and age is controlled for in all methodologically sound analyses of hypertension related factors. But even this is not consistent. Jenkins, Somervell, and Hames (1983) reported that only about half of the 175 men in their longitudinal study increased their BP with age. Their findings indicate the BP increases with age may also be influenced by other than biological factors. In this study, anxiety and hostility correlated with concurrent BP levels but not with BP increases over years.

Relative weight (or body mass index), salt intake, smoking, and alcohol consumption involve health behaviors which can also contribute to physiological changes leading to hypertension. They are also influenced and modified by psychosocial factors.

Psychophysiological Mechanisms

Though there is still a great deal of discussion concerning the physiology of hypertension development and maintenance, there is extensive evidence that behavioral factors play a major role.

Obrist and Light have described the tendency of certain individuals, principally those with parental hypertension, to react with a greater heart rate and systolic blood pressure response mediated partially by the beta-adrenergic branch of the sympathetic nervous system. Fredrikson's research and review of the literature substantiate this.

Since a parental history of hypertension seems to be associated with this behavioral hyperreactivity, it could be concluded that this reaction pattern involves, to a great extent, an inherited trait. However, the findings of Manuck and others seem clearly to indicate that this hyperreactivity is also associated with specific ways of perceiving the situation. In Manuck's study, only those subjects with a parental history, who *also* experienced anxiety and anger, were hyperreactive. In other words, reactivity must be seen in a context. In the behavioral tests of physiological reactivity where stressors such as mental arithmetic, stroop, and cold pressor are used, the terms active and passive apply fairly well, though the act of continuing to hold one's hand in painfully cold water can hardly be thought of as a totally passive act. However, many of the situations with which an individual has to cope in real life also involve his emotions and require emotional coping. The examples cited were submissiveness, inhibited power motivation, aggression inhibition, etc. Here hypertensives varied markedly in their physiological reaction patterns.

Older theories held that borderline hypertension was characterized by an increase in cardiac output, and that, in established hypertension, cardiac output was normal but peripheral vascular resistance increased. The increased vascular resistance in established hypertension is attributed to muscle hypertrophy in the vessels and a resulting increase in the wall-to-lumen ratio during contraction. However, we now know that only in some cases of borderline hypertension is there an increase in cardiac output. Julius and Esler (1975) cited one study where only 30% of the borderline patients had cardiac output values two standard deviations above the mean for normal subjects. The above mentioned differences in reaction patterns explain why this is so.

We know from animal research that, for instance, submissive behavior and aggressive behavior correspond to different physiological reaction patterns. The first is characterized by the pituitary adrenal cortical system, and the second by the sympathetic adrenal medullary system. Both of these can lead to rises in blood pressure. Detailed descriptions of these processes can be obtained in Sterling and Eyer (1981). Knardahl (1983), Abboud (1982), Henry (1976, 1982), and Folkow (1982). The multifactorial etiology of hypertension means that different weights and combinations of factors can combine to cause a variety of bodily changes whose end symptom is elevated blood pressure. There are borderline hypertensives with increased cardiac output and those with increased peripheral resistance, borderline hypertensives with low renin and those with high renin. More research is needed in order to specify which combinations of etiological factors coincide with these different psychophysiological reaction patterns.

Though there is still controversy concerning borderline hypertension, there seems to be a fair amount of agreement concerning established hypertension. Guyton (1974) has stated that the renal-body fluid volume mechanism for pressure control is a feedback control system which has infinite gain, i.e., will always return blood pressure to normal if it is not malfunctioning. In other words, chronic blood pressure elevation must involve this mechanism in some way. Folkow (1982) concurs, saying that, as primary hypertension advances, the reset kidneys more and more tend to dominate the situation and to counteract normalization. The kidneys are affected by volume mechanisms and by sympathetic innervation. Renal sympathetic innervation influences renin release, renal blood flow, and glomerular filtration rate, as well as increases in reabsorbation of sodium in the proximal tubules (Knardahl, 1983). For blood pressure increases to become chronic, the kidneys must be involved.

TREATMENT

Only about 34% of patients gain control over their hypertension with medication (Rowland & Roberts, 1982). The reason for this is that the body tries to compensate for a forced change in one system by balancing with a compensatory change in others (Sterling & Eyer, 1981). Thus, diuretics, which stimulate salt and water secretion, provoke a compensatory increase in secretion of renin, angiotensin, aldosterone, and antidiuretic hormone. Propranolol, a beta-blocker for the sympathetic nervous system, blocks beta-receptors for vasodilation and allows the alpha-receptors for vasoconstriction to act without opposition.

Antivasoconstrictors such as reserpine and alpha methyl dopa cause vascular relaxation and a resulting fall in pressure. This, in turn, leads to compensatory increases in the renin-angiotensin-aldosterone system as well as in cardiac output.

These facts concerning pharmacological treatment, together with the now established importance of psychosocial factors in the etiology of hypertension, are two main reasons for the abundant research concerning behavioral treatment methods.

The main methods which have been tested in this area concern those aimed at reducing physical risk factors such as overweight (exercise, diet, etc.), those directly aimed at affecting blood pressure (biofeedback), and those aimed at reducing sympathetic discharge in the autonomic nervous system (e.g., biofeedback and relaxation), as well as stress management, which usually includes some kind of relaxation as well as helping the patient to deal with different types of stress in his life.

The biofeedback techniques involve feedback for blood pressure reductions (Kristt & Engel, 1975; Messerli, DeCarvalho, Christie, & Frohlich, 1979), feedback for reduction of frontalis muscle tension (McGrady, Yonker, Tan, Fine, & Woerner, 1981), and feedback for skin conductance (Patel & Datey, 1977). Often these are combined with relaxation techniques (Patel & Datey, 1977; Patel, 1975; Glasgow, Gaarder, & Engel, 1982).

Most of the studies using biofeedback alone show rather small reductions: 4–9 mm Hg systolic and 1–6 mm Hg diastolic. However, there are exceptions to this: Benson, Shapiro, Tursky, and Schwartz (1971) achieved a systolic reduction ranging from 16 to 34 mm Hg; Kristt and Engel (1975) achieved 18 mm Hg systolic and 8 mm Hg diastolic. And Kallinke, Kulick, and Heim (1982) achieved systolic reductions of 19 mm Hg.

But the best results with biofeedback have been achieved using it together with relaxation. In three studies, Patel (1973, 1975, 1977) and her colleagues attained reductions of 25/14, 20/14, and 28/15 mm Hg, combining biofeedback and relaxation or yoga.

Many of the earlier studies did not use adequate follow-up periods to see if reductions could be maintained. But follow-up periods are now included in almost all studies.

Those studies using only relaxation have generally tended to use Jacobsson's progressive relaxation although autogenic training has also been employed. Not all of them have been successful, but in general their reductions are of the same magnitude as those with biofeedback and biofeedback combinations (Bali, 1979; Jacob, Fortmann, Kraemer, Farquhar, & Agras, 1985).

Exercise alone has also been tried as a behavioral treatment measure, due among other things to the fact that overweight contributes to blood pressure increase. In one such study, Cade et al. (1984) reported a 15 mm Hg reduction in mean blood pressure after several months of exercise.

Stress management is a combination of relaxation and behavioral methods for reducing stress and is a newer form of treatment. Here also promising blood pressure reductions have been achieved: 16 mm Hg systolic and 7 mm Hg diastolic after 10 sessions and a 3-month follow-up (Knox, Theorell, Malmberg, & Lindquist, 1986), and 18mm Hg systolic and 8 mm Hg diastolic after eight sessions and a 6-month follow-up period (Crowther, 1983); 22 mm Hg systolic and 11 mm Hg diastolic in hypertensives after 8 months (Patel, Marmut, & Terry, 1981).

The purpose of stress management methods is to use relaxation to effectuate a reduction of sympathetic discharge, together with behavioral techniques to deal with some of the psychosocial and physical risk factors involved in hypertension development. With regard to the causal factors discussed in this chapter, combined treatment makes the most sense and should be developed further to refine and fit the different types of psychophysiological subgroups seen in borderline hypertension. In this context, it is important to note that lack of social support, which has been shown to be important in the etiology of hypertension, is also important for treatment compliance. In the Edgecombe County blood pressure control program (Williams et al., 1985) women who dropped out of treatment had less social support on the job, less spouse approval, and less perceived access to supportive structures.

The one positive aspect that the behavioral treatment methods have in common is that, unlike pharmacological measures, they have no side effects. The magnitude of reduction in many of these studies was not great, in others quite substantial. But Marzuk (1985) points out that even small blood pressure reductions can result in a significant improvement in mortality rate. As understanding of the specifics of psychophysiological reaction patterning in hypertension grows, treatment methods will be able to focus on specific subgroups of hypertensives, and their effectiveness should increase substantially.

SUMMARY AND CONCLUSIONS

Despite the prevalence of primary hypertension, about 90% of all diagnosed cases are still labeled as essential, that is, of unknown origin. Research has shown that there is a certain genetic predisposition. The rest can be attributed to psychosocial and environmental factors. Though there is still a great deal of controversy concerning which factors have the most etiological relevance, the following conclusions can be drawn from current research:

1. The etiology of essential hypertension is complex, and there is more than one pathway leading to chronically elevated blood pressure; that is, borderline hypertensives can be divided into subgroups according to their physiology.
2. Individual and situational factors are equally important in terms of causality and can only be interpreted correctly when observed in relation to each other.
3. The following variables have been repeatedly reported to influence blood pressure: high dietary salt intake; overweight; occupational status; level of education; high-stress living area; race; working environment factors such as travel stress, decision latitude, and employment security; lack of social support; coping strategies involving aggression inhibition; inhibited power motivation; low assertiveness; and submissiveness.
4. In order to achieve a clearer understanding of the etiological mechanisms involved in high blood pressure, path analysis models are needed to test hypotheses concerning effects of specific factors and combinations of factors on the physiological substrates of systolic and diastolic blood pressure elevation. The intimate interactions between nervous, vascular, and hormonal autoregulatory mechanisms mean that a disturbance in one automatically effects changes in the others. Methods which include blood pressure as the only physiological measure are looking only at the end symptom of a complicated disease process and risk a gross underestimation of effects.
5. Treatment measures combining relaxation and behavioral techniques to deal with psychosocial and physical risk factors involved in hypertension development show the most promise. Future research in this area should gear these techniques to specific subgroups of hypertensives and include a large range of physiological measures so that treatment effects can be interpreted with greater accuracy.

REFERENCES

Abboud, F. M. (1982). The sympathetic system in hypertension. *State-of-the-Art-Review Hypertension*, *4*(suppl II), 208–225.

Alfredsson, L., Karasek, R. A., & Theorell, T. (1982). Myocardial infarction risk and psychosocial work environment: An analysis of the male Swedish working force. *Social Science and Medicine*, *16*, 463–467.

Baer, P. E., Collins, F. H., Bourianoff, G. G., & Ketchel, M. F. (1979). Assessing personality factors in essential hypertension with a brief self-report instrument. *Psychosomatic Medicine, 41*, 321–330.

Bali, L. R. (1979). Long-term effect of relaxation on blood pressure and anxiety levels of essential hypertensive males: A controlled study. *Psychosomatic Medicine, 41*, 637–646.

Beard, M. T. (1982). Trust, life events, and risk factors among adults. *Advances in Nursing Science, 4*, 26–43.

Benson H., Shapiro, D., Tursky, B., & Schwartz, G. E. (1971). Decreased systolic blood pressure through operant conditioning techniques in patients with essential hypertension. *Science, 173*, 740–742.

Cade, R., Mars, D., Wagemaker, H., Zauner, C., Packer, D., Privette, M., Cade, M., Peterson, P., & Hood-Lewis, D. (1984). Effect of aerobic exercise training on patients with systemic arterial hypertension. *The American Journal of Medicine, 77*, 785–790.

Cochrane, R. (1973). Hostility and neuroticism among unselected essential hypertensives. *Journal of Psychosomatic Research, 17*, 215–218.

Crowther, J. H. (1983). Stress management training and relaxation imagery in the treatment of essential hypertension. *Journal of Behavioral Medicine, 6*, 169–187.

Dressler, W. W. (1983). Blood pressure, relative weight, and psychosocial resources. *Psychosomatic Medicine, 45*, 527–536.

Eide, R. (1982). *Psychosocial factors and indices of health risks*. Unpublished thesis, Institute of Somatic Psychology, University of Bergen, Norway.

Folkow, B. (1982). Physiological aspects of primary hypertension. *Physiological Reviews, 62*, 347–504.

Fredrikson, M. (1986). Behavioral aspects of cardiovascular reactivity in essential hypertension. In T. D. Dembroski, T. H. Schmidt, & C. Blumchen (Eds.), *Biological and psychological factors in cardiovascular disease* (pp. 418–446). Berlin: Springer.

Fulton, W. (1980). Blood pressure in blacks and whites: Life stress and personality *Dissertation Abstracts International, 41*, 1912–B.

Gentry, W. G., Chesney, A. P., Gary, H. E., Hall, R. P., & Harburg, E. (1982). Habitual anger-coping styles: I. Effect on mean blood pressure and risk for essential hypertension. *Psychosomatic Medicine, 44*, 195–202.

Glasgow, M. S., Gaarder, K. R., & Engel, B. T. (1982). Behavioral treatment of high blood pressure: II. Acute and sustained effects of relaxation and systolic blood pressure biofeedback. *Psychosomatic Medicine, 44*, 155–170.

Goldberg, E. L., Comstock, G. W., & Graves, C. G. (1980). Psychosocial factors and blood pressure. *Psychological Medicine, 10*, 243–255.

Guyton, A. C., Cowley, A. W., Coleman, T. G., DeClue, J. W., Norman, R. A., & Manning, R. D. (1974). Hypertension: A disease of abnormal circulatory control. *Chest, 65*, 328–338.

Handkins, R. E., & Munz, D. C. (1978). Essential hypertension and self-disclosure. *Journal of Clinical Psychology, 34*, 870–875.

Harburg, E., Erfurt, J., Hauenstein, L. S., Chape, C., Schall, W. J., & Schork, M. A. (1973). Socio-ecological stress, suppressed hostility, skin colour and black–white male blood pressure. *Psychosomatic Medicine, 35*, 276–296.

Harburg, E., Blakelock, E. H., Jr., & Roeper, P. J. (1979). Resentful and reflective coping with arbitrary authority and blood pressure: Detroit. *Psychosomatic Medicine, 41*(3), 189–202.

Heiburg, A., Magnus, P., Berg, K., & Nance, W. I. (1981). Blood pressure in Norwegian twins. In L. Gedda, P. Paris, & W. E. Nance (Eds.), *Twin research 3: Epidemiological and clinical studies* (pp. 163–168). New York: Alan R. Liss, Inc.

Henderson S., Duncan-Jones, P., Byrne, D. G., & Scott, R. (1980). Measuring social relationships: The Interview Schedule for Social Interaction. *Psychology in Medicine, 10*, 723–734.

Henry, J. P. (1976). Understanding the early pathophysiology of essential hypertension. *Geriatrics, 31*, 59–72.

Henry, J. P. (1982). The relation of social to biological processes in disease. *Social Science and Medicine, 16*, 369–380.

Holmes, T. H., & Rahe, R. H. (1967). The social adjustment rating scale. *Journal of Psychosomatic Research, 11*, 213–218.

Insel, P. M., Fraser, G. E., Phillips, R., & Williams, P. (1981). Psychosocial factors and blood pressure in children. *Journal of Psychosomatic Research. 25*, 505–511.

Iselius, L. (1983). *Genetic epidemiology of some major risk factors for coronary heart disease.* Unpublished doctoral dissertation, Department of Clinical Genetics, Karolinska Hospital, Stockholm, Sweden.

Jacob, R. G., Fortmann, S. P., Kraemer, H. C., Farquhar, J. W., & Agras, W. S. (1985). Combining behavioral treatments to reduce blood pressure. *Behavior Modification, 9*, 32–54.

Jenkins, C. D., Tuthill, R. W., Tannenbaum, S. I., & Kirby, C. (1979). Social stressors and excess mortality from hypertensive diseases. *Journal of Human Stress*, pp. 29–40.

Jenkins, C. D., Somervell, P. D., & Hames, C. G. (1983). Does blood pressure usually rise with age . . . or with stress? *Journal of Human Stress, 9*, 4–12.

Julius, S., & Esler, M. (1975). Automatic nervous cardiovascular regulation in borderline hypertension. *The American Journal of Cardiology, 36*, 685–696.

Kallinke, D., Kulick, B., & Heim, P. (1981). Behaviour analysis and treatment of essential hypertensives. *Journal of Psychosomatic Research, 26*, 541–549.

Karasek, R. A., Schwartz, J., & Theorell, T. (1982). *Job characteristics, occupation and coronary heart disease. Phase I* (pp. 1–145). New York: Columbia University, Department of Industrial Engineering and Operations Research.

Knardahl, S. (1983). Psychological pathogenesis of arterial hypertension. In H. Ursin, & R. Murison (Eds.), *Biological and psychological basis of psychosomatic disease.* New York: Pergamon Press.

Knox, S., Theorell, T., Svensson, J. & Waller, D. (1985).The relation of social support and working environment to medical variables associated with elevated blood pressure in young males: a structural model. *Social Science and Medicine, 21*, 525–531.

Knox, S., Theorell, T., Svensson, J., & Waller, D. (1984). Subjective description and "objective" classification of jobs in relation to blood pressure level and blood pressure variations. In W. V. Eimeren, R. Engelbrecht, & Ch.D. Flagle (Eds.) *Third International Conference*. Berlin: Springer-Verlag.

Knox, S., Theorell, T., Malmberg, B. G., & Lindqvist, R. (1986). Stress management in the treatment of essential hypertension in primary health care. *Scandinavian Journal of Primary Health Care, 4*, 1–7.

Kristt, D. A., & Engel, B. T. (1975). Learned control of blood pressure in patients with high blood pressure. *Circulation, 51*, 370–378.

LaPensee, K. T. (1981). Stress, illness, and coping in a rural Connecticut town. *Dissertation Abstracts International, 43*, 856–A.

Lee, S. G., Carstairs, G. M., & Pickersgill, M. J. (1971). Essential hypertension and the recall of motives. *Journal of Psychosomatic Research, 15*, 95–105.

Light, K. C. (1981). Young psychophysiologist award address, 1980. Cardiovascular responses to effortful active coping: Implications for the role of stress in hypertension development. *Psychophysiology, 18*, 216–225.

Magnusson, D. (1982). Situational determinants of stress: An international perspective. In L. Goldgerg & S. Breznits (Eds.), *Handbook of stress*. New York: The Free Press.

Manuck, S. B., Morrison, R. L., Bellack, A. S., & Polefrone, J. M. (1984). Behavioral factors in hypertension: Cardiovascular responsivity, anger, and social competence. In M. Chesney, S. Goldston, & R. Rosenman (Eds.), *Anger, hostility and behavioral medicine*. New York: Hemisphere.

Marmot, M. G., & Khaw, K. T. (1982). Epidemiological aspects of hypertension. Implications for population studies of the age trend in blood pressure. *Contributions to Nephrology, 30*, 101–107.

Marzuk, P. M. (1985). Biofeedback for hypertension. Position paper. *Annals of Internal Medicine, 102*, 709–715.

Mayer, V. H. (1972). Interkorrelationen von Blutdruck und Aggressivität. *Zeitschrift für Klinische Psychologie und Psychotherapie, 20*, 363–371.

McClelland, D. C. (1979). Inhibited power motivation and high blood pressure in men. *Journal of Abnormal Psychology, 88*, 182–190.

McGrady, A. V., Yonker, R., Tan, S. Y., Fine, T. H., & Woerner, M. (1981). The effect of biofeedback-assisted relaxation training on blood pressure and selected biochemical parameters in patients with essential hypertension. *Biofeedback Self-Regulation, 6*, 343–353.

Messerli, F. H., DeCarvalho, J. G. R., Christie, B., & Frohlich, E. D. (1979). Systemic haemodynamic effects of biofeedback in borderline hypertension. *Clinical Science, 57(suppl 5)*, 437s–439s.

Meyer, E., Derogatis, L. R., Miller, M., & Reading, A. (1978). Hypertension and psychological distress. *Psychosomatics, 19*, 160–163, 167–168.

Myers, H. F., & Miles, R. E. (1981). Life events stress, subjective appraisal and somatization in hypertension: A pilot study. *Journal of Human Stress, 7*, 17–27.

Novaco, R. W., Stokols, D., Campbell, J., & Stokols, J. (1979). Transportation, stress and community psychology. *American Journal of Community Psychology, 7*, 361–380.

Obrist, P. A. (1976). The cardiovascular-behavioral interaction—as it appears today. *Psychophysiology, 13*, 95–106.

Okamoto, K. (Ed.). (1972). *Spontaneous hypertension. Its pathogenesis and complications.* Tokyo, Japan: Igaku Shoin.

Osti, R. M. A., Trombini, G., & Magnani, B. (1980). Stress and distress in essential hypertension. *Psychotherapy and Psychosomatics. 33*, 193–197.

Patel, C. (1975). 12-month follow-up of yoga and biofeedback in the management of hypertension. *Lancet, 1*, 62–64.

Patel, C. H. (1973, November 10). Yoga and bio-feedback in the management of hypertension. *The Lancet*, pp 1053–1055.

Patel, C. H., & Datey, K. K. (1977). Relaxation and biofeedback techniques in the management of hypertension. *Angiology, 27*, 401–405.

Patel, C. H. (1977). Biofeedback-aided relaxation and meditation in the management of hypertension. *Biofeedback and Self-Regulation, 2*, 1–41.

Patel, C., Marmot, M. G., & Terry, D. J. (1981). Controlled trial of biofeedback-aided behavioural methods in reducing mild hypertension. *British Medical Journal, 282*, 2005–2008.

Perini, C., Amann, F. W., Bolli, P., & Buehler, F. R. (1982). Personality and adrenergic factors in essential hypertension. *Contributions to Nephrology, 30*, 64–69.

Rowland, M., & Roberts, J. (1982). *Blood pressure levels and hypertension in persons aged 6–74 years: United States, 1976–80.* National Center for Health Statistics, Advance Data from Vital and Health Statistics, No. 84, DHHS Pub. No., 82–1250. Hyattsville, MD: U.S. Dept. of Health and Human Services.

Schalling, D., & Svennson, J. (1984). Blood pressure and personality. *Personality and Individual Differences, 5,* 41–51.

Schill, T. R. (1972). Aggression and blood pressure responses of high- and low-guilt subjects following frustration. *Journal of Consulting and Clinical Psychology, 38,* 461.

Siegel, J. M., Matthews, K. A., & Leitch, C. J. (1983). Blood pressure variability and the Type A behavior pattern in adolescence. *Journal of Psychosomatic Research, 27,* 265–272.

Sterling, P., & Eyer, J. (1981). Biological basis of stress-related mortality. *Social Science and Medicine, 15E,* 3 42.

Theorell, T., Alfredsson, L., Knox, S., Perski, A., Svensson, J., & Waller D. (1984). On the interplay between socioeconomic factors, personality, and work environment in the pathogenesis of cardiovascular disease. *Scandinavian Journal of Work Environment and Health, 10,* 373–380.

Theorell, T., Svennson, J., Knox, S., & Ahlborg, B. (1982). Blood pressure variations across areas in the greater Stockholm region: Analysis of 74,000 18-year-old men. *Social Science and Medicine, 16,* 469–473.

Theorell, T., Svensson, J., Knox, S., Waller, D., & Alvarez, M. (1986). Young men with high blood pressure report few recent life events. *Journal of Psychosomatic Research, 30,* 243–249.

Warr, P. (1985, October). *The Psychological impact of continuing unemployment: Some longitudinal data and a general model.* Paper presented at the World Health Organization Meeting on Vulnerability among long-term unemployed, Ljubljana.

Weiner, H. (1979). *Psychobiology of essential hypertension.* New York: Elsevier.

Weyer, G., & Hodapp, V. (1977). Persönlichkeitseigenschaften bei Essentiellen Hypertonikern. *Zeitschrift für Kliniche Psychologie, 6,* 70–78.

Why does blood pressure rise with age? (1981). [Editorial]. *Lancet, 2,* 289–290.

Williams, C. A., Beresford, S. A. A., James, S. A., LaCroix, A. Z., Strogatz, D. S., Wagner, E. H., Kleinbaum, D. G., Cutchin, L. M., & Ibrahim, M. A. (1985). The Edgecombe County high blood pressure control program:III. Social support, social stressors, and treatment dropout. *American Journal of Public Health, 75,* 483–486.

6

Behavioral Management and Rehabilitation After Acute Myocardial Infarction

Peter G. F. Nixon

Cardiac Department,
Charing Cross Hospital (Fulham)
London, England

"Knowledge dispels fear."

INTRODUCTION

The prospect of myocardial infarction faces everyone in middle age these days. It is a breakdown caused by overwork and various kinds of social disruption (Eyer, 1980). It occurs when the victim is exhausted and least well fitted for this major attack upon his ability to cope and adapt. He needs to withdraw from the demands of his environment to sleep and rest, and learn how to become successful at living, but he has an inherent inability to hold back when other people need him. Nor do we in medicine provide what he needs: we do not give him a license to go off duty and sort himself out before the breakdown, but provide coronary-care units to pick up the pieces afterwards. We occupy ourselves with relatively unimportant risk factors and suppress the symptoms of the approaching breakdown with palliative drugs and surgery. We forget that myocardial infarction is not necessarily a product of atheroma. It certainly bears no simple relationship to the appearances of the coronary arteries: In some cases these arteries are scarcely diseased, and dynamic factors related to failure of coping are responsible for the heart attack (Freeman & Nixon, 1985a,b). In most cases the arteries are significantly narrowed by atheroma, but the same degrees of narrowing do not prevent other individuals from enjoying good health (Baroldi, Mariani, & Falzi, 1978). In our management we treat the dynamic case in the same way as the atherogenic and neglect the psychosocial causes. In our culture we have even forgotten how to look after exhaustion and illness in the home (Osmond, 1980).

The purpose of this chapter is to describe the real needs of patients after myocardial infarction and to suggest rational responses in the biopsychosocial framework (Engel, 1982) of clinical practice.

AXIOMS, MODELS, AND PARADIGMS

The predicament of the coronary patient is that he cannot do what he wants, and the harder he struggles the more he suffers and fails. Rehabilitation teaches him that rest can break these vicious circles of struggle and defeat, bring him into acceptance, and enable him to train for improvement of cardiac function and coping ability. Its management requires familiarity with working concepts of homeostasis and the physiology of arousal.

HOMEOSTASIS

The internal milieu does not remain constant during effort. There is hardly an organ or physiological process that is not involved in one way or another (Asmussen, 1976). The derangement of the internal milieu partly depends upon the nature, intensity, and duration of the effort. For example, physical activity brings familiar changes in heart rate and blood pressure, but it is less well known that stressful conditions can raise the plasma cholesterol 60% above its base line, or the effort of adapting to widowhood depress the immune function for nearly a year. The derangement of the internal milieu also depends upon the power of the homeostasis, the organism's self-regulating system, to recover and maintain a stable and orderly equilibrium internally during the effort of coping and adapting to changes in the outside environment. This power to keep the internal milieu within healthy limits varies from person to person. It is high in hardiness (Kobasa, Maddi, & Kahn, 1982) and low in exhaustion. It requires time and adequate conditions in order to be effective. For example, a soldier "played out by continuous work, disturbed sleep and continuous strain" would become grossly unfit and suffer from tachycardia and hypertension (Lewis, 1918), because his self-regulating mechanisms had not been given the chance to produce a normal internal milieu. In those days it was recognized that sleep and rest were required for the recovery of homeostasis. Homeostasis is much affected by arousal.

The Physiology of Arousal

Nowadays the word *arousal* is used clinically in the sense of Hebb's (1955) "general drive state" or Lader's (1975) behavioral continuum extending from drowsiness at one extreme, through alertness and conditions of excitement, to the extremes of revulsion, rage, panic, and ecstasy at the other. Kahneman (1973) saw it as a reflection of what the individual is doing and the effort he is investing plus what is happening to him and the stress to which he is exposed.

The Treadwheel Model

The treadwheel (Figure 6.1) is a useful model for teaching relationships between effort and arousal in cardiac rehabilitation. One figure is clearly well and in control. He fits his social milieu and enjoys the social assets required for high and sustained effort (Cassel, 1976). He has an adequate flow of information for prediction and, where necessary, for avoidance and escape (Weiss, 1972). Fitness and stamina are adequate.

The other figure is going down into exhaustion, ill-health, and defeat, possibly outstripping the competence of his coronary arteries and laying the foundation of a heart attack. As he goes down out of control, he suffers periods of rage, fear, and fruitless struggling, alternating with periods of defeat, despair, and wanting to give up (Engel, 1974). The rage, fear, and furious struggling sets up high levels of arousal of the primitive sympatho-adrenomedullary defense and control system (S-AM), and the defeat and despair are linked with hyperarousal of the pituitary-adrenocortical conservation-withdrawal system (P-AC) (Henry & Meehan, 1981; Henry, 1982).

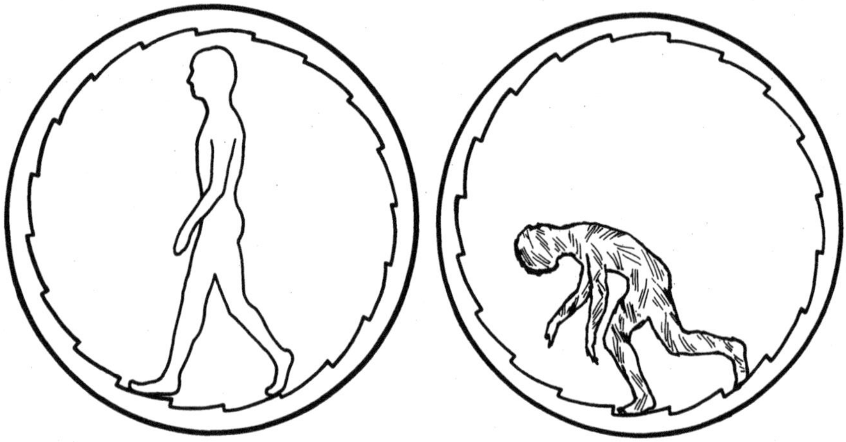

FIGURE 6.1. The treadwheel is a useful image for considering the factors which determine the ability to cope with heavy effort over long periods of time, and the consequences of success or failure.

The hyperarousal of these two systems sooner or later outstrips the ability of the homeostasis to maintain a normal milieu and sets up a catabolic condition (Sterling & Eyer, 1981; Kagan, 1982) characterized by an excess of aldosterone, cortisol, antidiuretic hormone, catecholamines, growth hormone, thyroid-stimulating and thyroid hormones. The recognized consequences of this catabolic condition include systolic and diastolic hypertension, increased tissue demands for oxygen, increased heart rate and stroke volume, and increased serum uric acid, cholesterol and free fatty acids, plasma glucose, platelet adhesiveness, and blood viscosity (see Table 6.1). Constriction of the peripheral resistance and the capacitance vessels of the body can occur, and it is thought that this catabolic internal milieu can damage the arteries and impair left ventricular function. Eventually, a point of instability is reached where a small increment of catabolic change can produce the catastrophe of vascular occlusion (Oliva, 1981). The coup de grace sometimes takes the form of a fatal arrhythmia or an attack of coronary vasospasm induced by hyperventilation at a time when the homeostatic defenses are reduced by exhaustion (Nixon, 1982a,b, 1984; Freeman & Nixon, 1985a,b).

There are many contributors to this hypothesis, and important sources include Friedman and Rosenman (1974), Buell and Eliot (1980) and the publications by Raab (1969), Levi (1972), Kagan and Levi (1974), Groen (1976), Henry and Meehan (1981), Sterling and Eyer (1981), Karasek, Russell and Theorell (1982), and Kagan (1982).

Table 6.1.
Catabolic and Anabolic Processes (Sterling & Eyer, 1981)

Hormonal pattern during arousal	
Catabolic hormones increase	Anabolic hormones decrease
Cortisol	Insulin
Epinephrine	Calcitonin
Glucagon	Testosterone
Growth hormone	Estrogen
Antidiuretic hormone	Prolactin
Renin	Luteinising hormone
Angiotensin	Follicle stimulating hormone
Aldosterone	Gonadotropin releasing hormone (GnRH)
Eythropoietin	Prolactin releasing hormone (PRH)
Thyroxin	
Parathormone	
Melatonin	

Anabolic and catabolic states

Anabolic state
- Increased synthesis of protein, fat, carbohydrate (growth, energy storage)
- Decreased breakdown of protein, fat, carbohydrate (growth, energy storage)
- Increased production of cells for immune system (white blood cells of thymus and bone marrow)
- Increased bone repair and growth
- Increase in sexual processes (cellular, hormonal, psychological)

Catabolic state (arousal)
- Halt in synthesis of protein, fat, carbohydrate
- Increased breakdown of protein, fat, carbohydrate (energy mobilisation)
- Elevated blood levels of glucose, free fatty acids, low density lipoprotein, cholesterol (for energy)
- Increased production of red blood cells and liver enzymes (for energy)
- Decreased repair and replacement of bone
- Decreased repair and replacement of cells with normally high turnover (gut, skin, etc)
- Decreased production of cells for immune system (thymus shrinks, circulating white cells decrease)
- Decreased sexual processes
- Increased blood pressure, cardiac output
- Increased salt and water retention

The patient whose heart has been damaged by these processes is less well able to withstand the neuroendocrine consequences of rage and frustration, and more vulnerable to heart failure when despair, hopelessness, and discouragement cause salt and water retention (Sodeman & Burch, 1938; Chambers & Reiser, 1953; Barnes & Schottstaedt, 1960; Perlman, Ferguson, Bergum, Isenberg, & Hammarsten, 1971).

One of the most important determinants of left ventricular performance at its compliance. A healthy left ventricle working under normal conditions fills easily, with little rise of diastolic pressure (see Figure 6.2).

Its being overdistended or stiffened compels it to work with higher diastolic pressure and increased wall tension. These changes increase the myocardial demands for oxygen extravagantly and, where coronary narrowings are present, invite ischaemia, or failure of quick and coordinated diastolic relaxation, systolic dysfunction, and arrhythmia. In the earlier stages of coronary heart disease the patient presents wide variations of left ventricular performance. There are times when he can make effort in a normal fashion, and periods when he is grossly disabled. The bad periods correspond clinically with exhaustion and hyperarousal, which activate the dynamic causes of angina such as loss of left ventricular compliance and hyperventilation-induced restriction of the coronary lumen (Freeman & Nixon, 1985a, b). Recovery can be brought about by sleep and rest. In the later stages of disease it is not so easy to induce remissions, because of the left ventricle becomes permanently stiffened by fibrous tissue replacement of the myocardium that has been destroyed by repeated ischaemic injury (Raab, 1971; Freeman & Nixon, 1985a,b). This is an excellent reason for advising the patient to avoid the sorts of effort which induce ischaemia.

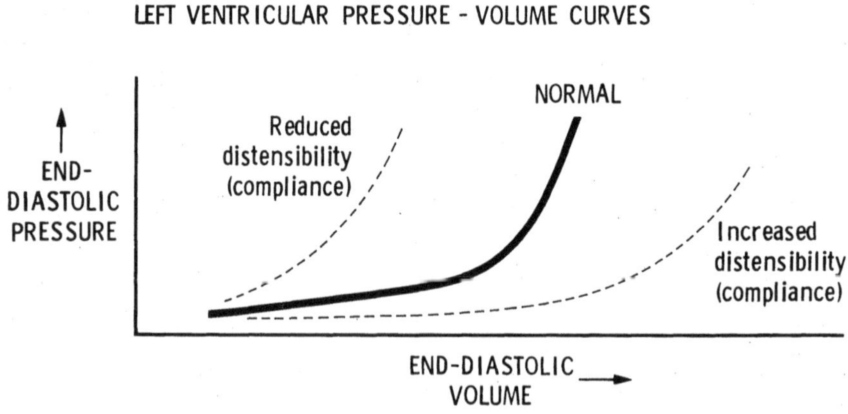

FIGURE 6.2. A diagram of left ventricular pressure volume relationships. Normally, a large volume is accepted with a minimal rise of pressure. In angina pectoris and coronary spasm the distensibility is reduced by temporary and/or permanent changes in the ventricle and even small increments of filling cause a steep rise of pressure. The mechanical disturbances precede the onset of pain and ECG abnormalities.

Henry's Model

Henry (1982, 1983) drew the axis of sympatho-adrenomedullary arousal (S-AM) vertically, from relaxation at the lower pole to the extremes of struggle and rage at the upper (Figure 6.3); and the axis of pituitary-adrencortical arousal, from well-being on the left to distress and defeat on the right. The black-shaded area of the upper-right quadrant represents the excursions of effort and defeat that homeostasis can accommodate and still keep the internal milieu within the healthy range. The stippled area represents the levels of effort and defeat that overwhelm the homeostasis and produce destructive catabolic activity. It is suggested that prolonged violation of homeostasis close to the S-AM axis may present as hypertension, close to the P-AC axis as loss of immune competence, and, in the intermediate zone, as coronary heart disease. The lower-left quadrant of well-being and relaxation is regarded as anabolic, favoring tissue repair and the re-creation of defenses. A list of the major catabolic and anabolic pro-

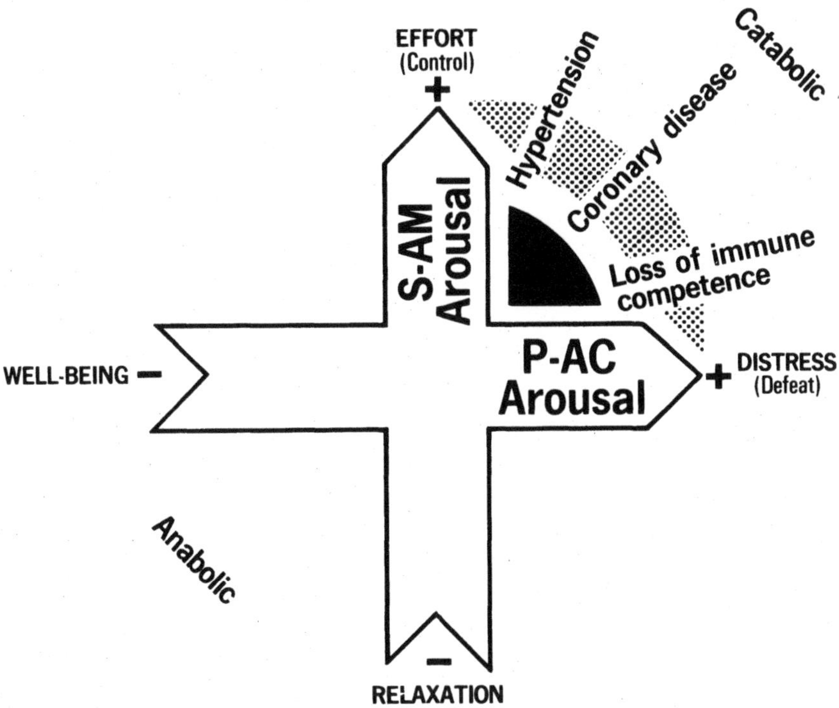

FIGURE 6.3. Henry's axes of sympatho-adrenomedullary (S-AM) and pituitary-adrenocortical arousal (P-AC).

cesses has been provided by Sterling and Eyer (1981) (see Table 6.1). Henry's model is persuasive: It invites us to prescribe conditions of relaxation and well-being, not only in accordance with commonsense and Hippocratic tradition, but also to reduce myocardial damage and provide the best possible conditions of anabolism for healing.

The Human Function Curve

The practice of rehabilitation involves a variety of practitioners from many disciplines of medicine, complementary medicine, nursing, and the auxiliary professions. They must understand each other and cooperate, but the language of conventional medicine is inadequate. A map or guide is required to mark the position of the patient and the direction of his course at any given moment. I have used the *human function curve* (HFC), a performance-arousal curve, as a model for this purpose (see Figure 6.4; Nixon, 1976, 1982a,b, 1984).

It allows the patient to be seen as enjoying health function, as healthy tired, as exhausted, ill, or verging (P) upon a catastrophic change or breakdown. The spectrum is shown as a curve related to performance and arousal (struggle, effort). On the upslope arousal increments increase performance, but on the downslope reduce it. The

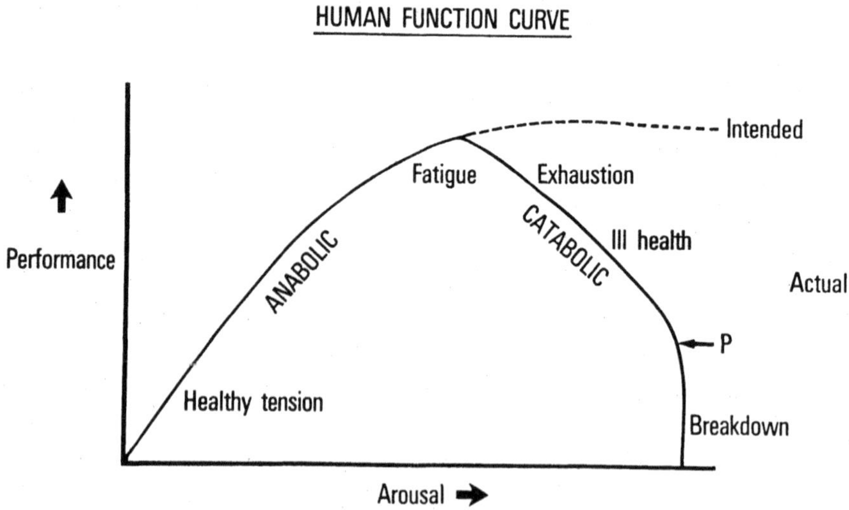

FIGURE 6.4. The human function curve. Performance relates to coping ability and efficiency. Arousal relates to effort and, at the higher levels, to struggle. P. represents the "catastrophic cliff edge" of instability, where little further arousal is required to precipitate a breakdown.

curve is shown with a peaked top, because most coronary patients can pinpoint the time or event which marked their "going over the top" from healthy function into exhaustion and preinfarction ill health. The "intended" dotted line is drawn to emphasize the fact that patients on the downslope produce their own deterioration: The struggle to close the gap between the actual performance and the intended achievement increases arousal, reduces performance, further disorganizes the internal milieu, and promotes illness.

Some individuals have high curves and others low. A high curve permits great performance, whereas as low curve invites exhaustion, ill health, and premature coronary breakdown. The handicaps which produce low coping curves in cardiac patients are commonly educational and psychosocial: migration (*British Medical Journal*, 1976), failure at school (Jenkins, 1978; Weinblatt et al., 1978), poor mothering (Montagu, 1971; Henry & Stephens, 1977), poverty and struggle in childhood (Forsdahl, 1977; Taylor, 1975), loneliness (Lynch, 1977); overwhelming coping burdens with lack of support, satisfaction, and appreciation (Cassell, 1976), and loss of prediction and control of life events (Weiss, 1972).

The curve also enables us to picture the intrinsic and extrinsic drives which can get out of hand, produce morbid shifts to the right, and increase the risk of exhaustion, ill health, and coronary breakdown. The intrinsic drives include high levels of anger, anxiety, exhaustion, and tension (Nixon & Bethell, 1974), sociopsychological exhaustion (Paffenbarger, Wolf, Notkin, & Thorn, 1966), lack of assertion skills (Harburg et al., 1964), restlessness and guilt about relaxation (Russek, 1967), inability to be satisfied by achievement (Arlow, 1945), and the Type A problems of anger, anxiety, aggression, acceleration, haste, hostility, irritation, and impatience (Friedman & Rosenman, 1974).

The extrinsic causes of morbid shifts to the right that have been associated with excessive coronary mortality include blizzards (Glass & Zack, 1979), bereavement (Parkes, Benjamin, & Fitzgerald, 1969), financial hardship (Brenner, 1971), and waves of unemployment (Bunn, 1979). A high Life Change Score making us struggle to adapt more rapidly and efficiently than we are able is a well-recognized contributor to ill health (Rahe & Ransom, 1978), and the harmful cardiovascular effects of information-input overloading have been described by Lipowski (1975). Karasek and his colleagues (1982) have described the effects of the combination of excessive life demands with inadequate control of the environment; and Ruberman, Weinblatt, Goldberg, and Chaudhary (1984), the dangers of high stress levels with social isolation.

THE RECOGNITION OF POSITION ON THE HUMAN FUNCTION CURVE

Diagnosis of Health Function and Fatigue

The characteristics have been described elsewhere (Nixon, 1976). The main point about healthy tiredness is that it is self-limiting. The individual accepts it and takes steps to recover as soon as possible. He is not caught up in vicious circles of sleep loss, deteriorating performance, and increasing arousal.

Diagnosis of Exhaustion

Lipowski's (1975) list of the effects of information-input overloading provides a useful basis of classification for cardiological work. The brain's signal handling becomes less efficient, fewer problems are solved by our "automatic pilots," and we become more easily aroused—hot and bothered—about more things. Thus the heart is given more work to do, and the product of the heart rate and blood pressure becomes greater for a given amount of effort.

Performance is impaired by loss of energy and stamina, loss of speed and accuracy of response, and increasing feelings of resentment and paranoia. Vigilance and restlessness increase. Discriminative powers deteriorate, and the subject becomes less capable of managing his time and resources efficiently. Judgment is impaired. The loss of leadership qualities compels more reliance to be placed on rank and seniority. Reducing adaptability causes defenses to be erected against change and a tendency to dwell in the past instead of in the future. There is a temptation to sit around eating, drinking, and talking too much instead of getting on with the task in hand. Aggression flares up and destroys the goodwill of potential allies. Maladaptive coping habits are commonly adopted. They include acquiescence in sleep derivation, denial of major problems, and indulgence in exhausting displacement activities. People in this phase of exhaustion are prone to hurl themselves into ill-judged physical effort, producing the risk of myocardial infarction and cardiac arrest. Total failure of coping is very close when the patient feels desperately trapped, unable to carry on and unable to opt out. Feeling trapped, he is likely to hyperventilate, and the hyperventilation can trigger off coronary arterial spasm and fatal arrhythmia.

Social disorganization occurs when the subject stops listening to others. He loses insight, becomes impossible to live with or work with, and neurotic traits get out of hand.

Neurohumorally, it is thought that S-AM and P-AC activity can rise to extremely high levels, and phaeochromocytoma-like levels of catecholamine activity have been recorded. It becomes extremely difficult for the body's self-regulating mechanisms (homeostasis) to withstand the catabolic assults and maintain a healthy internal milieu (see Figure 6.5).

An important cause of the catabolic disintegration found in exhaustion is defective habituation (Gruzelier, Nixon, Liddiard, Pugh, & Baxter 1986). This finding supports Eliasson and Atterhog's (1982) description of discrete neuronal mechanisms as opposed to generalized sympathoadrenal discharges.

A great danger of the downslope is sleep disorder. Apart from setting up vicious circles that encourage catabolic disarray in general (Adam & Oswald, 1984), it has specific associations with failure of

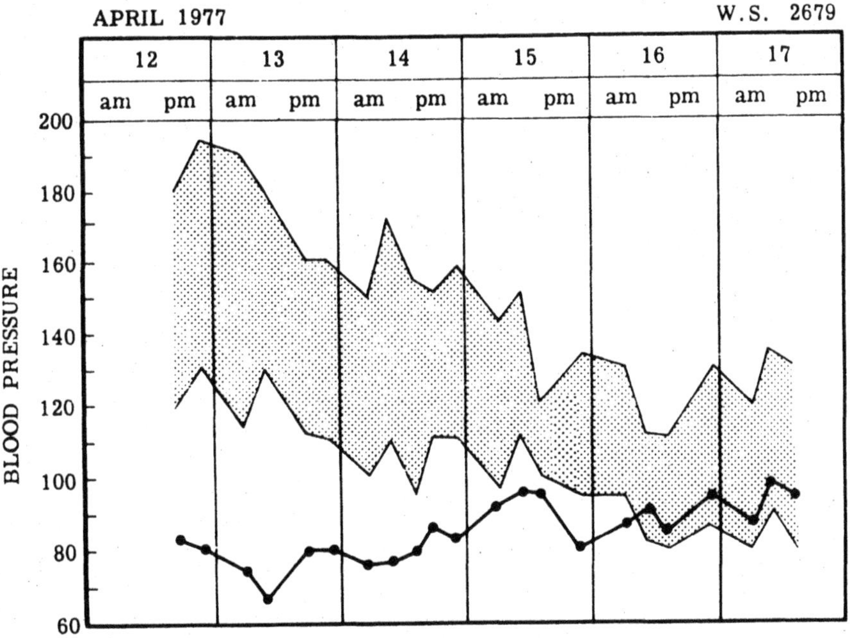

FIGURE 6.5. Businessman aged 54 years. The blood pressure (stippled area) and heart-rate (0-0-0) changes during a sleeping-resting regimen prescribed for recovery from a period of homeostasis violation induced by exhausting effort and loss of sleep during a business tour in the Middle East. From April 12 to 14, the sleep required hypnotics, but from April 15 to 17, it occurred naturally. Afterwards the blood pressure returned to its customary level of $^{110}/_{60}$ and remained there. Without a sleeping-resting regimen in such cases, the blood pressure usually remains raised, becomes resistant to hypotensive drug therapy, and increases.

recovery from angina pectoris (Mackenzie, 1908; Freeman & Nixon, 1985b).

DIAGNOSIS OF ILL HEALTH

The ill health that inevitably occurs when the exhausted press onwards and downwards towards P can take many forms. The fruits of disabling anger, social disruption, alcoholic bouts, automobile and industrial accidents, loss of resistance to infection, flare-ups of psychosomatic or psychiatric illness, and the various syndromes of chronic habitual hyperventilation are commonplace, but the cardiovascular disorders are a natural choice for people whose life is a perpetual struggle to close the gap between their actual performance and the level of achievement they think is intended of them, particularly when they possess a highly responsive arousal system and the will to force themselves beyond the limits of physiological tolerance. Their period of greatest danger comes when they are defeated and cut off, or lose their place in the pecking order (Henry, 1983).

The commonest cardiovascular forms of ill health encountered in cardiac rehabilitation are:

1. Loss of fitness and stamina. Deconditioning.
2. Hyperventilation disorders: effort syndrome or da Costa's syndrome.
3. Ectopic beating and arrhythmia.
4. Catabolic disorders, e.g., hypertension (Figure 6.5), hyperglycaemia, hyperlipidaemia, hyperuricaemia, and increased blood coagulability.
5. Electrolyte shifts and fluid retention conducive to arrhythmia (potassium loss) or heart failure (sodium retention). Magnesium depletion.
6. Coronary syndromes such as angina pectoris, acute coronary insufficiency, recurrences of mycardial infarction and cardiac arrest where the highly aroused demands put upon the heart outstrip the competence of the coronary circulation. Atheromatous coronary lesions can range from the most severe to the most trivial in these cases, and need not even be present. The heart can suffer ischaemic injury from coronary vasospasm, intravascular thrombosis, and, probably, from catecholamine toxicity (Freeman & Nixon, 1985a, b; Baroldi et al., 1978, James, 1983).

The disposition to violate the homeostasis and produce illness of these sorts is far from peculiar to coronary patients. The ordinary activities of everyday life can produce increased catecholamine secretion, sometimes approaching the level found in phaeochromocytoma. The catecholamine secretion roughly parallels the degree of arousal (Kagan & Levi, 1974), and the disorders listed above are commonplace. Nevertheless, coronary patients seem particularly keen to thrust themselves through exhaustion into catabolic ill health and to deny responsibility. Some see it as a joy and others as a duty, but each illness breeds more obstacles to recovery (Byrne, Whyte, & Butler, 1981), and so particular care and discipline are required to prevent their lurching from one infarction to another at ever-shortening intervals.

Breakdown

Once the individual comes close to P, the point of breakdown on the HFC, it may take very little extra arousal to precipitate a sudden and drastic change, just as an overloaded camel may require very little straw to break its back! These sudden changes that break continuity are mathematically the subject of catastrophe theory, and Postle (1980) uses the HFC to illustrate the theory's application to medical problems. It does provide opportunities for anticipation and prevention not offered by the binary system of thought, common in medicine, which attempts to force the patients into "nondiseased" or "diseased" pigeon holes.

Human breakdown takes many forms (Cullen et al., 1984), Behavioral, psychiatric, and psychosomatic breakdown is usually recognized for what it is, but the concept is less often used these days in cardiology. Irrespective of whether arrival at P presents with angina pectoris, coronary insufficiency, myocardial infarction, cardiac arrest, or a dangerous arrhythmia, the patient's general condition is profoundly disturbed. The chances are that he has been exhausted for a year or more but has been concealing, denying, or rationalizing the deterioration of performance. He is highly aroused and low in coping ability. He suffers from disrupted social relationships and inadequate support, and is handicapped by childhood poverty and a hard life. Devoid of effective responses for dealing with his new predicament, and helplessly dependent upon whatever medical system he has fallen into, his body has been violated by lengthy periods of catabolic abuse, and his heart is in urgent need of anabolic conditions for healing.

These behavioral changes of the downslope that provide the opportunity for anticipation and prevention have usually been present for a year or more before the infarction (Nixon & Bethell, 1984; Appels, 1983).

Hyperventilation commonly precipitates the cardiac catastrophe (see Figure 6.6). It destabilizes the acid–base balance, and hence, the equilibrium of the autonomic nervous system and the potassium and calcium homeostasis. These effects are a common cause of illness in every day life (Lum, 1976; Magarian, 1982), but in the exhausted state they seem to be capable of triggering coronary arterial spasm and thereby causing acute myocardial ischaemia, infarction, and sudden death (Freeman & Nixon, 1985a,b). The spasm may damage the intima and cause stenosis (Marzilli, Goldstein, Trivella, Paulumbo, & Maseri, 1980). In atheromatous coronary heart disease, the hyperventilation-induced coronary spasm may fracture a plaque and cause thrombotic

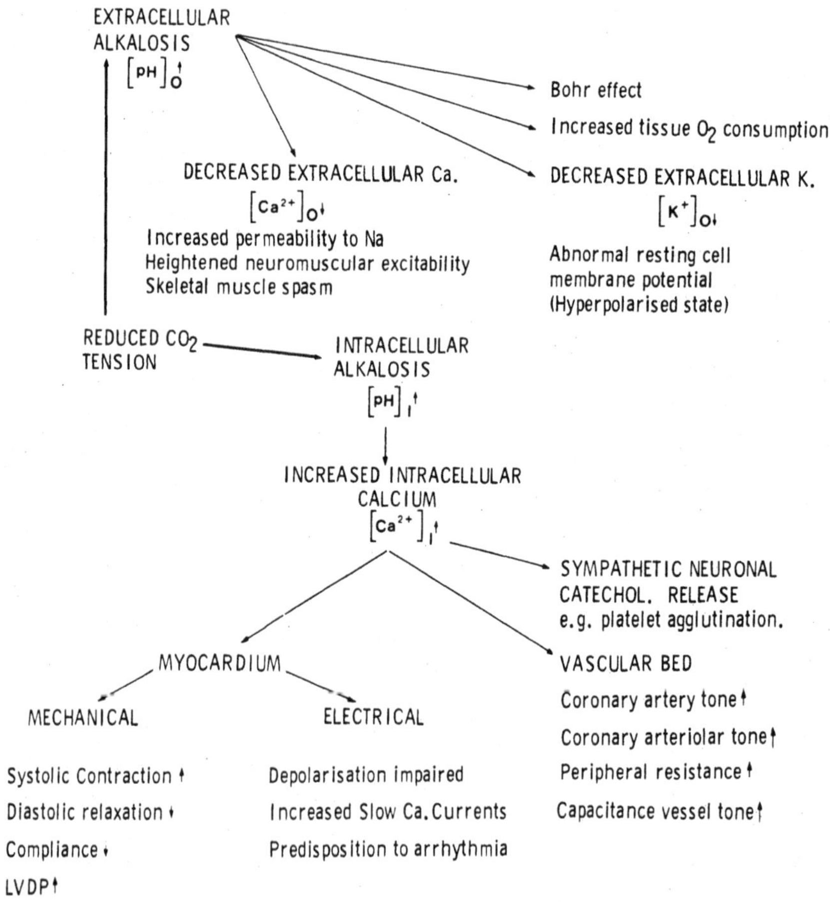

FIGURE 6.6. The mechanisms by which hyperventilation, causing a fluctuating reduction of the blood CO2 tension, induces vasomotor instability and disturbances of function (courtesy of Abdul Hamid Al-Abbasi, 1982).

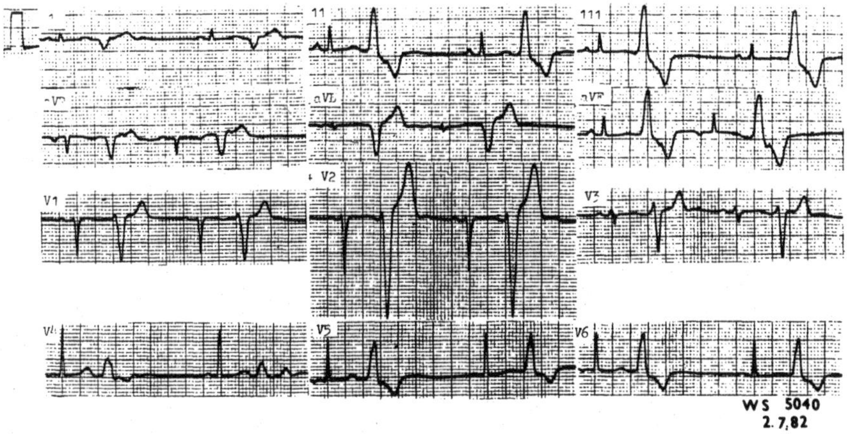

FIGURE 6.7. An example of right ventricular ectopy induced by hyperventilation in an exhausted patient. Note small R wave V1, left bundle branch block appearance in V6 and right axis.

occlusion. Right ventricular ectopy is a common product of hyperventilation in coronary care units (Figure 6.7) and may cause ventricular fibrillation. A well-trained nurse will prevent this by calming the patient and teaching him to breathe as he should.

Current Cardiological Policies

If the HFC is used as a paradigm for examining contemporary cardiological practice, it does suggest that we may be using drugs and bypass operations to palliate the symptoms of living on the downslope. Ill-time risk factor intervention might increase arousal and precipitate a breakdown, one reason for risk factor intervention trials failing to show the hoped-for reduction of death rate. The paradigm suggests that we pay too little attention to getting patients off the downslope before breakdown, too little to preventing recurrence of breakdown, and almost none to the creation of high curves and hardiness.

PRINCIPLES OF MANAGEMENT

"It is almost as if something inside the patient refused to get well until the doctor had really listened to what was wrong and taught the patient to outwit its influence" (Groddeck, 1977).

The purpose of cardiac rehabilitation is to enable the patient to take care of himself and make the best of his resources, and we have found ourselves moving away from the idea that exercise is its most important intervention. We are inclining to the view that exercise is something which can be taken up for pleasure and benefit in most cases when the exhaustion and high arousal states have been dealt with by counselling and other measures, and when the patient can support the effort required by the activities of daily living (ADL). The disappointing reports of exercise-based cardiac rehabilitation have been reviewed recently (Nixon, Al-Abbasi, King, & Freeman, 1986). I have deliberately given much space to models and paradigms in this chapter, because policy for rehabilitation is not yet laid down, and their use enables a wide variety of therapists to help the patient achieve a measure of control over his internal milieu and live a reasonably free life after breakdown.

The Setting for Cardiac Rehabilitation

The heart is clearly subordinate to the brain and sensitive to the processes of the mind. At the same time, the processes of the mind and the coping ability are influenced by the individual's perception of his heart's condition. A reductionist or mechanistic attitude towards heart disease which ignores these relationships does not favor the processes of rehabilitation. Rehabilitation is encouraged by an integrated or biopsychosocial approach to cardiological problems: competent clinical craftmanship and an efficient technical service, combined with humane and compassionate treatment which respects the patient's dignity, his sense of values, and his cultural canons. The cardiologist must work with the patient in a cooperative way, as a trainer, agreeing upon the objects of therapy with him and making a joint effort to achieve them. He is sensitive to suffering and distress and minimizes the interventions which threaten the intactness of the individual and his relationships with his people. He is aware that the recovery of healthy function may be impossible if illness and medical interventions make the patient incapable of occupying a satisfactory position in his society. The care he provides reduces the patient's needs for vigilance which, like suffering and depersonalization, can cause exhaustion and loss of resistance to disease. The cardiologist pays close attention to the family and deals as best he can with denial and their feelings of fear, anger, and guilt. He is aware of their hopes and anxieties, and reinforces their ability to deal with the heart attack in their midst. The biopsychosocial approach can accommodate the idea of myocardial infarction as a breakdown, and respond by integrating the best of conventional technology with the best possible training for healthy patterns of coping and adapting (Cousins, 1983).

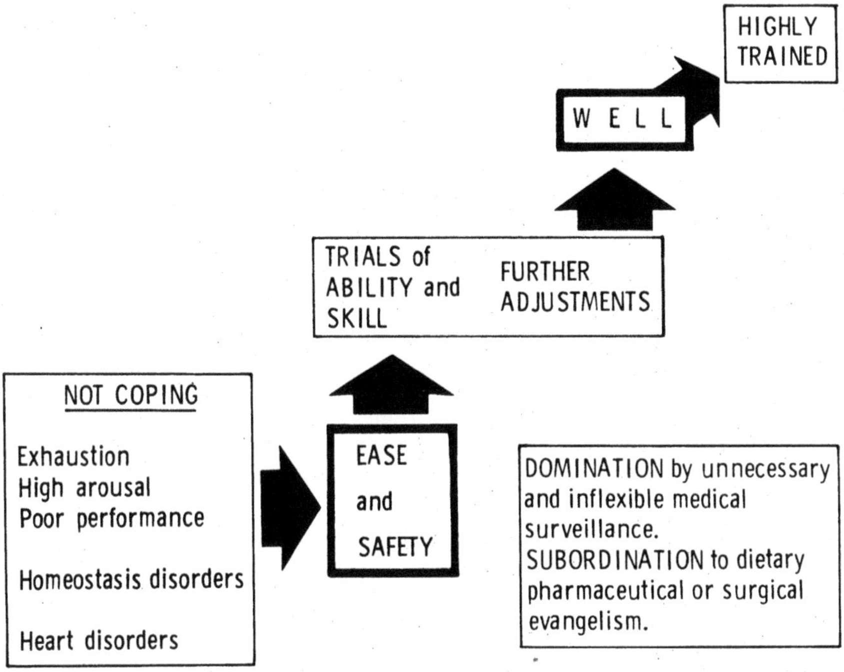

FIGURE 6.8. A flow diagram showing the described pathway (broad arrows) from cardiovascular ill health and breakdown to the highly trained condition of rehabilitation. The freedom of the patient to avoid being trapped in the bottom right-hand box may depend more upon the philosophy of his cardiologist and the prevailing culture than upon the condition of his heart.

The Flow Diagram of Management and Rehabilitation

Figure 6.8 indicates the progression through the various phases of recovery.

The provision of ease and safety takes the patient out of a catabolic milieu and provides him with anabolic conditions for recovery: out of the treadwheel of effort (see Figure 6.1) and off the downslope of HFC (see Figure 6.4). When he is ready, he is helped to make trials of his coping ability and skill and reach a point where he is well: able to make the best of himself and avoid recurrence of exhaustion and illness. If he wishes, he can be provided with the training to achieve hardiness and a "high-level wellness" (Kobasa et al., 1982; Reed, 1984).

Phase 1 (a). Ease and Safety

This is essentially a nursing phase. I employ a sleeping-resting regimen (Nixon, Taylor, Morton, & Bromfield, 1968) in which great care is taken to overcome the exhausting effects of pain, fear and distress, and the arrhythmic consequences of hyperventilation. Sedation with promethazine and diazepam is employed in the smallest effective dosage to help the patient to sleep like a "pink, well-fed baby" between meal times and at night. The nurses are trained to avoid disturbing the sleeping-resting regimen unnecessarily: Observations, care of the breathing, leg exercises, and other functions can be carried out when the patient is awake. The sleeping-resting regimen is continued until the patient is comfortable and relaxed and can waken without hyperventilating when he looks around and realizes where he is.

The sleeping-resting regimen has many uses. It expands the amount of anabolic time available in each 24-hour period and reduces vigilance and arousal. It reduces the demands upon the heart and coronary circulation and helps to recover autonomic stability. It can bring the patient through the modes of denial, rage, bargaining, and depression so quickly that he reaches acceptance long before his family. Our nurses are trained, not only to provide the regimen in hospital, but to organize and manage it by telephone at the patient's home where he may need it later, for 2 or 3 days perhaps, to recover from the effects of ill-judged activity.

The management of this stage is a major determinant of the patient's career after myocardial infarction. Handled well, it can provide confidence and optimism. Handled badly, it can increase arousal and vigilance and aggravate the risk of catastrophe, regress the patient to a state of incompetence, and produce undesirable dependence upon medical systems. Deprivation of dignity and respect cause resentment and set the patient's mind against cooperation in training. The seed is sown for the maladaptive forms of behavior, which can be more of a handicap than the pathological changes in the heart itself (Byrne et al., 1981). Too short an investment in this periods may well result in a higher mortality during the second and third years (West & Henderson, 1979). Evans (1983, p. 218; capitalization not in original) has written: "in uncomplicated cases a walk around the ward on the twelfth day appears to do no harm, the patient having rested for a full nine days and remaining in care in hospital for 21 days, but THERE IS NO SOUND BASIS FOR EARLIER AMBULATION."

Phase 1 (b). The Beginning of Training

The patient is passive during the sleeping-resting regimen, but begins to take a more active part in his recovery when he reaches the mode of acceptance, and is usually ready to consider his predicament. At the beginning of this stage he meets a trainer. The trainer's earlier moves are protective, and establish a relationship which can be used afterwards to encourage modification of illness behavior. Verbal methods or massage can be employed to teach relaxation and control of hyperventilation. The patient learns to take his own pulse rate in order to assess his responses to effort. The trainer helps the patient to understand the hospital and avoid the pitfalls of becoming "a difficult case." He or she may negotiate with the staff on the patient's behalf. She helps him to make a success of this new and unwanted experience, meets his family, and helps them towards acceptance. In a good unit with high morale the staff is all aware of the patient's needs, and its functions are flexible and interchangeable. As the patient moves out of nursing dependence, the trainer takes a stronger role. His or her professional background may be that of occupational therapist or counsellor trained in cardiological crisis intervention. The cardiac infarction is a crisis and must not be wasted, or the patient and those around him will lose the opportunity for making desirable changes of behavior and relationships.

The trainer must cope with surges of hopelessness, denial, rage, and resignation which come with the coronary predicament, and keeping the patient on course will be easier when he or she can draw from a store of goodwill created in the earliest days of the illness. There is much to be done before the patient is free to enjoy his convalescence. The tasks include assessment, education, and the prescription of effort.

The assessment takes account of the patient's assets and handicaps (high or low HFC) and his intended level of activity. Motivation and readiness for effort are considered. The circumstances at home are weighed up in the knowledge that most urban families no longer know how to conduct illness (Osmond, 1980). Domestic tension may be too high for convalescence or recovery to be feasible, and so the spouse may need to be rested or eased into a more comfortable condition for providing support. Hitherto rebellious children often turn out to be remarkably supportive if the crisis is well used.

The educational aspects of the work include helping the patient to recover respect for fatigue instead of remaining oblivious to it, and become articulate about feelings of rage or despair in order to deal with them instead of bottling them up. Survival may depend upon awareness of the influences which caused the breakdown and ability to outwit them. He will need to learn about the cardiological consequences of "people poisoning" (tension created by people he cannot escape), conflicting hierarchical demands, and righteous indignation. Getting upset is a personal choice and steps must be taken to avoid exercising it too often.

The treadwheel (See Figure 6.1) and HFC (See Figure 6.4) models are freely used, because they provide many patients with a flash of insight into their predicament, and a common-sense pathway out of it.

The prescription of effort is important. No patient knows his capacity after suffering preinfarction ill health, myocardial infarction, and deconditioning by bedrest. Most will strive to do too much too soon and defeat themselves, re-creating the vicious circles of frustration and despair that caused the illness. Most will assume that they should be able to do more with each passing day and make themselves ill with frustration when they fail. A few are trapped into low levels of activity by thoughts of sudden death: Fear and anger keep them low on the downslope of the HFC.

It is easy enough for the patient to learn to check his heart rate and responses to effort, and use them as a guide to activity (see Figure 6.9), but it can be extremely difficult for him to understand the degree to

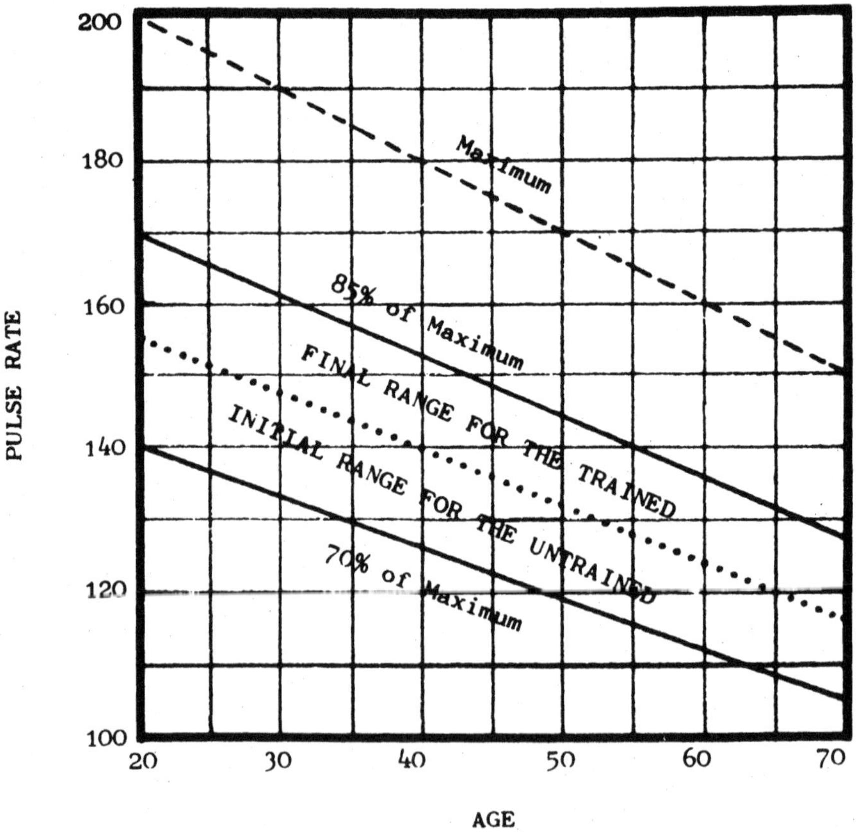

FIGURE 6.9. Heart rate and age chart. Activities prescribed for untrained patients keep the heart rates below the 70% of maximum.

which they can be influenced by certain physiological variables. We refer to these variables by the acronym SABRES and teach our patients to employ them as tools for obtaining the best possible performance in the shortest time (Nixon, 1984).

S = SLEEP—awareness of the quantity and quality required, and how to get it.
A = AROUSAL—awareness and modulation of rage and struggle, despair and defeat.
B = BREATHING—awareness and control in place of hyperventilation's inappropriate upper chest movement, sighing, and irregularities of rate and depth.
R = REST—achieving the ability to be still and calm when required.
E = EFFORT—recognizing and respecting the limits of beneficial physical and mental effort, and the onset of healthy tiredness. Stopping before the onset of myocardial ischaemia.
S = SELF-ESTEEM—linked with confidence. Restored by close support and the successful mastery of the physiological variables.

The patient learns SABRES by heart in order to foresee and outwit failures of performance which otherwise might seem capricious and undeserved. He learns that the "bad days" which threaten a relapse come from sleeplessness, ungoverned arousal, disordered breathing, restlessness, exhausting overactivity, and loss of confidence—not being in control of the internal environment. The "good days," offering as much as a tenfold increase of performance, come from being well slept, emotionally in control, enjoying the benefit of well-chosen activity and adequate rest, and feeling like a "winner."

Convalescence begins when the patient leaves hospital with enough information and support to carry him safely forward for 2 or 3 weeks.

Phase 2 (a). Convalescence

Convalescence is much more than a retreat. It is the gateway to recovery from the deconditioning processes of illness and hospitalization to the reestablishment of tolerable domestic and social relationships and to the reassertion of autonomy. The prudent therapist assumes that the patient will soon become forgetful of fatigue, unable to put self-interest before social demands, and dissatisfied by anything less than self-defeating amounts of activity. His burdens of explanation (Finlayson & McEwan, 1977) are heavy, and he will avoid them by taking on too much activity too soon in order to prove to those around him that they have no right to pry into his habits. He is defenseless against the people who can arouse him to a level which thrusts him onto the downslope of the HFC.

In order to outwit these hazards, we offer a program that provides little opportunity for self-defeat, and a briefing that caters for as many activities of daily living (ADL) as possible. SABRES are kept in mind when the trainer discusses effort, exercise, play, food and drink, sleep, sex, tension, the restriction of visitors, and the need to control a tendency to hyperventilate when emotionally upset.

Before the start of the convalescence, the patient and the family are reassured that their trainer will remain warm, friendly, approachable, and accessible by telephone—a valuable friend and ally in the strange, hard new world of infarction.

Phase 2 (b). After Convalescence

The cardiologist and the trainer meet the patient after convalescence and start the series of negotiations and compromises which will bring him freedom: When he can do what he wants or tolerate compromise, he will no longer be a patient.

The gap between his actual performance and his intended level of activity is assessed, and note made of handicaps which might make his goals difficult or impossible. Particular attention is paid to influences in his social milieu which might raise his arousal and thrust him "over the top" of the HFC before he can organize his defenses. He might not want to go back to the life that was "killing" him. Motivation must be developed and coupled with discipline and body awareness for rehabilitation to be successful.

Many obstacles to success will be found. Commonly encountered are impatience with the time requirements of training for effective rehabilitation. Many cannot be still: Boredom will be their cry. Some are adrenalin addicted and given to breaking the rules in order to enjoy the arousal induced by risk taking. Pride and denial may make one man feel above the biological imperatives which govern lesser mortals, while a psychopathic urge for gratification in the short term may deprive another of the chance to cultivate staying power. Many are tempted off course by evangelists with unbalanced views about diet, exercise, or the magical effects of pharmaceutical palliatives and surgical "cures." The processes of finding and returning to an optimum level of ADL necessarily involve the patient in making an audit of the effort required to support the various domains of his life: He cannot immediately afford all their demands and must rank them in order of priority. It is essential to avoid the "Icarus syndrome" of attempting too much too soon and crashing defeated, because this is certain to maintain catabolic levels of arousal. The patient needs to be convinced that recovery is possible and the program rational and prudent. It may be helpful to use imagery such as "we can teach you to use this breakdown as a means of breaking through or breaking out into a better way of life," or show him the similarity between his predicament and that of Hackett (1977, p. 49; emphasis my own), wounded at Arnhem: "I had gone into the battle as fit as a prize-fighter and certainly owed to this reserve of physical strength much of the resistance I had been able to offer to the stresses of the last few weeks. There was not much left to draw on. I was soon to fall so low that *it would take much time and care to creep back up again.*"

The patient will find that good days of high performance are interrupted by bad days of greatly restricted ability. He must be taught that the phases of deterioration are not due to chance or relapse of disease, but to variations of the cardiac reserves which must be analyzed in terms of SABRES and countered intelligently. Recovery is assisted by methods which enable the patient to get to know his body better and become more friendly with it: our occupational therapists and counsellors are ably reinforced by masseuses and hypnotists, remedial gymnasts, dance therapists, and osteopaths. They are especially helpful where the patient is unwilling to "let go" of exhausting levels of vigilance and tension.

During this phase of exploring and returning to an optimum level of ADL, the patient is encouraged to walk. He is taught that distance is much more important than speed. If he can learn to walk for two or three miles at an untiring pace, he will be able to add speed later, but if he hastens into fatigue, pain, or breathlessness he will never improve himself. He practices taking his heart rate and keeping his activity within the prescribed limits of 60%–70% of maximum (see Figure 6.9; Nixon, Carruthers, Taylor, Bethell, & Grabau, 1976).

The cardiologist checks that this level of effort can be enjoyed without symptoms of overexertion and without the production of arrhythmia or ischaemia before he delegates the management of daily effort to the trainer. Once the patient can hold a firm position on the upslope of the HFC and avoid being dragged over the top into exhaustion, it is reasonable to begin an exercise training program to hasten the removal of deconditioning and recover fitness and stamina at the best possible rate. The physical aspects of the training consist of about half an hour of individually prescribed exercise carried out two or three times a week. The prescription of the exercise is based on the observation of the patient and his pulse rate, and the watchword is "train, don't strain." The desirable level is 60%–70% of the individual's maximum, well below the amount which causes pain and distress or silent ischaemia. The patient soon learns that tension and tiredness have a great effect upon his progress, and he learns to assert his right to the conditions of life which enable him to continue to improve himself even if it cuts across the demands of those nearest and dearest to him.

Well-tested exercise prescriptions have been published widely. Our own (Nixon et al., 1976) are consistent with Kavanagh's (1980) practice and the recommendations of the American Heart Association (Erb, Fletcher, & Sheffield, 1980). Since we began in 1965, we have carried out the bulk of exercise training in a gymnasium that is not close to the hospital and has no doctor in attendance: There has been no need of hospital support or medical attendance, and there is much to be said for training patients to be well at a distance from the sick house. The training provided before the start of an exercise program enables the patient to manage effort without running into pain, and so trinitrin and its derivatives are not required. We do not accept patients for training if they profess a need for betablockade: the restriction of the heart rate's response to exercise removes a most useful guide to training, the various side-effects are undesirable, and a supposed dependence upon a pharmaceutical palliative is not required by a patient who is learning to be well.

Group rehabilitation provides the assets of the fellowship and psychological support, but care must be taken to avoid self-defeating competition. I visited a German residential rehabilitation unit on the day a priest died after getting up at 5 a.m. to double the amount of exercise effort he could put into the day: By doing this, he thought he would get well in half the time it took his competitors.

It is a good idea to have a relaxing holiday before returning to work.

Phase 2 (c). Returning to Work

The patient returns to work when he is confident he can accommodate the change without becoming exhausted or driving himself into a catabolic mode. The time depends upon individual circumstances, but 3 months from the time of infarction is a common interval for making a start. The return to work should be a series of gradual steps, and I like patients to go to their jobs on Mondays, Wednesdays, and Fridays for a "running in" period of 1, or 2 months, keeping Tuesdays and Thursdays as buffer periods for working quietly at home, resting, or exercising according to the needs of the moment.

The trainer watches the position closely. He or she is alert to shifts over the top of the HFC, particularly where a sense of duty overrides common sense and self-interest, where there is inability to say "no" to the demands of others, and where lack of social assets and support make the patient too restless to do well. It is not necessary for the trainer and patient to meet frequently if telephone calls are made once or twice a week. With very little practice it is easy for the trainer to pick up the voice of exhaustion and defeat; and the knowledge that friendly surveillance is readily available helps the patient to keep on a favorable course.

Very little cardiological supervision is required, because there are no pills to prescribe, apart from sedation with Phenergan 10 mgm and Valium 5 mgm when circumstances threaten sleep deprivation, and the patient is most unlikely to be overtaxing his heart if he is on the upslope of HFC behaviorally.

Deterioration of the heart follows exhaustion. The first cardiac sign of deterioration is elicited by examining the apex beat of the heart when the patient is lying in the left lateral position. The normal left ventricle presents a thumb-nail area of systolic outward movement and a double, lup-dup, rhythm. The overdistended left ventricle present an enlarged area of systolic outward pulsation, and the left atrial contribution to its filling becomes powerful enough to provide a palpable and audible atrial triple rhythm (Figure 6.10).

In frank failure the atrial triple rhythm is replaced by an early diastolic third sound gallop. Thus the conventional palpation and auscultation of the heart become a useful field tool for rehabilitation, and graphic records can be taken with the apexcardiograph and phonocardiograph. The methods and interpretation have been described by Bethell and Nixon (1973a,b) and Nixon (1974).

The management of the return to work and the ability to avoid overloading have long been regarded as crucial steps: "when, above all, a man's circumstances are such as to allow him to take as much care of himself as he pleases, many years, even ten or a dozen, have been known to elapse between the first attack and the patient's death" (Latham, 1846, p. 409).

Phase 3. Staying Well

Staying well indicates that the patient can do whatever he needs or accept a healthy compromise with a familiar handicap. He is master enough of his circumstances or adaptable enough to avoid the downslope of the HFC with its attendant catabolic and arteriopathic disarray. He does not require cardiological supervision but should keep in friendly contact with his trainer for advice or assessment. The trainer

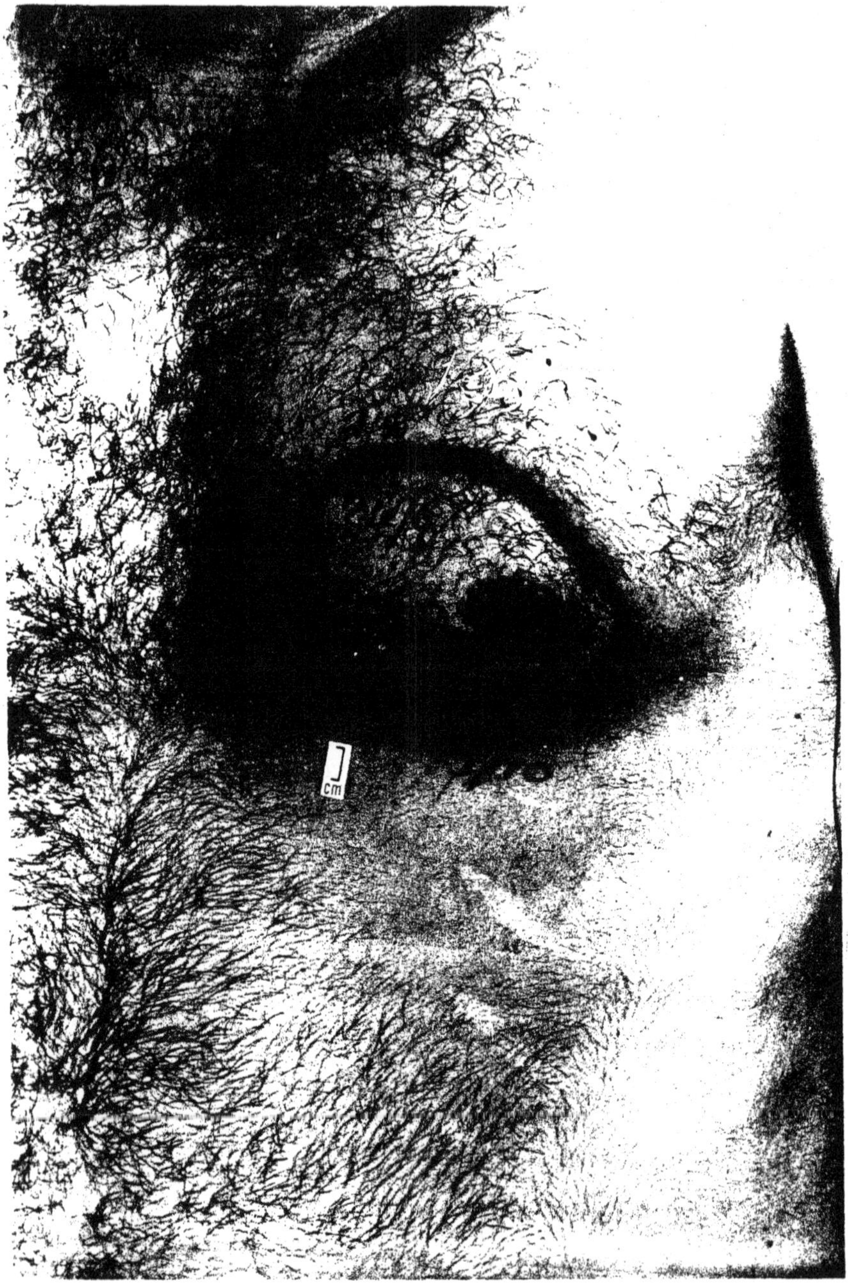

FIGURE 6.10. Male aged 34 years. The larger area outlined on September 24 is the area of palpable paradoxical left ventricular dyskinetic thrust found in a case of coronary heart disease with acutely progressive angina produced by a period of excessive effort. A sleeping-resting regimen restored the left ventricular pulsation to a normal area by October 5, and the patient recovered his former performance level.

will arrange for him to see the cardiologist whenever a consultation is desirable. In this way the cardiologist's services are employed when they are needed and not wasted in a "routine" follow-up clinic where the patient's appointments may never coincide with his needs. Moreover, the patient is much less likely to deny and withhold important information from a friendly trainer than from the doctor.

There is scarcely a patient who can avoid being driven into a corner sometimes and exhausted by the demands of life. The skillful ones will withdraw into a "bolt-hole bed" for a day or two, sleep long and well with doses of Phenergan 10 mgm and Valium 5 mgm, and extricate themselves from the predicament before the vicious circles of sleeplessness and catabolic arousal can take hold.

Phase 4. Becoming Highly Trained

A well-managed myocardial infarction is a well-managed crisis that can provide a breakthrough to a happier and more comfortable life. Many patients feel healthy for the first time they can remember and wish to capitalize on this achievement by becoming superfit. The safe pathways to high levels of endurance after infarction, such a marathon running, have been described by Kavanagh (1980). In the survival stakes the prizes go to those with hardiness (Kobasa et al., 1982), well-developed social assets, and the ability to avoid distress (Ruberman et al., 1984).

Cardiac Surgery

The outcome of coronary artery bypass grafting (CABG) is disappointing from the point of view of ability to sustain physical effort (Nixon & Pugh, 1983) or return to former levels of work and recreation (CASS Principal Investigators, 1983). This is surprising, because there are many powerful "hidden persuaders" capable of reinforcing the benefits of surgical intervention. The placebo effect can be strong and last for several years (Preston, 1977). Cognitive dissonance can induce the patient to change his habits and strive to make a success of a painful and costly operation (Totman, 1979). The coronary patient's burdens of explanation, his ability to find room and time for manoeuvre, and his inability to change role (Finlayson & McEwan, 1977) can disappear at the first stroke of the knife. Inadequacies of treatment and education in the preoperative period can be made good by an enthusiastic surgical team's commitment to success, particularly where suggestion leads the patient to believe that he is now receiving a "cure" for his "disease" I suppose the failure of patients to return to work or remain gainfully employed (McIntosh & Garcia, 1978) must either be a sign that they use the operation as a rite of passage into a preferred position of life, or an indication that their therapists do not know how to provide a return ticket!

It is our practice to offer coronary arteriography and consider surgical treatment where careful training has not dealt with disablement. As Braunwald (1983, p. 1183) wrote after the CASS (1983) trial,

> most important, however, the results of CASS suggest that it is not mandatory to operate on patients with multivessel disease who are asymptomatic or whose angina is not intractable, in an effort to prolong survival or prevent myocardial infarction: it is certainly possible to defer surgery in such patients. If CABG prolongs life or prevents myocardial infarction in only a small subset of patients with coronary-artery disease, such as those with severe obstruction of the left main coronary artery, it follows that coronary angiography can be limited to patients who, on clinical examination and non-invasive exercise stress testing, are considered to be at high risk.

The phrase "failure of full medical treatment" is commonly used as an excuse for bypass grafting where pharmaceutical preparatins have been prescribed without any attempt to teach the patient to recover healthy function. It is important to understand exactly what the speaker has in mind when the phrase is employed, because the surgeon rarely sends the patient back for more adequate treatment. It is useful to remember that "a man seems to be able to get along very well on about a quarter of his coronary circulation" (Osler, 1910), and that "patients who can climb a flight of stairs can be treated medically for there is no good evidence that surgery will prolong their lives" (Hamptom, 1984).

In 1983, Jenkins et al. drew attention to their finding, in a group of 204 candidates for bypass graft surgery, that behavioral and psychological factors were stronger predictors of angina pectoris than severity of coronary obstruction. There surely cannot be a stronger case for adequate preoperative assessment and a biopsychosocial approach to management. A treadmill test and a coronary arteriogram are not enough.

If open-heart surgery is required, the patient returns to his trainer to learn to make the best of his operation.

CONCLUSION

Throughout the Victorian period and into the 1940s the cardiologist relied upon behavioral management and rehabilitation for improving the condition of his patients. He had no alternative. Close attention was paid to the removal of exhaustion and the avoidance of angina. Rest, sleep, mental attitudes, bodily comfort, diet, massage, and exercise were important topics at the consultation (Mackenzie, 1908). During the 1914–1918 War, Sir Thomas Lewis and Sir James Mackenzie provided cardiac rehabilitation at an especially established unit in London, and each lived and worked for 20 years after the onset of his own angina pectoris. In those days a good prognosis was expected when a man was able to work and yet provide his heart with the conditions required for healthy function. After the 1940s these perspectives were lost, displaced by commitment to drugs and operations, risk factor manipulation, and preoccupation with technology. Doctors no longer thought about the clinical and behavioral consequences of living in a catabolic fashion at the limits of endurance, far beyond the ability of homeostasis to maintain a stable and orderly condition of the internal milieu. But that phase is ending with the realization that a "comprehensive programme of treatment involves both the full utilization of medical science and the full development of the human healing system. The fact that the belief system can be a vital activator of the healing system may serve as an open door to an auspicious future in medical research and practice" (Cousins, 1983).

REFERENCES

Adam, K., & Oswald, I. (1984). Sleep helps healing. *British Medical Journal, 289,* 1400–1401.

Appels, A. (1983). The year before myocardial infarction. In T. M. Dembrowski, T. H. Schmidt, & G. Blumchen (Eds.), *Biobehavioural bases of coronary heart disease.* Basel, Switzerland: Karger.

Arlow, J. A. (1945). Identification mechanisms in coronary occlusion. *Psychosomatic Medicine, 7,* 195–209.

Asmussen, E. (1976). In R. Passmore & J. S. Robson (Eds.), *A companion to medical studies* (Vol. 1, pp. 45–51). Oxford: Blackwell Scientific Publications.

Barnes, E., & Schottstaedt, W. W. (1960). The relation of emotional state to renal excretion of water and electrolytes in patients with congestive heart failure. *American Journal of Medicine, 29,* 217–27.

Baroldi, G., Mariani, G., & Falzi, G. (1978). Degree of coronary obstruction in patients with coronary heart disease compared with "control" population. In A. Maseri, G. A. Klassen, & M. Lesch (Eds.), *Primary and secondary angina.* New York: Grune and Stratton.

Bethell, H. J. N., & Nixon, P. G. F. (1973a). Understanding the atrial sound. *British Heart Journal, 35,* 229–235.

Bethell, H. J. N., & Nixon, P. G. F. (1973b). Examination of heart in supine and left lateral positions. *British Heart Journal, 35,* 902–907.

Braunwald, E. (1983). Effects of coronary-artery bypass grafting on survival. Implications of the randomised coronary artery surgery study. *New England Journal of Medicine, 309,* 1181–4.

Brenner, M. H. (1971). Economic changes and heart disease mortality. *American Journal of Public Health, 61,* 606–11.

British Medical Journal [Editorial]. (1976). *Migrants and Cardiovascular Disease, 1,* 1423–1424.

Buell, J. C., & Eliot, R. S. (1980). Psychosocial and behavioral influences in the pathogenesis of acquired cardiovascular disease. *American Heart Journal, 100,* 723–740.

Bunn, A. R. (1979). Ischaemic heart disease mortality and the business cycle in Australia. *Australian Journal of Public Health, 69,* 772–781.

Byrne, D. G., Whyte, H. M., & Butler, K. L. (1981). Illness behaviour and outcome following survived myocardial infarction: A prospective study. *Journal of Psychosomatic Research, 25,* 97–107.

CASS principal investigators and their associates. (1983). Coronary artery surgery study (CASS): A randomised trial of coronary artery bypass surgery. Quality of life in patients randomly assigned to treatment groups. *Circulation, 68,* 951–60.

Cassel, J. (1976). The contribution of the social environment to host resistance. *American Journal of Epidemiology, 104,* 107–123.

Chambers, W. N., & Reiser, M. F. (1953). Emotional stress in the precipitation of congestive heart failure. *Psychosomatic Medicine, 15,* 38–60.

Cousins, N. (1983). The healing heart. *International Journal of Cardiology, 3,* 56–65 and 219–229.

Cullen, J., Siegrist, J., Wegmann, H. M., Ballieux, R. E., Fielding, J. F., & L'Abbate, A. (1984). *Breakdown in human adaptation to stress: Towards a multidisciplinary approach.* Boston, MA: Martinus Nijhoff.

Eliasson, K., & Atterhog, J. H. (1982). Psychological stress—circulatory and catecholamine changes in men with T-wave aberrations. *Contributions to Nephrology, 30,* 70–77.

Engel, G. L. (1974). Memorial lecture: The psychosomatic approach to individual susceptibility to disease. *Gastroentenology, 67,* 1085–1093.

Engel, G. L. (1982). Biopsychosocial model and medical education. *New England Journal of Medicine, 306,* 802–5.

Erb, B. D., Fletcher, G. G., & Sheffield, L. T. (1980). Standards for supervised cardiovascular exercise maintenance programs. *Circulation, 62,* 669A–673A.

Evans, D. W. (1983). Early ambulation after myocardial infarction. *Journal of the Royal College of Physicians, 17,* 217–219.

Eyer, J. (1980). Social causes of coronary heart disease. *Psychotherapy and Psychosomatics, 34,* 75–87.

Finlayson, A., & McEwan, J. (1977). *Coronary heart disease and patterns of living.* London: Croom Helm.

Forsdahl, A. (1977). Are poor living conditions in childhood and adolescence an important risk factor for arteriosclerotic heart disease? *British Journal of Preventive and Social Medicine, 31,* 91–95.

Freeman, L. J., & Nixon, P. G. F. (1985a). Chest pain and the hyperventilation syndrome—some aetiological considerations. *Postgraduate Medical Journal, 61,* 957–961.

Freeman, L. J., & Nixon, P. G. F. (1985b). Dynamic causes of angina pectoris. *American Heart Journal, 110,* 1087–1092.

Friedman, M., & Rosenman, R. H. (1974). *Type A behaviour and your heart.* London: Wildwood House.

Glass, R. I., & Zack, M. M. (1979). Increase in deaths from ischaemic heart disease after blizzards. *Lancet, 1,* 485–487.

Groddeck, G. (1977). *The meaning of illness.* London: The Hogarth Press.

Groen, J. J. (1976). Psychosomatic aspects of ischaemic (coronary) heart disease. In O. W. Hill (Ed.), *Modern trends in psychosomatic medicine* (Vol. 3). London: Butterworths.

Gruzelier, J. H., Nixon, P. G. F., Liddiard, D., Pugh, S., & Baxter, R. (1986). Retarded habituation and lateral asymmetries in electrodermal activity in cardiovascular disorders. *International Journal of Psychophysiology, 3,* 219–226.

Hackett, General Sir John. (1977). *I was a stranger.* London: Chatto and Windus.

Hampton, J. R. (1984). Coronary artery bypass grafting for the reduction of mortality: An analysis of the trials. *British Medical Journal, 289,* 1166–70.

Harburg, E., Julius, S., McGinn, N. F., McLeod, J., & Hoobler, W. W. (1964). Personality traits and behavioural patterns associated with systolic blood pressure levels in college males. *Journal of Chronic Diseases, 17,* 405–414.

Hebb, D. O. (1955). Drives and the C.N.S. (conceptual nervous system). *Psychological Review, 62,* 243–254.

Henry, J. P. (1982). The relation of social to biological processes in disease. *Social Science and Medicine, 16,* 369–380.

Henry, J. P. (1983). Coronary heart disease and arousal of the adrenal cortical axis. In T. M. Dembroski, T. H. Schmidt, & G. Blumchen (Eds.), *Biobehavioural bases of coronary heart disease.* Basel, Switzerland: Karger.

Henry, J. P., & Meehan, J. P. (1981). Psychosocial stimuli, physiological specificity, and cardiovascular disease. In H. Weiner, M A. Hofer, & A. J. Stunkard (Eds.), *Brain, behaviour and bodily disease.* New York: Raven Press.

Henry, J. P., & Stephens, P. M. (1977). *Stress, health, and the social environment.* New York, Heidelberg, Berlin: Springer-Verlag.

James, T. N. (1983). Chance and sudden death. *Journal of the American College of Cardiology, 1,* 164–183.

Jenkins, D. C. (1978). Low education: A risk factor for death. *New England Journal of Medicine, 299,* 95–97.

Jenkins, D. C., Stanton, B., Klein, M. D., Savageau, J. A., & Harken, D. E. (1983). Correlates of angina pectoris among men awaiting coronary bypass surgery. *Psychosomatic Medicine, 45,* 141–153.

Kagan, A. (1982). Introduction to the role of psychosocial stressors in ischaemic heart disease. In Kellerman (Ed.), *Psychological problems before and after myocardial infarction.* Basel, Switzerland: Karger.

Kagan, A. R., & Levi, L. (1974). Health and environment—Psychosocial stimuli: A review. *Social Science and Medicine, 8,* 225–241.

Kahneman, D. (1973). *Attention and effort.* Englewood Cliffs, NJ: Prentice-Hall, Inc.

Karasek, R. A., Russell, S. R., & Theorell, T. (1982). Physiology of stress and regeneration in job related cardiovascular illness. *Journal of Human Stress, 8,* 29–42.

Kavanagh, T. (1980). *The healthy heart program.* Toronto, Canada: Van Nostrand Reinhold.

Kobasa, S. C., Maddi, S. R., & Kahn, K. H. (1982). Hardiness and Health: A prospective study. *Journal of Personality and Social Psychology, 42,* 168–177.

Lader, M. (1975). Psychophysiological methods and parameters. In L. Levi (Ed.), *Emotions. Their parameters and measurement.* New York: Raven Press.

Latham, P. M. (1846). *Diseases of the heart* (Vol. 2). London: Longman, Brown, Green & Longmans.

Levi, L. (1972). *Stress and distress in response to psychosocial stimuli.* Oxford, England: Pergamon Press.

Lewis, T. (1918). *The soldier's heart and the effort syndrome.* London: Shaw & Sons.

Lipowski, Z. J. (1975). Sensory and information inputs overload: Behavioural effects. *Comprehensive Psychiatry, 16,* 199–221.

Lum, L. C. (1976). The syndrome of habitual chronic hyperventilation. In O. W. Hill (Ed.), *Modern trends in psychosomatic medicine* (Vol. 3). London: Butterworths.

Lynch, J. J. (1977). *The broken heart.* New York: Basic Books, Inc.

Mackenzie, J. (1908). *Diseases of the heart.* London. Hodder & Stoughton.

McIntosh, H. D., & Garcia, J. A. (1978). The first decade of aortocoronary bypass grafting. *Circulation, 57,* 405–431.

Magarian, G. J. (1982). Hyperventilation syndrome: Infrequently recognized common expressions of anxiety and stress. *Medicine, 61,* 219–236.

Marzilli, M., Goldstein, S., Trivella, M. G., Paulumbo, C., & Maseri, A. (1980). Some clinical considerations regarding the relation of coronary vasospasm to coronary atherosclerosis; A hypothetical pathogenesis. *American Journal of Cardiology, 45,* 483.

Montagu, A. (1971). *Touching: The human significance of the skin.* New York: Columbia University Press.

Nixon, P. G. F. (1974). Noninvasive techniques in angina pectoris. In O. Paul (Ed.), *Angina pectoris* (pp. 50–73). New York: Medcom Press.

Nixon, P. G. F. (1976). The human function curve. *The Practitioner, 217,* 765–769, 935–944.

Nixon, P. G. F. (1982a). Are there clinically significant prodromal signs and symptoms of impending sudden death? *Practical Cardiology, 8,* 175–183.

Nixon, P. G. F. (1982b). Stress and the cardiovascular system. *Practitioner, 226,* 1589–1598.

Nixon, P. G. F. (1984). Stress, life-style and cardiovascular disease. A cardiological odyssey. *British Journal of Holistic Medicine, 1,* 20–29.

Nixon, P. G. F., Al-Abbasi, A. H., King, J. C., & Freeman, L. J. (1986). Hyperventilation in cardiac rehabilitation. *Holistic Medicine, 1,* 5–13.

Nixon, P. G. F., & Bethell, H. J. N. (1974). Preinfarction ill health. *American Journal of Cardiology, 33,* 446–449.

Nixon, P. G. F., Carruthers, M. E., Taylor, D. J. E., Bethell, H. J. N., & Grabau, W. (1976). British pilot study of exercise therapy: II. Patients with cardiovascular disease. *British Journal of Sports Medicine, 10,* 54–61.

Nixon, P. G. F., & Pugh, S. E. (1983). Coronary artery bypass surgery. *Lancet, 1,* 242.

Nixon, P. G. F., Taylor, D. J. E., Morton, S. D., & Bromfield, M. (1968). A sleep regimen for acute myocardial infarction. *Lancet, 1,* 726–728.

Oliva, P. B. (1981). Pathophysiology of acute myocardial infarction. *Annals of Internal Medicine, 94,* 236–250.

Osler, W. (1910). Angina pectoris. *Lancet, 1,* 839–844.

Osmond, H. (1980). God and the doctor. *New England Journal of Medicine, 302,* 555–558.

Paffenbarger, R. S., Jr., Wolf, P. A., Notkin, J., & Thorn, M. C. (1966). Chronic disease in former college students. 1: Early precursors of fatal coronary heart disease. *American Journal of Epidemiology, 83,* 314–328.

Parkes, C. M., Benjamin, B., & Fitzgerald, R. G. (1969). Broken heart: A statistical study of increased mortality among widowers. *British Medical Journal, 1,* 740–743.

Perlman, L. C., Ferguson, S., Bergum, K., Isenberg, E. L., & Hammarsten, J. F. (1971). Precipitation of congestive heart failure: social and emotional factors. *Annals of Internal Medicine, 75,* 1–7.

Postle, D. (1980). *Catastrophe theory* Glasgow, Scotland: William Collins Sons & Co. Ltd.

Preston, T. A. (1977). *Coronary artery surgery: A critical review.* New York: Raven Press.

Raab, W. (1969). Myocardial electrolyte derangement: crucial feature of pluricausal, so-called coronary, heart disease. *Annals of New York Academy of Sciences, 147,* 627–686.

Raab, W. (1971). Cardiotoxic biochemical effects of emotional-environmental stressors—fundamentals of psychocardiology. In L. Levi (Ed.), *Society, stress and disease* (pp. 331–337). London: Oxford University Press.

Rahe, R. H., & Ransom, J. A. (1978). Life change and illness studies: and future directions. *Journal of Human Stress, 4,* 3–15.

Reed, K. L. (1984). *Models of practice in occupational therapy.* Baltimore, MD & London: Williams & Wilkins.

Ruberman, W., Weinblatt, E., Goldberg, J. D., & Chaudhary, B. S. (1984). Psychosocial influences on mortality after myocardial infarction. *New England Journal of Medicine, 311,* 552–559.

Russek, H. I. (1967). Role of emotional stress in the etiology of clinical coronary heart disease. *Diseases of the Chest, 52,* 1–9.

Sodeman, W. A., & Burch, G. C. (1938). The precipitating cause of congestive heart failure. *American Heart Journal, 15,* 22–27.

Sterling, P., & Eyer, J. (1981). Biological basis of stress-related mortality. *Social Science and Medicine, 15E,* 3–42.

Lord Taylor, (1975). Poverty, wealth, and health, or getting the dosage right. *British Medical Journal, 2,* 207–211.

Totman, R. (1979). *Social causes of illness.* London: Condor Books, Souvenir Press (E & A) Ltd.

Weinblatt, E., Ruberman, W., Goldberg, J. D., Frank, C. W., Shapiro, S., & Chaudhary, B. S. (1978). Relation of education to sudden death after myocardial infarction. *New England Journal of Medicine, 229,* 60–65.

Weiss, J. M. (1972). Influence of psychological variables on stress-induced pathology. In *Physiology, Emotions and Psychosomatic Illness* (Ciba Foundation, Symposium 8). Amsterdam, Holland: Elsevier-Excerpta Medica.

West, R. R., & Henderson, A. H. (1979). Randomised multicentre trial of early mobilization after uncomplicated myocardial infarction. *British Heart Journal, 42,* 381–385.

7

"Vascular" Headache Syndromes and their Treatment*

Peter D. Drummond

Psychology Section
Murdoch University
Perth, West Australia

In recent years biofeedback procedures, progressive muscular relaxation and other stress management techniques have become established as viable alternatives to pharmacological treatment of headache. In this chapter, developments in clinical, psychological, and physiological assessment of migraine, tension-vascular, and cluster headache will be reviewed, followed by a discussion of the rationale and effectiveness of various forms of treatment.

* I wish to thank Professor J. W. Lance for his critical appraisal of the manuscript, the National Health and Medical Research Council of Australia, and the J. A. Perini and Basser Trusts, for their financial support.

ASSESSMENT OF HEADACHE

Clinical Assessment

The major headache syndromes were outlined by the Ad Hoc Committee on Classification of Headache (1962). Several categories of head pain arising from inflammation or structural changes were defined (for example, lesions causing displacement of normal tissue, pain due to systemic infections or cranial inflammation, or headache due to abrupt rises in blood pressure). Such diseases are uncommon but can be lethal, so a neurological and general physical examination should be carried out before medical or psychological treatment is begun.

The major clinical categories of benign recurrent headache are listed in Table 7.1, and the various subtypes of migraine are presented in Table 7.2. These tables contain descriptions, rather than definitions, of clinically recognized headache categories. Patients sometimes report symptoms from more than one category or a few symptoms from only one category. Presumed differences in etiology separate the categories and provide a conceptual guide for medical management of headache. Apart from lower-half headache, where the site of pain defines the category, the major difference among subtypes of migraine lies in the nature and time course of neurological symptoms in relation to the onset of head pain (Table 7.2). Such symptoms reflect disturbances in the cerebral cortex (classical and hemiplegic migraine), brainstem (vertebrobasilar migraine), cranial nerves (ophthalmopolegic migraine), and hypothalamus (premonitory migraine).

Cluster headache is considered to be separate from migraine or tension headache because of its distinctive time course, site, and autonomic features. The independence of cluster headache was verified on clinical grounds in a recent computer analysis of the objectivity of diagnoses in 600 patients with benign recurrent headache (Drummond & Lance, 1984a). Of 58 patients diagnosed clinically as having cluster headache, all but four were assigned to this category by an objective classification procedure (discriminant analysis) in which the time course, site of headache, and nature of associated symptoms were used as variables. Factor analysis confirmed that features of cluster headache (frequently recurring unilateral facial pain associated with a drooping eyelid, watering eye, and running nostril on the affected side) were usually reported together. Cluster headache is a comparatively rare condition; its prevalence has been estimated to be only 2.4 per 1000 individuals (Kudrow, 1980). Approximately 85% of cluster headache patients are male (Kudrow, 1980).

Table 7.1.
Clinical Categories of Benign Recurrent Headache

	Time Course	Location	Symptoms
migraine	lasts hours or days with complete remission for days, weeks or months	often unilateral in temple, forehead, or behind the eye	neurological prodrome in classical migraine; constant or throbbing pain; nausea; vomiting; sensitivity to light
tension	episodic, daily, or continuous pain	usually bilateral across forehead, temples, back of neck, vertex, or behind eyes	sensation of pressure, tightness or constriction without accompanying migrainous symptoms
tension-vascular (combined, mixed)	episodic, daily, or continuous mild pain with intermittent severe episodes	severe pain often unilateral, mild pain unilateral or bilateral in forehead, temples, eyes, or back of neck	mixture of migrainous and tension headache symptoms
posttraumatic	episodic, daily, or continuous pain	unilateral or bilateral; may be localized to the site of injury	features of migraine or tension headache beginning after head injury
cluster	one or more attacks per day lasting minutes or hours for several weeks or months with weeks or months of remission (episodic cluster) or without remission for at least 1 year (chronic cluster)	always unilateral behind eye, temple, upper or lower jaw, spreading to the back of the neck	rapid onset over several minutes, ipsilateral eye bloodshot, watering, nostril blocked or running, eyelid drooping, pupil constricted (one-third of patients)

Table 7.2.
Clinical Subgroups of Migraine

	Time Course of Symptoms	Symptoms
premonitory symptoms	1–24 hours before headache	predictable changes in mood; hunger, particularly a craving for sweet food; change in alertness; may precede classical or common migraine
classical	during the hour before headache	sharply defined transient neurological disturbances commonly involving vision, but also affecting speech, sensation, or movement in some instances
hemiplegic	before or during headache	weakness or paralysis down one side of the body
ophthalmoplegic	during headache	weakness or paralysis of the muscles controlling eye movement
vertebrobasilar	during headache	symptoms of brainstem disturbance such as dizziness, faintness, incoordination, double vision, loss of consciousness, or slurred speech
lower-half	during headache	recurrent pain in the cheek or jaw
common	before or during headache	no focal neurological symptoms

Defining other clinical categories of benign recurrent headache is more difficult. In our analysis, almost 15% of patients diagnosed clinically as having common migraine, tension-vascular, or tension headache were assigned by objective computer classification to some other category (Drummond & Lance, 1984a), thus demonstrating considerable clinical overlap of categories. Symptoms commonly regarded as migrainous (infrequent headache associated with gastrointestinal disturbances, sensory hyperacuity, facial pallor, and cold extremities) were reported most often by patients diagnosed as having classical or common migraine. These symptoms were reported less often by tension-vascular patients, and least of all by tension headache patients. Thus the number, rather than the nature, of common migraine symptoms apparently was used clinically to define these categories.

Epidemiological studies of headache symptoms in the general community have questioned the validity of the migraine–tension headache dichotomy, because a "migraine syndrome" that fits with clinical descriptions cannot be separated from other forms of headache (Waters, 1973; Kaganov, Bakal, & Dunn, 1981). Instead, the number of migrainous features and symptoms of "idiopathic" or "essential" headache (aching pain, tightness or pressure in the neck, vertex, or forehead) were found to increase in proportion to the rating of headache severity. Considerable overlap of migraine and muscle contraction symptoms is typical (Kaganov et al., 1981), thus suggesting that migraine and tension headache may share some mechanisms.

Symptoms associated with the patient's most severe attacks are usually given greatest priority in clinical diagnosis despite great variation in headache severity and symptomatology from one attack to another. For example, of 40 patients with a history of classical migraine who had a headache at the time of examination, only seven actually had focal neurological symptoms with that particular episode (Drummond & Lance, 1984b). Headache in the other 33 patients resembled common migraine, tension-vascular, or tension headache. In another investigation of symptoms in 726 patients who presented with acute headache, more than 30% of patients were not assigned a diagnosis by the clinician, apparently because symptoms were intermediate between migraine and tension headache (Diehr, Wood, Barr, Wolcott, Slay, & Tompkins, 1981). Subsequent analyses identified subgroups of patients with headache of rapid onset, eye pain, and symptoms of upper respiratory tract infection. Other categories seemed to reflect a particular style of answering questions: Some patients reported almost every symptom, whereas others described very few symptoms. Only 8% of patients were classified as having classical migraine, whereas 26% formed a tension headache category (Diehr, Diehr, Koepsell, Wood, Beach, Wolcott, & Tompkins, 1982). Common migraine and tension-vascular categories could not be differentiated by Diehr et al. (1982). These findings illustrate the difficulty of separating patients into migraine and tension headache categories on the basis of presenting symptoms, and also emphasize the need for a thorough neurological and physical examination to rule out structural or inflammatory causes of headache.

In summary, clinical assessment focuses on the time course and site of headache, and the nature of symptoms associated with the attack. This is usually enough to identify cluster headache, but it may be more difficult to categorize other types of headache which form a continuum in symptomatology from migraine to tension headache. Headache with features both of common migraine and of tension headache is often described as *mixed* or *combined* headache. Because these terms presuppose the existence of two independent headache mechanisms, the more general term *tension-vascular* headache is used in this review. Tension headache is used in preference to *muscle contraction* headache because the contribution of the scalp and neck muscles to head pain has not been demonstrated conclusively (Pikoff, 1984). The mechanism and behavioral treatment of tension headache is reviewed elsewhere in this series.

Psychological Assessment

More than 60% of migrainous patients believe that an emotional upset, worry, or some other psychological factor can precipitate headache (Selby & Lance, 1960; Drummond, 1985a). A prospective analysis of emotional state around the time of headache indicated that over 50% of attacks coincided with some form of emotional stress (anxiety, overwork, other emotional strain, anger, resentment, or relief from strain) (Henryk-Gutt & Rees, 1973). During migraine, patients typically feel drowsy and fatigued (Dalkvist, Ekbom, & Waldenlind, 1984; Harrigan, Kues, Ricks, & Smith, 1984), and frustrated at not being able to carry on with normal activity (Harrigan et al., 1984). Feeling trapped or hemmed in, coupled with feelings of lethargy and exhaustion, were found to be the best predictors of impending headache (Harrigan et al., 1984). As well as emotional factors, susceptibility to headache may also be increased by consumption of certain foods or alcohol, hunger, changes in weather and exercise patterns, or hormonal variations associated with puberty, menstruation, and taking oral contraceptives (Lance, 1982).

It has long been suspected that migraine sufferers have certain personality traits which increase their emotional response to psychological stress. Psychometric studies using the Minnesota Multiphasic Personality Inventory (MMPI) have demonstrated a "conversion V" configuration on the "neurotic triad" of subscales in adult headache sufferers (Harrison, 1975). In this configuration, scores are high on the hypochondriasis and hysteria subscales and somewhat lower on the depression subscale. Children with migraine also appear to be more anxious and cautious than other children, but whether this is a predisposing factor, or develops in response to repeated episodes of head pain, is uncertain (Hoelscher & Lichstein, 1984).

Recent studies have emphasized the progression of psychological disturbance, particularly neuroticism and depression, from cluster headache and migraine to tension-vascular and tension headache. For instance, Kudrow and Sutkus (1979) found such robust differences between headache types in the hypochondriasis, depression, and hysteria subscales of the MMPI that headache diagnoses could be assigned accurately to 75% of males and 67% of females using MMPI criteria alone. Migraine and cluster headache groups were essentially normal, whereas tension-vascular and tension headache groups appeared to have hysterical concern over minor bodily symptoms and were moderately depressed. Scores on many MMPI subscales were elevated for patients with posttraumatic or *conversion* headache. Since Kudrow and Sutkus relied on the patient's rating of the severity of headache to differentiate conversion from tension headache, the difference between these two clinical subtypes is probably quantitative rather than qualitative. Posttraumatic headache sometimes forms part of a "workers-compensation syndrome," which may explain why MMPI scores were elevated in this group.

The MMPI criteria proposed by Kudrow and Sutkus (1979) were used by Andrasik, Blanchard, Arena, Teders, and Rodichok (1982a) to classify patients into clinical categories but this was unsuccessful for tension-vascular and tension headache patients. Andrasik et al. pointed out that the degree of psychological distress may depend on the population being studied. Whereas half of their patients were self-referred and the other half referred by a physician, patients studied by Kudrow and Sutkus (1979) were all drawn from a neurology outpatients clinic.

In a more detailed presentation of their findings, Andrasik, Blanchard, Arena, Teders, Teevan, and Rodichok (1982b) described differences among headache and nonheadache groups in five clinical subscales of the MMPI, the Psychosomatic Symptom Checklist, and the State-Trait Anxiety Inventory. Psychological disturbance was least in cluster headache patients, followed by migraine and tension-vascular headache, and was most apparent in those with tension headache. None of the headache groups showed marked elevations on any of the tests, although certain individuals in each group (including the control group) sometimes exceeded normal limits. Patients in the migraine group appeared to be preoccupied with vague bodily symptoms; those with tension-vascular headache reported mild depression and worry as well, while tension headache patients usually showed all of these features and were resentful and inflexible in outlook.

Higher scores for tension-vascular than for episodic migraine patients on the hypochondriasis, depression, hysteria, and psychasthenia subscales of the MMPI were reported by Weeks, Baskin, Rapoport, Sheftell, and Arrowsmith (1983). These investigators cautioned that scores may have been elevated by MMPI items relating more closely to the consequences of daily headaches than to true psychopathology. For instance, questions dealing with frequent headache, neck pain, nausea, and lethargy could inflate scores on the hypochondriasis and hysteria subscales. This should be kept in mind when selecting scales for psychological assessment of headache patients.

A history of depressive episodes is often associated with frequent headache in settings both clinical (Drummond, 1985a; Couch, Ziegler, & Hassanein, 1975) and nonclinical (Ziegler, Rhodes, & Hassanein, 1978). The relationship between headache and depression was clearly demonstrated by Garvey, Schaffer, and Tuason (1983), who reported that headache frequency increased during depression in patients with a major depressive disorder but returned to previous levels during the nondepressed period. In some patients depression is probably a consequence of headache rather than a predisposing factor. The transformation of episodic into constant headache may be associated with hypertension, oral contraceptives, and medication overuse (particularly ergotamine tartrate) as well as psychological factors (Mathew, Stubits, & Nigam, 1982).

In summary, a strong relationship between psychological disturbance and frequent or continuous headache has been demonstrated. Little permanent psychological disturbance appears to be associated with cluster headache or episodically recurring migraine, although emotional reactions may precede or accompany individual attacks.

VASCULAR CHANGES DURING HEADACHE

The current concept of migraine is that pain arises from distension of pain-sensitized scalp arteries. An increase in amplitude of pulsation of the frontal branch of the superficial temporal artery during migraine was first demonstrated by Tunis and Wolff (1953). Greater variation in pulse amplitude was observed during the headache-free period in 10 headache sufferers selected from a pool of 75 subjects than in nonheadache controls, and pulse amplitude increased early in the course of the migraine attack. These observations were questioned by other researchers who could find no relation between pulse amplitude and headache; they emphasized the difficulty of obtaining a reproducable pulse wave which altered greatly with small changes in position and pressure of application of the displacement transducer (Brazil & Friedman, 1956; Heyck, 1969). A recent investigation using photoplethysmography to measure temporal pulse amplitude met with similar negative results (Feuerstein, Bortolussi, Houle & Labbe, 1983).

The rate of clearance of ^{24}Na, injected into the skin of the temples, demonstrated that blood flow through frontotemporal regions was greater during than between migraine episodes, particularly on the side of headache (Elkind, Friedman, & Grossman, 1964). Similarly, clearance of inhaled ^{133}Xe from the extracerebral compartment was found to be greater during than between migraine episodes (Sakai & Meyer, 1978), indicating that extracranial blood flow increased during headache. To account for the paradoxical association between facial pallor and increased scalp blood flow during migraine, Heyck (1969) proposed that blood shunts directly from scalp arteries to veins, thus bypassing the capillary bed in the skin.

The calibre of microscopic blood vessels in the conjunctiva of the eye was seen to increase during headache in some patients but to decrease in others (Blau & Davis, 1970). Vascular changes in the eye are not comparable with changes in other parts of the scalp, because conjunctival vessels stem from the internal carotid artery supplying the brain, whereas branches of the external carotid artery, such as the superficial temporal artery, perfuse the scalp. Even so, the findings of Blau and Davis suggest that the direction and extent of vascular changes during migraine may differ from one individual to another.

This hypothesis was investigated in our study of thermographic and pulse amplitude changes during unilateral migraine and tension-vascular headache (Drummond & Lance, 1983, 1984b). A subgroup of one-third of patients reported a significant reduction in pain during compression of the superficial temporal artery proximal to the site of pain, implying a relationship between arterial distension and pain; in this subgroup, heat loss and pulse amplitude from the frontotemporal region was usually greater on the side of headache. These findings indicate that distension of pain-sensitized scalp arteries was a source of pain in only a minority of patients during unilateral headache. Although such attacks were associated with migrainous features such as nausea and vomiting more frequently than attacks which did not respond to arterial compression, an extracranial vascular component was not detected by thermography or vascular compression for many headaches with clinical features of migraine (Drummond & Lance, 1984b).

Modern theories of migraine have swung away from the view that the intra- and extracranial circulations are of primary importance. Sicuteri (1967) postulated that the primary event in migraine was a release of catecholamines causing vasoconstriction and then reactive microvascular dilatation with the release of pain-producing substances such as substance P, histamine, and bradykinin. A decrease in circulating levels of the monoamine vasoconstrictor serotonin during migraine was thought to encourage vasodilatation (Anthony, Hinterberger, & Lance, 1967), but it has since been suggested that this fall may mirror a depletion of serotonin in brainstem centres where it acts as a neurotransmitter and influences perception of pain (Sicuteri, 1976).

Marked changes in hunger, particularly a craving for sweet food, water balance, alertness, and emotional swings sometimes anticipate migraine by up to 24 hours, suggesting that migraine is preceded by a hypothalamic disturbance (Herberg, 1975). A spread of neural disturbance to centers in the brainstem controlling vasomotor and gastrointestinal functions could initiate cerebral vascular changes and nausea.

For instance, stimulating the locus coeruleus in monkeys produced vascular changes resembling those of classical migraine in that flow through the internal carotid circulation decreased whereas external carotid blood flow increased (Lance, Lambert, Goadsby, & Duckworth, 1983). Lance et al. (1983) postulated that low frequency firing of the locus coeruleus could constrict the cortical microcirculation or directly inhibit cortical neuronal activity, thus initiating a wave of depression of neural activity spreading forward from the occipital cortex, accompanied by reduced blood flow. This would account for the prodrome of classical migraine (Lauritzen, Olsen, Lassen, & Paulson, 1983). An increase in firing rate of the locus coeruleus could then initiate extracranial vascular dilatation, whereas a secondary "fatigue" phase may disrupt neighboring centers controlling perception of pain. A slightly different hypothesis was put forward by Amery (1982), who proposed that the primary event in migraine was an insufficient supply of oxygen in cerebral tissue,which caused a release and depletion of serotonin within the brainstem and subsequent initiation of the biochemical and vascular changes of migraine.

Headache may also be sustained, at least in part, by a shortage of naturally occurring morphine-like substances (endorphins and enkephalins) which may act as "analgesic neurotransmitters" in the central nervous system (Anselmi, Baldi, Casacci, & Salmon, 1980). During the headache-free interval, levels of beta-endorphin in the cerebrospinal fluid were found to be lower than control levels in common migraine patients, particularly when acute headache was accompanied by daily low-grade pain (Nappi et al., 1985). Reduction of beta-endorphin levels in the blood of migrainous patients during the headache-free interval is not consistent (Nappi et al., 1985; Fettes, Gawel, Kuzniak, & Edmeads, 1985; Bach, Jensen, Blegvad, Fenger, Jordal, & Olesen, 1985), but these levels may not reflect endorphin activity in the central nervous system.

These neural theories of migraine emphasize that headache in the migraine–tension headache continuum may not necessarily result from cerebral vascular disturbances. In contrast to the findings in classical migraine, no significant focal or global reduction of cerebral blood flow was observed during spontaneous attacks of common migraine (Lauritzen & Olesen, 1984) or attacks induced by red wine (Olesen, Tfelt-Hansen, Henricksen, & Larsen, 1981). Although extracranial vasodilatation was associated more frequently with migraine than with tension-vascular headache, such changes did not appear to be an essential requirement for migraine (Drummond & Lance, 1984b).

Unlike migraine, cluster headache is usually associated with a unilateral increase in blood flow through the facial areas in which pain is experienced. A consistent unilateral increase in corneal temperature, intraocular pressure, and amplitude of intraocular pulsation indicated that blood flow through the eye increased during cluster headache (Hørven & Sjaastad, 1977). Superficial temporal artery and supraorbital pulsations increased more on the painful side in some patients (Drummond & Anthony, 1985), and greater heat loss from the orbit and cheek on the affected side sometimes spread above the eye, down the nose, and to the temple (Drummond & Lance, 1984c). Despite the strong association between extracranial vasodilatation and cluster headache, these changes are probably secondary phenomena because they usually develop after the onset of pain (Drummond & Lance, 1984c).

AUTONOMIC ACTIVITY IN MIGRAINE

The mechanism through which emotional reactions initiate headache probably involves the autonomic nervous system, either centrally within the brainstem and hypothalamus, or peripherally through monoaminergic actions on the circulation or other end-organs. If the trigger zone for headache is located within the hypothalamus and brainstem, a disruption to the normal rhythm of neural activity could initiate an attack. This could account for the multitude of factors which appear to precipitate migraine and tension-vascular headache, including emotional stress, overload of the special senses (flashing lights, loud noises), hormonal variations during the menstrual cycle, and hypoglycaemia (Lance, 1982).

Emotional reactions initiate changes in autonomic nervous system activity that prepare the individual for muscular action. Whether these autonomic changes differ from normal in headache sufferers will now be reviewed, concentrating first on reactions of the blood vessels of the scalp, and then on responses in other physiological systems.

Extracranial Vascular Responses

Wolff (1953) observed that migrainous patients responded to discussion of threatening topics with dilatation and distension of cranial arteries, whereas responses were minimal in nonheadache subjects. Wolff suggested that reactivity of the cranial vasculature was greater in migrainous patients than in controls.

This hypothesis was tested experimentally by studying changes in temporal pulse amplitude after light exercise (a Harvard step test) (Drummond & Lance, 1981). Increases were greater on the habitually affected side in patients subject to unilateral migraine or tension-vascular headache, but this increase did not significantly exceed that of nonheadache control subjects. Changes in temporal pulse amplitude were also studied during a battery of tests designed to activate the autonomic nervous system, including isometric exercise, rebreathing carbon dioxide, exposure to heat and cold, head-up and head-back tilt, and mental arithmetic (Drummond, 1982a). An attempt was made to induce a "stress" response during mental arithmetic by urging the subject to work faster and by pointing out mistakes. The average increase in temporal pulse amplitude during mental arithmetic (corrected for simultaneous increases in systolic blood pressure and heart rate) was greater in the migraine group than in nonheadache controls, although subsequent individual examination of responses demonstrated that this was due to large increases in a minority of migrainous subjects (Drummond, 1985b). Changes in pulse amplitude during other tests did not differ consistently between the migraine and control groups (Drummond, 1982a).

In a further experiment, pulse amplitude responses during mental arithmetic and after light exercise were analyzed in relation to signs of involvement of the extracranial vasculature during headache (temporary relief during compression of the superficial temporal artery, or an increase in heat loss from the affected frontotemporal region) (Drummond, 1984). The increase during both tests was greater in patients who had previously shown some sign of extracranial vasodilatation during headache, suggesting the scalp arteries dilated readily both during and between headache episodes in a subgroup of migrainous patients. Scalp arteries could be inherently responsive in such patients, or this could develop in response to repeated episodes of vasodilatation during headache. Alternatively, vasomotor centers in the brainstem could be activated readily both during and between headache episodes.

Paradoxically, other extracranial vascular measures indicate greater cutaneous vasoconstriction in migrainous subjects than in nonheadache controls during psychological stress. For example, skin temperature of the temples and cheeks increased less in migrainous subjects than in nonheadache controls during mental arithmetic tests (Drummond, 1982a, 1985b). Changes in temporal pulse amplitude correlated significantly with changes in systolic blood pressure and heart rate during mental arithmetic (Drummond, 1982a), suggesting that the increase in temporal pulse amplitude was due, at least in part, to an increase in cardiac output. By contrast, changes in facial temperature were unrelated to changes in blood pressure, heart rate, or pulse amplitude, indicating that the increase in facial temperature during mental arithmetic was a local response.

Vascular pulsations from the earlobe were found to decrease more in migrainous subjects than in controls following mental arithmetic tests and ischaemic arm pain (Gannon, Haynes, Safranek, & Hamilton, 1981). Since the earlobe consists mainly of skin, these findings indicate that cutaneous vasoconstriction was greater in migrainous subjects. The change in the DC component of photoplethysmograph signals from the fingers and temples during a single session of biofeedback, relaxation, or control procedures was studied by Price and Tursky (1976). The change in the DC component is thought to reflect a change of blood volume in the tissue from which the recording is being taken. Marked differences between migrainous and nonmigrainous subjects developed in both measurement sites regardless of the experimental condition; digital and temporal blood volumes increased in control subjects, while digital blood volume remained constant and temporal blood volume decreased progressively in migraine sufferers. These findings indicate that migrainous subjects responded to the demands of the experimental procedures with constriction in the microcirculation of the temples.

In contrast to microvascular reactions, there is no strong evidence that large scalp arteries constrict more readily in migrainous subjects than in controls. Temporal pulse amplitude decreased more in migrainous than in control subjects in response to 90 dB tones, but this difference was significant only on the right side and only when the test was repeated during a second session (Ellertsen & Hammerborg, 1982). In a similar experiment by Bakal and Kaganov (1977), velocity of blood flow through superficial temporal arteries decreased in headache patients and increased in controls. However, the difference was of sufficient magnitude to achieve statistical significance for the left side only, and could thus have been a chance result. Morley (1985) observed a greater reduction in temporal pulse amplitude in migrainous subjects than in controls while anticipating an unpleasantly loud noise, but had difficulty interpreting this finding, since constriction was greater on the nonsymptomatic side, particularly during the final few seconds of measurement.

Whether vascular reactions differ between migrainous subjects and controls is influenced strongly by the nature of the stimulus. For example, during tests where temporal pulse amplitude did not change from baseline (or decreased), responses were unrelated to the migrainous predisposition, whereas during mental arithmetic, where pulse amplitude increased, responses were of greater magnitude in migrainous subjects (Drummond, 1982a). Others have reported that silent rehearsal of mental arithmetic or imagining threatening scenes did not induce changes in temporal pulse amplitude in controls or in migrainous subjects, presumably because of the low level of stimulation these tests provided (Feuerstein, Bush, & Corbisiero, 1982; Thompson & Adams, 1984). Significant increases in temporal pulse amplitude during mental arithmetic were reported by Andrasik, Blanchard, Arena, Saunders, and Barron (1982c) and by Passchier, van der Helm-Hylkema, and Orlebeke (1984), although no differences between headache categories and control groups were detected. Individual differences in vascular reactivity within categories of headache may account for these negative results.

Other Autonomic Responses

One view of migraine is that it forms part of a generalized deficiency in regulation of vascular tone. This hypothesis was tested by Appenzeller, Davison, and Marshall (1963), who heated the trunk of the body and measured the extent of reflex vasodilatation in the hands of migrainous patients and nonheadache controls. The absence of reflex vasodilatation in migrainous patients reported by Appenzeller et al. was not confirmed by French, Lassers, and Desai (1967) or by Hockaday, MacMillan, and Whitty (1967), who suggested that vasoactive medication such as ergotamine tartrate could have influenced Appenzeller's results. Further experiments supporting the view that peripheral vasodilatation was impaired in migraine (Elliott, Frewin, & Downey, 1974; Downey & Frewin, 1972) were criticized on methodological grounds by Morley (1977), who pointed out deficiencies in statistical methods, selection of experimental and control groups, and procedural limitations.

Price and Clarke (1979) aimed to establish whether conditioned modification of autonomic responses was impaired in migrainous subjects. They studied the acquisition of classically conditioned vasoconstriction in the hands, and found that the digital blood vessels of migrainous subjects constricted to all stimuli, whereas control subjects gradually acquired conditioned vasoconstriction. These findings led to the conclusion that migrainous subjects react to stimuli with a more persistent increase in sympathetic nervous system activity than do nonheadache subjects. This hypothesis was not confirmed in experiments comparing cardiovascular and electrodermal responses of migrainous and tension-vascular subjects with those of controls during conditions of stress and relaxation (Cohen, Rickles, & McArthur, 1978;

Gannon et al., 1981; Anderson & Franks, 1981; Drummond, 1982a, Andrasik et al., 1982c). Furthermore, Thompson and Adams (1984) could find no consistent change in resting levels or responses in cardiovascular or electrodermal variables with the development of headache.

Impairment of the autonomic nervous system appears to be greater in the head than in other parts of the body in headache sufferers. For example, pharmacological investigations have demonstrated a sympathetic nervous system deficit in the pupils of migraine and cluster headache patients (Fanciullacci, 1979), which can sometimes be observed clinically during cluster headache as pupillary constriction on the affected side. Unilateral impairment of sympathetic nervous system function was found to persist between bouts of cluster headache despite restoration of pupil symmetry under normal conditions (Fanciullacci, Pietrini, Gatto, Boccuni, & Sicuteri, 1982). In migraine, pharmacological exploration indicated a deficiency of noradrenaline in sympathetic neurones innervating the iris with consequent hypersensitivity to noradrenaline-like compounds. Fanciullacci (1979) speculated that this deficiency could mirror neurotransmitter impairment in neural pathways in the brainstem involved in the production of headache.

Other symptoms frequently reported by migraine patients point to a deficiency of autonomic regulation in the head. For example, dizziness or faintness on changing posture quickly, which is usually attributed to a transient fall in blood pressure in vessels supplying the brainstem, is more common in headache sufferers than in nonheadache controls (Drummond, 1982b; Raskin & Knittle, 1976). These symptoms indicate diminished autonomic control of intracranial blood vessels in at least some migrainous patients. Impairment of the vestibular apparatus, which detects linear and acceleratory rotation of the head, was observed in up to 80% of migrainous patients (Kuritzky, Toglia, & Thomas, 1981). This impairment could be associated with the high prevalence of vomiting in childhood, travel sickness, and vertigo in migrainous patients (Selby & Lance, 1960; Kuritzky, Ziegler, & Hassanein, 1981; Kayan & Hood, 1984; Drummond, 1985a). Vestibular problems could stem from disruption of brainstem neurotransmitters also involved in the production of headache or, alternatively, they could result from prolonged brainstem ischaemia during migraine. An increased prevalence of ice-cream headache (brief head pain on ingesting cold food or drinks) and icepick-like pains (momentary stabbing head pain) was observed in migrainous patients (Raskin & Knittle, 1976; Raskin & Schwartz, 1980; Drummond, 1985a), the site of transient pain coinciding with the site of headache in 30% to 40% of patients

(Drummond & Lance, 1984d). Such findings suggest that the neurovascular reflexes involved in headache may persist in an excitable state between headache episodes, although whether this is a primary mechanism or secondary to repeated episodes of head pain is unknown.

BEHAVIORAL TREATMENTS

The major nonpharmacological treatments for migraine include biofeedback-assisted constriction of scalp arteries, hand temperature biofeedback, and muscular relaxation in combination with other methods of stress management. Opinion is divided over the value of biofeedback training for migraine. For example, a comprehensive review of the relevant literature led Jessup, Neufeld, and Merskey (1979) to conclude that controlled research on hand-warming biofeedback, with or without autogenic relaxation, failed to support the specific benefit of these treatments for reducing migraine symptoms. Holmes and Burish (1983) also concluded their review by stating that there was no sound evidence to support the use of biofeedback as a treatment for migraine. On the other hand, Adams, Feuerstein, and Fowler (1980) and Blanchard, Andrasik, Ahles, Teders, and O'Keefe (1980) reviewed essentially the same literature and were cautiously optimistic about the value of biofeedback.

The results of many studies in this area are difficult to interpret, because acquisition of voluntary control over physiological functions was often not demonstrated, suitable procedures to control for nonspecific effects were not included, only one or two subjects were studied, or subjective estimates of "improvement" were used by the clinician or patient. The acquisition of physiological self-control without feedback is necessary if the patient is to prevent the onset of headaches in normal situations. Teaching the patient when to use physiological self-control strategies, and the maintenance of these skills, has been overlooked in the majority of studies (Haber, Thompson, Raczynski, & Sikora, 1983; Johansson & Ost, 1982). Without this assessment, it is impossible to determine whether biofeedback procedures provide more than general psychological support (or just a "placebo effect") in the treatment of migraine. Many patients suffer from tension and tension-vascular headaches as well as migraine. Although similar physiological mechanisms may underlie these different clinical manifestations of headache, until this has been demonstrated, the specificity of treatment effects should be studied separately for each type of headache if more than one type is described.

Constriction of Scalp Arteries

Drugs such as ergotamine tartrate are thought to alleviate migraine by preventing dilatation of pain-sensitized scalp arteries (Graham & Wolff, 1938). The development of biofeedback techniques to condition autonomic activity introduced the possibility of nonpharmacological regulation of tone in these vessels.

The first assessment of voluntary constriction of scalp arteries as a treatment for migraine was carried out by Friar and Beatty (1976). In their study, nine patients were trained to decrease superficial temporal artery pulse amplitude, while a control group was given feedback of digital pulse amplitude. After eight sessions of training, the acquisition of voluntary control was assessed without feedback. Patients trained to decrease superficial temporal artery pulsations demonstrated an average decrease in pulse amplitude of 20% during the final four trials of this assessment session, whereas control subjects showed systematic reductions only in finger pulse amplitude. A count of the number of migraine episodes lasting more than 3 hours during the 30 days after treatment indicated that biofeedback for superficial temporal artery pulse amplitude was superior to that for finger pulse amplitude in reducing the frequency of attacks. Friar and Beatty concluded that voluntary constriction of the superficial temporal artery had a specific treatment effect.

More recent findings have questioned the specificity of trained vasoconstriction as a treatment for migraine. For example, Bild and Adams (1980) found that decreases in the number of hours per week with headache during the 6 weeks after training were similar in patients who learned to constrict the superficial temporal artery or to relax the frontalis muscles. Four biofeedback procedures (forehead cooling, frontalis electromyograph (EMG) relaxation, enhancement of electroencephalograph (EEG) alpha activity, and vasoconstriction of the superficial temporal artery) were compared by Cohen, McArthur, and Rickles (1980). All four procedures resulted in a reduction of about 20% in headache frequency but no change in the intensity or duration of attacks. A modest training effect was demonstrated for all variables except EEG-alpha, but voluntary control without feedback was not tested. A more direct test of the specificity of trained vasoconstriction was carried out by Gauthier, Doyon, Lacroix, and Drolet (1983). Therapeutic gains did not differ between groups trained to increase or decrease superficial temporal artery pulse amplitude, thus arguing against a specific treatment effect.

The failure to confirm the findings of Friar and Beatty (1976) may stem from the different criteria used to select subjects. Of the

19 subjects in Friar and Beatty's study, 18 reported that the vasoconstrictor ergotamine tartrate was effective in relieving headache. This selection criterion was not used in later investigations. In our thermographic studies, extracranial vasodilatation in the frontotemporal region was detected more frequently in migrainous and tension-vascular patients responsive to ergotamine tartrate than in other patients (Drummond & Lance, 1984b). Further investigations should aim to determine whether trained vasoconstriction of the superficial temporal artery provides a specific treatment effect in this subgroup of patients.

Hand Warming

Sargent, Walters, and Green (1973) introduced hand temperature biofeedback training in combination with suggestions of warmth and relaxation (autogenic training) as a treatment for migraine. They alleged that voluntarily increasing hand temperature decreased sympathetic nervous system activity, which reduced the frequency and severity of migrainous episodes and sometimes prevented the onset of headache or abolished the attack shortly after its onset. This investigation created a great deal of clinical interest in hand temperature training as a possible treatment for migraine, but was criticized on scientific grounds for the absence of control conditions, for using global clinical judgments of headache improvement instead of more objective indices, for not providing data concerning changes in hand temperature, and for not investigating the effects of biofeedback and autogenic training separately (Holmes & Burish, 1983).

The majority of later studies have not confirmed that hand temperature training exerts a specific effect on headache activity. Control or comparison procedures included false hand temperature biofeedback (Mullinix, Norton, Hack, & Fishman, 1978), biofeedback training to decrease hand temperature (Largen, Mathew, Dobbins, & Claghorn, 1981; Kewman & Roberts, 1980; Turin & Johnson, 1976), progressive muscular relaxation (Daly, Donn, Galliher, & Zimmerman, 1983; Lacroix, Clarke, Bock, Doxey, Wood, & Lewis, 1983; Blanchard, Theobald, Williamson, Silver, & Brown, 1978) and frontalis EMG biofeedback (Lake, Rainey, & Papsdorf, 1979; Daly et al., 1983; Cohen et al., 1980; Lacroix et al., 1983). Except for the findings of Turin and Johnson (1976), where the control group consisted of only three subjects, and those of Lacroix et al. (1983), where subjective self-ratings of improvement were used to assess therapeutic success, hand temperature training showed no specific treatment effect. Nonetheless, headache activity often decreased significantly both during hand temperature training (Kewman & Roberts, 1980; Blanchard et al., 1978; Turin & Johnson, 1976; Daly et al., 1983; Lacroix et al., 1983; Cohen et al., 1980) and comparison procedures (Kewman & Roberts, 1980; Daly et al., 1983; Lacroix et al., 1983; Blanchard et al., 1978, Lake et al., 1979; Cohen et al., 1980). Although the aim of these studies was to test the specificity of hand temperature training, this was not possible in some instances because of insufficient group sizes (Largen et al., 1981; Mullinix et al., 1978; Turin & Johnson, 1976) or because voluntary control over hand temperature was not attained by the majority of subjects (Lake et al., 1979). Except for the study of Lacroix et al. (1983), hand temperature control without feedback was not assessed, so whether laboratory-trained skills can be applied in everyday situations is unknown.

A definitive evaluation of the specificity of hand temperature training should include an assessment of control without feedback in a variety of environmental conditions to ensure that the patient is capable of regulating hand temperature in everyday situations. The use of double-blind methodology is also important when assessing the specificity of treatment gains in disorders such as headache (Kewman & Roberts, 1980). Ambient temperature may be important both for providing optimum conditions for learning vasomotor control and for the maintenance of control outside the laboratory. For example, in our laboratory hand temperature measured thermographically was found to decrease from an initial level of 34.6°C to 29.3°C ($p < .001$) over the course of 4 hours in six healthy young male nonsmokers who sat quietly in a room maintained at 22°C (unpublished observations). Thus, in cool conditions, it may be more difficult to increase hand temperature voluntarily than in warmer surroundings.

An interesting study by Elmore and Tursky (1981) shed some light on the physiological mechanisms involved in voluntarily increasing hand temperature. They demonstrated that an increase in hand temperature, approaching 3°C during the ninth training session, was associated with a transient doubling in amplitude of arterial pulsations from the finger, thus indicating that a brief increase in blood flow was sufficient to maintain the increase in hand temperature throughout the session. If the operative component of hand temperature training is this brief increase in blood flow, as postulated by Sargent et al. (1973), it would be more appropriate to provide feedback for changes in finger pulse amplitude than hand temperature.

Although a specific treatment effect has yet to be demonstrated, hand temperature training appears to promote nonspecific treatment gains. Table 7.3 shows the percentage of patients who demonstrated

Table 7.3.
Clinical Improvement After Hand Temperature Training, Control Conditions, and While Taking Placebo Medication

	Definition of Clinical Improvement	Type of Control	Total (*N*)	Control Conditions Positive Response (*N*)	Total (*N*)	Hand Temperature Positive Response (*N*)
Medication Placebo						
Lance et al. (1970)	−50% (freq.)	double blind	50	16		
Weber et al. (1972)	−50% (freq. or sev.)	double blind	19	2		
Ludvigsson (1974)	−33% (freq.)	double blind	28	7		
Total (N)			97	25		
(percent)				(26%)		
Hand Temperature						
Turin et al. (1976)	−33% (freq.)	decrease temp.	3	0	7	4
Mullinix et al. (1978)	−33% (sev. x hours)	false feedback	5	2	6	2
Lake et al. (1979)	−33% (sev. x hours)	waiting list	6	1	12	6
" "	" "	EMG feedback	6	6	—	—
Largen et al. (1980)	−33% (freq. or sev.)	decrease temp.	5	2	6	6
Daly et al. (1983)	−50% (2 of 3 indices)	relaxation	11	6	10	8
" "	" "	EMG feedback	10	7	—	—
Lacroix et al. (1983)	no headaches	relaxation	9	2	9	4
" "	" "	EMG feedback	9	3	—	—
Total (N) (percent)				29 (45%)[a]	50	30 (60%)[b]

[a]Comparison with medication placebo: $\chi^2(1) = 5.76$ ($p < .05$)
[b]Comparison with medication placebo: $\chi^2(1) = 15.08$ ($p < .001$)

clinically significant improvement in headache activity after hand temperature training and control procedures. For comparison, percentage improvement during the placebo condition of three double-blind placebo-controlled medication trials is also presented. Clinical improvement after hand temperature training and comparison procedures far outweighed those observed in medication placebo studies, suggesting that psychological treatment provided more than the usual expectancy effect.

Spontaneous remission of symptoms, relaxation, and achieving a sense of control over headache could contribute to nonspecific improvement (Blanchard et al., 1978; Cohen et al., 1980; Kewman & Roberts, 1980). Because patients usually seek treatment when headaches are severe, Blanchard et al. (1978) included a no-treatment waiting list condition to assess the degree of spontaneous remission of symptoms. These patients showed a significant decrease in the frequency of headaches after 10 weeks of recording their headache activity but no improvement otherwise. Patients who received hand temperature biofeedback training improved more than waiting list patients on a headache index, ratings of intensity, and duration of moderate or severe headaches. Lake et al. (1979) also included a waiting list group in their comparison of changes in headache activity from pretreatment to 3 months after biofeedback treatment. Although 6 of 12 patients who had received hand temperature training showed at least 33% reduction in headache activity, this was not significantly greater than in the waiting list, where one of six patients improved. Kewman and Roberts (1980) found no differences between groups trained to raise or lower hand temperature and a waiting list group on measures of headache severity, number of symptoms, medication consumption (which all decreased significantly during and after treatment), headache frequency, or minutes of headache (which showed no significant change over treatment). When patients were grouped according to whether or not they had demonstrated hand temperature control, members in the waiting list showed as much improvement as those who had learned to increase or decrease hand temperature. From these studies, it may be concluded that headache activity sometimes improves in patients who simply record the frequency and severity of attacks, although the degree of improvement is usually less than in patients given more extensive treatment. The maintenance of treatment gains 1 year after hand temperature training argues against transient spontaneous remission of symptoms being the only operative factor (Silver, Blanchard, Williamson, Theobald, & Brown, 1979).

Therapeutic gains after progressive muscular relaxation training are similar to those of hand temperature training (Blanchard et al.,

1980). To determine whether these two procedures were equivalent, 14 migraine and 14 tension-vascular patients who had not improved after 10 sessions of relaxation training were treated with hand temperature biofeedback (Blanchard, et al., 1982a). Of these 28 patients, 15 showed a reduction in headache activity of more than 50% after thermal biofeedback, suggesting that the effectiveness of the two procedures depended on different factors. The active ingredient in the positive response to hand temperature training was not clear, because examination of physiological changes in a subset of patients indicated that therapeutic success was not related to the degree of hand temperature control (Blanchard, et al., 1982b). A cumulative effect of biofeedback training on headache activity was reported by Gamble and Elder (1983). A comparison of the effectiveness of different combinations of three treatments (biofeedback trained cooling of the temple, frontalis relaxation with EMG biofeedback, and progressive muscular relaxation) indicated that a combination of the two biofeedback procedures was superior to relaxation training.

Other Behavorial Treatments

The absence of specific treatment effects associated with hand temperature feedback suggests that therapeutic gains could be due to a sense of control over headache which sometimes develops during hand temperature training. In other words, a positive attitude toward headache control may be enough to prevent headaches from developing. This positive frame of mind is encouraged during psychological treatment, where patients are taught to regulate emotional reactions through physical and mental relaxation.

Clinical trials demonstrated that approximately two-thirds of patients reported major improvements in frequency, severity, or duration of migrainous episodes after a course of relaxation training (Warner & Lance, 1975; Hay & Madders, 1971; Paulley & Haskell, 1975). Because these trials were not controlled for the rate of spontaneous remission of symptoms or for nonspecific treatment effects, the value of the relaxation exercises themselves could not be determined. Relaxation alone was not associated with headache improvement in a controlled investigation by Mitchell and Mitchell (1971) and was associated with a reduction in headache activity of more than 50% in only 30% of migrainous patients and 22% of tension-vascular patients (Blanchard et al., 1982a). On the other hand, an earlier investigation by Blanchard et al. (1978) indicated that therapeutic gains after relaxation training exceeded those associated with self-recording headache activity, and improvement was maintained one year after treatment (Silver et al., 1979).

The application of behavior therapy techniques to the treatment of migraine was systematically explored by Mitchell and Mitchell (1971). Migrainous subjects who had completed a program of muscular relaxation, desensitization to imagined threatening situations, and assertive therapy reported greater reductions in headache frequency and duration than others who received relaxation or desensitization alone, or who just recorded headache activity for the duration of treatment. Mitchell and Mitchell argued that the success of the combined treatment package was due to the inclusion of procedures designed to bring about changes in the subject's disturbing life patterns, whereas relaxation training and systematic desensitization merely focused on modifying the subject's response to environmental stresses. Mitchell and White (1977) further investigated the therapeutic effectiveness of training subjects to record headache activity, recognize and record stress cues, achieve physical and mental relaxation through progressive muscular relaxation training and self-desensitization to threatening situations, and improve self-confidence and control over disruptive emotional states. Headache frequency decreased from 13.7 per month before treatment to 2.3 per month during a 3-month follow-up in the three subjects who completed all four stages of treatment. Decreases from 13.8 headaches per month to 6.2 per month were noted in three subjects who completed the first three stages of treatment, but headache activity remained unchanged in the other six subjects, who only recorded stress cues and/or migrainous symptoms.

When headache loses its episodic character and recurs daily or near-daily, the main stress in the patient's life may be the headache itself. In other words, thoughts and feelings associated with constant headache may influence perception of pain and maintain the disorder. The effectiveness of procedures designed to interrupt this vicious circle was investigated in 45 chronic headache sufferers who had been diagnosed as having migraine, tension-vascular, or tension headache (Bakal, Demjen, & Kaganov, 1981). Treatment consisted of seven sessions of biofeedback-assisted relaxation training and five sessions during which patients were taught to reduce their emotional response to headache through attention focusing, imagery production and thought management. Average daily headache hours, headache index, and medication usage decreased significantly after treatment, and improvement was maintained in the 20 patients who were followed up 6 months later. Hours of headache per day were reduced by half in those patients who reported less than 15 hours of head pain per day before treatment, but other patients with continuous or near continuous pain during waking hours showed little improvement. The implication that modifying the emotional response to headache is beneficial must be accepted cautiously, because Bakal et al. did not separate the effects of physical and psychological relaxation, and did not investigate the rate of spontaneous remission of symptoms for a time period equivalent to treatment.

Imagining pleasant scenes may promote muscular relaxation and may help divert attention away from emotionally disturbing situations. The specific and nonspecific effects of imagery training on headache activity were studied by Brown (1984). To investigate nonspecific effects of the treatment procedure, subjects in a control group were told that relaxing scenes would be presented by slide at subliminal levels of awareness to "unlearn" subconscious stressful thoughts. These subjects were actually shown unfocused vacation slides presented for 0.1 second. Despite similar expectation for improvement, subjects in the control condition showed little change in headache activity, whereas subjects given imagery training reported significant headache improvement. In addition, pain tolerance while holding an arm in cold water increased after imagery training but remained the same in the control group. Subjects who frequently used their imagery strategy to interrupt anxious thoughts or simply to practice reported most headache improvement. Brown suggested that imagery training provided a means of coping with headache which may have increased the expectation that headache could be controlled. Thus, positive thoughts or action may help prevent the onset of headache.

OTHER TREATMENT APPROACHES

Medical Management

Various pharmaceutical agents are useful in the prevention and treatment of migraine. Ergotamine tartrate is generally recommended as the most useful drug in relieving the pain of migraine, although it does not help every patient and in one double-blind trial was found to be no more effective than placebo medication (Waters, 1970). Since ergotamine tartrate constricts extracranial arteries, therapeutic effects may be greatest in patients whose headache is accompanied by extracranial vasodilatation (Lance, 1982).

Prophylactic medications include agents which antagonize the action of serotonin (methysergide, pizotifen), antagonists of adrenaline and noradrenaline (propranolol, timolol), drugs which block the movement of calcium into smooth muscle (verapamil), and tricyclic antidepressants (amitriptyline) (Lance, 1982). All of these drugs have been shown to have some therapeutic benefit for migraine, and occasionally prevent migraine completely, but benefits are often mitigated by unpleasant side-effects.

Manipulation of Diet

The influence of diet on migraine is controversial. Cheese, chocolate, oranges, and red wine are said to provoke migraine, although double-blind administration of tyramine or phenylethylamine, which were thought to be the active agents in some of these foods, triggered migraine no more frequently than placebo foods (Moffett, Swash, & Scott, 1972, 1974). Headache frequency was not reduced when migrainous patients were placed on a tyramine-free diet (Medina & Diamond, 1978), although greater success with an elimination diet was obtained by Monro, Brostoff, Carini, and Zilkha (1980).

The relationship between migraine and food allergy in children was studied by Egger, Carter, Wilson, Turner, and Soothill (1983). After 3 or 4 weeks on a simple diet, excluded foods were reintroduced singly each week to identify foods which provoked migraine. The response to one of the foods which had provoked symptoms when reintroduced into the diet was then tested in a double-blind, placebo-controlled crossover trial. Egger et al. identified 55 foods which were associated with an increase in headache activity when reintroduced into the diet, and most children reacted to more than one food (24 different foods in one instance). Excluded foods provoked symptoms more frequently than placebo foods when administered double-blind. Before the diet was commenced, most children had behavioral problems, gastrointestinal complaints, and other symptoms of allergic disorder. These all decreased substantially after the diet was modified. While these results are encouraging, the effect of modifying diet on headache activity in other age ranges, and in patients without a clear allergic disorder, requires further investigation.

Acupuncture

At present, there is no strong evidence that acupuncture has any long-term therapeutic benefit for migraine. The effect of acupuncture in preventing migraine was compared with standard medical treatment by Loh, Nathan, Schott, and Zilkha (1984). Sixteen of 41 patients reported "moderate" or "great" improvement after several sessions of acupuncture spanning 3 months, compared with only 4 of 36 patients treated medically. These findings must be interpreted cautiously, because placebo effects were not controlled.

A more rigorous examination of the effect of acupuncture on headache activity was carried out by Dowson, Lewith, and Machin (1985), who used mock transcutaneous nerve stimulation as a placebo treatment. During the 4 weeks after treatment, frequency of headache was reduced at least 50% in 32% of patients who had received acupuncture weekly for 6 weeks, and in 26% of the placebo treatment group.

CONCLUSIONS AND CLINICAL SUGGESTIONS

To date, little attempt has been made to tailor treatment to suit the requirements of the individual patient. How might this be accomplished?

The aim of assessment is to provide a rational basis for treatment. The first step should be to take a systematic headache history. Various questionnaires have been used experimentally to gather headache data (Ziegler, Hassanein, & Couch, 1982; Arena, Blanchard, Andrasik, & Dudek, 1982; Peck & Attfield, 1981), but most clinicians prefer to use a semistructured interview because this minimizes misinterpretation of questions. It is important to establish whether the patient has more than one type of headache, the total length of the headache history, the frequency and usual duration of pain, the usual time of onset of the attack, and the location and description of pain (Lance, 1982). The patient is then questioned about symptoms which precede or accompany headache, environmental or psychological factors which seem to precipitate or aggravate headache, and methods used previously to control or relieve pain (Drummond & Lance, 1984a; Drummond, 1985a). Questionnaires dealing specifically with associated symptoms (Tyler, 1984) and quality of pain (Hunter, 1983; Allen & Weinmann, 1982) can be used for detailed assessment.

The headache history is generally sufficient to identify patients with cluster headache. Although the etiology of cluster headache remains obscure, this disorder is usually controlled rapidly with medication (Lance, 1982). In over 70% of patients, individual attacks are relieved or abolished within 10 to 15 minutes by breathing 100% oxygen at 10 litres per minute (Kudrow, 1980). There is little evidence of psychological disturbance in the majority of cases, and attempts to treat cluster headache with relaxation and other behavorial methods have been unsuccessful (Blanchard, Andrasik, Jurish, & Teders, 1982c). It therefore seems appropriate to treat cluster headache medically.

Attention should next be focused on psychological factors. Psychological assessment should include measures of neuroticism and depression, and may also include measures of assertiveness and social readjustment (Andrasik et al., 1982b). Psychopathology is traditionally assessed with the MMPI, but shorter questionnaires such as the Beck Depression Inventory, the State-Trait Anxiety Scale, and Eysenck's Personality Inventory may be more convenient in clinical practice. Whether anxiety and depression are of primary importance or secondary to frequent or severe headache should be investigated. The clinician should also enquire about the patient's health and social background to assess problems with family, acquaintances, work, study, or financial situation.

Instructing the patient to record headache activity for several weeks before starting treatment provides useful baseline data for the evaluation of treatment effectiveness. Details of intensity, location, associated symptoms and medication usage are recorded in a headache diary (Bakal et al., 1981). Rating headache intensity presents the problem of subjectivity because most descriptions of pain contain an emotional component which may confuse intensity ratings. To circumvent this problem, ordered lists of adjectives commonly used to describe the sensory (intensity component) and reactive (emotional) aspects of pain could be used to provide indices of change over the course of treatment (Heft, Gracely, Dubner, & McGrath, 1980). Behavioral response to headache may also provide some indication of headache severity. This type of scale could range from "no effect on normal activity" to "interfered with normal activity" to "complete disruption of normal activity."

The validity of trigger factors cited during initial assessment should also be studied during the pretreatment baseline. For psychological factors, this could take the form of mood rating scales (Harrigan et al., 1984) or other self-monitored measures of emotional state. The usefulness of these records depends on the patient's willingness and ability to record events accurately, and on the effectiveness of preliminary training on accurate self-monitoring. Interviews with family or other household members could help validate self-report measures and also establish whether the patient received special attention or narcotic medication, avoided unpleasant duties, or received other secondary gains because of headache.

Assessment of extracranial vascular reactions during and between headache episodes aims to establish whether extracranial vasodilatation is associated with pain in individual cases. Such patients may respond selectively to vasoconstrictive medication or to trained constriction of scalp arteries, although this requires experimental confirmation.

The headache history, psychological assessment, prospective diaries, and extracranial vascular assessment should provide the clinician with enough information to define baseline headache activity and to plan appropriate treatment strategies. Treatment goals should be defined, and the patient should be encouraged to record headache activity and other treatment variables throughout treatment so that progress can be assessed objectively. If psychological problems are identified, standard behavior therapy programs may lead to substantial improvement in headache activity (Mitchell & Mitchell, 1971; Mitchell & White, 1977). If the headache itself appears to be the source of depression and anxiety, the patient should be encouraged to believe that the headache can be controlled. Since many patients are worried about the possibility of brain tumors, individual or group discussions of the physiology of headache may alleviate fears about structural causes of headache. If initial assessment and pretreatment records suggest no association between psychological state and headache, psychological treatment may be of little value, although imagery training or the nonspecific effects of hand temperature or relaxation training may still prove to be beneficial. This needs to be tested empirically.

Being able to predict clinical outcome may improve the efficiency of treating headache with behavioral methods. A step in this direction was made by Blanchard et al. (1983), who used a headache history, a 4-week headache diary, standard psychological tests, and laboratory measures of psychophysiological responses to stress to predict the outcome of relaxation therapy and hand temperature training. Information from the headache history alone correctly classified over 87% of migraine and tension-vascular patients as improved or unimproved, although no simple "rules-of-thumb" were identified. Psychological and psychophysiological measures provided less predictive power than the headache history, but even so, outcome for over 80% of migraine and tension-vascular patients was predicted correctly using psychological test scores. Treatment gains after a course of cognitive behavior therapy were analyzed in relation to clinical diagnosis, headache location, time course of headache, and associated symptoms (Bakal et al., 1981). The number of headache hours per day emerged as the only variable to predict clinical improvement; patients with almost continuous pain during waking hours showed little improvement. The prognostic significance of depression was examined by Jacob, Turner, Szekely, and Eidelman (1983). They reported that a low score on the Beck Depression Inventory was associated with a favorable outcome following relaxation training, and a high score with little improvement. These findings await cross-validation to identify the strongest predictors of headache improvement after behavorial treatment. Measures reflecting the mode of action of treatment may provide the best prediction of outcome. For example, therapeutic efforts to control emotional reactions would probably show greater benefit for intermittently or chronically anxious patients than for emotionally stable patients.

The introduction of self-help treatment packages promises to increase the availability of behavorial treatments for headache. Notable examples are the self-administered package of behavior therapy techniques described by Mitchell and White (1977), and the largely home-based, minimal-therapist-contact treatment program consisting of relaxation and hand temperature training, which proved to be more successful than a traditional clinic-based program in reducing headache activity (Jurish, Blanchard, Andrasik, Teders, Neff, & Arena, 1983). Treatment packages of this type could be introduced at little expense in materials or clinical time in standard headache clinics, where they would provide an alternative to, or supplement, pharmacological management of headache.

SUMMARY

In developing their classification system for headache, the Ad hoc Committee (1962) assumed that headache associated with symptoms of migraine had a vascular basis and was separate from tension headache, which was said to be caused by excessive contraction of scalp and neck muscles. In recent years the independence of migraine and tension headache has been questioned both on clinical and pathophysiological grounds; it now seems plausible that similar pain mechanisms may underly a continuum of headache symptomatology. Separate from this migraine–tension headache continuum is cluster headache, which forms an independent, clearly definable syndrome.

Extracranial vascular changes accompany a minority of migrainous episodes and the majority of attacks of cluster headache. However, the time course of pain onset and vascular changes in cluster headache suggests that vascular changes are secondary to pain. In a minority of migrainous patients, the readiness of extracranial blood vessels to dilate both during and between headache episodes indicates a disturbance in neural regulation of vasomotor tone or inherent exaggerated vascular reactivity. Controlled experimentation has been unable to support the view that migraine forms part of a general deficiency in regulation of vasomotor tone. However, migraine is often associated with symptoms of a deficiency of autonomic regulation in the head.

Behavioral treatments for migraine have focused on biofeedback-assisted constriction of scalp arteries, hand temperature biofeedback, and muscular relaxation in combination with other methods of stress management. Voluntary constriction of scalp arteries may provide specific treatment for the minority of patients who show extracranial vascular changes during headache. Hand temperature regulation appears to be associated with nonspecific treatment gains. If psychological problems accompany complaints of headache, behavior therapy programs incorporating muscular relaxation may lead to substantial improvement in headache activity.

REFERENCES

Ad hoc Committee on Classification of Headache. (1962). Classification of headache. *Journal of the American Medical Association, 179,* 717–718.

Adams, H. E., Feuerstein, M., & Fowler, J. L. (1980). Migraine headache: review of parameters, etiology and intervention. *Psychological Bulletin, 87,* 217–237.

Allen, R. A., & Weinmann, R. L. (1982). The McGill-Melzack Pain Questionnaire in the diagnosis of headache. *Headache, 22,* 20–29.

Amery, W. K. (1982). Brain hypoxia: The turning-point in the genesis of the migraine attack? *Cephalalgia, 2,* 83–109.

Anderson, C. D., & Franks, R. D. (1981). Migraine and tension headache: is there a physiological difference? *Headache, 21,* 63–71.

Andrasik, F., Blanchard, E. B., Arena, J. G., Teders, S. J., & Rodichok, L. D. (1982a). Cross-validation of the Kudrow-Sutkus MMPI classification system for diagnosing headache type. *Headache, 22,* 2–5.

Andrasik, F., Blanchard, E. B., Arena, J. G., Teders, S. J., Teevan, R. C., & Rodichok, L. D. (1982b). Psychological functioning in headache sufferers. *Psychosomatic Medicine, 44,* 171–182.

Andrasik, F., Blanchard, E. B., Arena, J. G., Saunders, N. L., & Barron, K. D. (1982c). Psychophysiology of recurrent headache: Methodological issues and new empirical findings. *Behavior Therapy, 13,* 407–429.

Anselmi, B., Baldi, E., Casacci, F., & Salmon, S. (1980). Endogenous opoids in cerebrospinal fluid and blood in idiopathic headache sufferers. *Headache, 20,* 294–299.

Anthony, M., Hinterberger, H., & Lance, J. W. (1967). Plasma serotonin in migraine and stress. *Archives of Neurology, 16,* 544–552.

Appenzeller, O., Davison, K., & Marshall, J. (1963). Reflex vasomotor abnormalities in the hands of migrainous subjects. *Journal of Neurology, Neurosurgery, and Psychiatry, 26,* 447–450.

Arena, J. G., Blanchard, E. B., Andrasik, F., & Dudek, B. C. (1982). The Headache Symptom Questionnaire: Discriminant classificatory ability and headache syndromes suggested by a factor analysis. *Journal of Behavioral Assessment, 4,* 55–69.

Bach, F. W., Jensen, K., Blegvad, N., Fenger, M., Jordal, R., & Olesen, J. (1985). Beta-endorphin and ACTH in plasma during attacks of common and classic migraine. *Cephalalgia, 5,* 177–182.

Bakal, D. A., & Kaganov, J. A. (1977). Muscle contraction and migraine headache: psychophysiologic comparison. *Headache, 17,* 208–215.

Bakal, D. A., Demjen, S., & Kaganov, J. A. (1981). Cognitive behavioral treatment of chronic headache. *Headache, 21,* 81–86.

Bild, R., & Adams, H. E. (1980). Modification of migraine headaches by cephalic blood volume pulse and EMG biofeedback. *Journal of Consulting and Clinical Psychology, 48,* 51–57.

Blanchard, E. B., Andrasik, F., Ahles, T. A., Teders, S. J., & O'Keefe, D. (1980). Migraine and tension headaches: A meta-analytic review. *Behavior Therapy, 11,* 613–631.

Blanchard, E. B., Andrasik, F., Arena, J. G., Neff, D. F., Jurish, S. E., Teders, S. J., Barron, K. D., & Rodichok, L. D. (1983). Nonpharmacologic treatment of chronic headache: Prediction of outcome. *Neurology, 33,* 1596–1603.

Blanchard, E. B., Andrasik, F., Neff, D. F., Arena, J. G., Ahles, T. A., Jurish, S. E., Pallmeyer, T. P., Saunders, N. L., Teders, S. J., Barron, K. D., & Rodichok, L. D. (1982a). Biofeedback and relaxation training with three kinds of headache: Treatment effects and their prediction. *Journal of Consulting and Clinical Psychology, 50,* 562–575.

Blanchard, E. B., Andrasik, F., Neff, D. F., Teders, S. J., Pallmeyer, T. P., Arena, J. G., Jurish, S. E., Saunders, N. L., Ahles, T. A., & Rodichok, L. D. (1982b). Sequential comparisons of relaxation training and biofeedback in the treatment of three kinds of chronic headache or, the machines may be necessary some of the time. *Behavior Research and Therapy, 20,* 469–481.

Blanchard, E. B., Andrasik, F., Jurish, S. E., & Teders, S. J. (1982c). The treatment of cluster headache with relaxation and thermal biofeedback. *Biofeedback and Self-Regulation, 7,* 185–191.

Blanchard, E. B., Theobald, D. E., Williamson, D. A., Silver, B. V., & Brown, D. A. (1978). Temperature biofeedback in the treatment of migraine headaches. A controlled evaluation. *Archives of General Psychiatry, 35,* 581–588.

Blau, J. N., & Davis, E. (1970). Small blood-vessels in migraine. *Lancet, 2,* 740–742.

Brazil, P., & Friedman, A. P. (1956). Craniovascular studies in headache. A report and analysis of pulse volume tracings. *Neurology, 6,* 96–102.

Brown, J. M. (1984). Imagery coping strategies in the treatment of migraine. *Pain, 18,* 157–167.

Cohen, M. J., McArthur, D. L., & Rickles, W. H. (1980). Comparison of four biofeedback treatments for migraine headache: Physiological and headache variables. *Psychosomatic Medicine, 42,* 463–480.

Cohen, M. J., Rickles, W. H., & McArthur, D. L. (1978). Evidence for physiological response stereotypy in migraine headache. *Psychosomatic Medicine, 40,* 344–354.

Couch, J. R., Ziegler, D. K., & Hassanein, R. S. (1975). Evaluation of the relationship between migraine headache and depression. *Headache, 15,* 41–50.

Dalkvist, J., Ekbom, K., & Waldenlind, E. (1984). Headache and mood: A time-series analysis of self-ratings. *Cephalalgia, 4,* 45–52.

Daly, E. J., Donn, P. A., Galliher, M. J., & Zimmerman, J. S. (1983). Biofeedback applications to migraine and tension headaches: A double-blinded outcome study. *Biofeedback and Self-Regulation, 8,* 135–152.

Diehr, P., Diehr, G., Koepsell, T., Wood, R., Beach, K., Wolcott, B., & Tompkins, R. K. (1982). Cluster analysis to determine headache types. *Journal of Chronic Diseases, 35,* 623–633.

Diehr, P., Wood, R. W., Barr, V., Wolcott, B., Slay, L., & Tompkins, R. K. (1981). Acute headaches: Presenting symptoms and diagnostic rules to identify patients with tension and migraine headache. *Journal of Chronic Diseases, 34,* 147–158.

Downey, J. A., & Frewin, D. B. (1972). Vascular responses in the hands of patients suffering from migraine. *Journal of Neurology, Neurosurgery, and Psychiatry, 35,* 258–263.

Dowson, D. I., Lewith, G. T., & Machin, D. (1985). The effects of acupuncture versus placebo in the treatment of headache. *Pain, 21,* 35–42.

Drummond, P. D. (1982a). Extracranial and cardiovascular reactivity in migrainous subjects. *Journal of Psychosomatic Research, 26,* 317–331.

Drummond, P. D. (1982b). Relationships among migrainous, vascular and orthostatic symptoms. *Cephalalgia, 2,* 157–161.

Drummond, P. D. (1984). Extracranial vascular changes during headache, exercise and stress. *Journal of Psychosomatic Research, 28,* 133–138.

Drummond, P. D. (1985a). Predisposing, precipitating and relieving factors in different categories of headache. *Headache, 25,* 16–22.

Drummond, P. D. (1985b). Vascular responses in headache-prone subjects during stress. *Biological Psychology, 21,* 11–25.

Drummond, P. D., & Anthony M. (1985). Extracranial vascular responses to sublingual nitroglycerin and oxygen inhalation in cluster headache patients. *Headache, 25,* 70–74.

Drummond, P. D., & Lance, J. W. (1981). Extracranial vascular reactivity in migraine and tension headache. *Cephalalgia, 1,* 149–155.

Drummond, P. D., & Lance, J. W. (1983). Extracranial vascular changes and the source of pain in migraine headache. *Annals of Neurology, 13,* 32–37.

Drummond, P. D., & Lance, J. W. (1984a). Clinical diagnosis and computer analysis of headache symptoms. *Journal of Neurology, Neurosurgery, and Psychiatry, 47,* 128–133.

Drummond, P. D., & Lance, J. W. (1984b). Facial temperature in migraine, tension-vascular and tension headache. *Cephalalgia, 4,* 149–158.

Drummond, P. D., & Lance, J. W. (1984c). Thermographic changes in cluster headache. *Neurology, 34,* 1292–1298.

Drummond, P. D., & Lance, J. W. (1984d). Neurovascular disturbances in headache patients. *Clinical and Experimental Neurology, 20,* 93–99.

Egger, J., Carter, C. M., Wilson, J., Turner, M. W., & Soothill, J. F. (1983). Is migraine food allergy? *Lancet, ii,* 865–869.

Elkind, A. H., Friedman, A. P., & Grossman, J. (1964). Cutaneous blood flow in vascular headaches of the migraine type. *Neurology, 14,* 24–30.

Ellertsen, B., & Hammerborg, D. (1982). Psychophysiological response patterns in migraine patients. *Cephalalgia, 2,* 19–24.

Elliott, K., Frewin, D. B., & Downey, J. A. (1974). Reflex vasomotor responses in the hands of patients suffering from migraine. *Headache, 13,* 188–196.

Elmore, A. M., & Tursky, B. (1981). A comparison of two psychophysiological approaches to the treatment of migraine. *Headache, 21,* 93–101.

Fanciullacci, M. (1979). Iris adrenergic impairment in idiopathic headache. *Headache, 19,* 8–13.

Fanciullacci, M., Pietrini, U., Gatto, G., Boccuni, M., & Sicuteri, F. (1982). Latent dysautonomic pupillary lateralization in cluster headache. A pupillometric study. *Cephalalgia, 2,* 135–144.

Fettes, I., Gawel, M., Kuzniak, S., & Edmeads, J. (1985). Endorphin levels in headache syndromes. *Headache, 25,* 37–39.

Feuerstein, M., Bortolussi, L., Houle, M., & Labbe, E. (1983). Stress, temporal artery activity, and pain in migraine headache: A prospective analysis. *Headache, 23,* 296–304.

Feuerstein, M., Bush, C., & Corbisiero, R. (1982). Stress and chronic headache: a psychophysiological analysis of mechanisms. *Journal of Psychosomatic Research, 26,* 167–181.

French, E. B., Lassers, B. W., & Desai, M. G. (1967). Reflex vasomotor responses in the hands of migrainous subjects. *Journal of Neurology, Neurosurgery, and Psychiatry, 30,* 276–278.

Friar, L. R., & Beatty, J. (1976). Migraine: management by trained control of vasoconstriction. *Journal of Consulting and Clinical Psychology, 44,* 46–53.

Gamble, E. H., & Elder, S. T. (1983). Multimodal feedback in the treatment of migraine. *Biofeedback and Self-Regulation, 8,* 383–392.

Gannon, L. R., Haynes, S. N., Safranek, R., & Hamilton, J. (1981). A psychophysiological investigation of muscle-contraction and migraine headache. *Journal of Psychosomatic Research, 25,* 271–280.

Garvey, M. J., Schaffer, C. B., & Tuason, V. B. (1983). Relationship of headaches to depression. *British Journal of Psychiatry, 143,* 544–547.

Gauthier, J., Doyon, J., Lacroix, R., & Drolet, M. (1983). Blood volume pulse biofeedback in the treatment of migraine headache: A controlled evaluation. *Biofeedback and Self-Regulation, 8,* 427–442.

Graham, J. R., & Wolff, H. G. (1938). Mechanism of migraine headache and action of ergotamine tartrate. *A. M. A. Archives of Neurology and Psychiatry, 39,* 737–763.

Haber, J. D., Thompson, J. K., Raczynski, J. M., & Sikora, T. L. (1983). Physiological self-control and the biofeedback treatment of headache. *Headache, 23,* 174–178.

Harrigan, J. A., Kues, J. R., Ricks, D. F., & Smith, R. (1984). Moods that predict coming migraine headaches. *Pain, 20,* 385–396.

Harrison, R. H. (1975). Psychological testing in headache: A review. *Headache, 14,* 177–185.

Hay, K. M., & Madders, J. (1971). Migraine treated by relaxation therapy. *Journal of the Royal College of General Practitioners, 21,* 664–669.

Heft, M. W., Gracely, R. H., Dubner, R., & McGrath, P. A. (1980). A validation model for verbal descriptor scaling of human clinical pain. *Pain, 9,* 363–373.

Henryk-Gutt, R., & Rees, W. L. (1973). Psychological aspects of migraine. *Journal of Psychosomatic Research, 17,* 141–153.

Herberg, L. J. (1975). The hypothalamus and aminergic pathways in migraine. In J. Pearce (Ed.), *Modern topics in migraine* (pp. 85–95). London: Heinemann.

Heyck, H. (1969). Pathogenesis of migraine. A contribution. *Research and clinical Studies in Headache, 2,* 1–28.

Hockaday, J. M., MacMillan, A. L., & Whitty, C. W. M. (1967). Vasomotor-reflex response in idiopathic and hormone-dependent migraine. *Lancet, 1,* 1023–1026.

Hoelscher, T. J., & Lichstein, K. L. (1984). Behavorial assessment and treatment of child migraine: Implications for clinical research and practice. *Headache, 24,* 94–103.

Holmes, D. S., & Burish, T. G. (1983). Effectiveness of biofeedback for treating migraine and tension headaches: A review of the evidence. *Journal of Psychosomatic Research, 27,* 515–532.

Hørven, I., & Sjaastad, O. (1977). Cluster headache syndrome and migraine. Ophthalmological support for a two-entity theory. *Acta Ophthalmologica, 55,* 35–51.

Hunter, M. (1983). The Headache Scale: A new approach to the assessment of headache pain based on pain descriptions. *Pain, 16,* 361–373.

Jacob, R. G., Turner, S. M., Szekely, B. C., & Eidelman, B. H. (1983). Predicting outcome of relaxation therapy in headaches: The role of 'depression'. *Behavior Therapy, 14,* 457–465.

Jessup, B. A., Neufeld, R. W. J., & Merskey, H. (1979). Biofeedback therapy for headache and other pain: An evaluative review. *Pain, 7,* 225–270.

Johansson, J., & Ost, L. (1982). Self-control procedures in biofeedback: A review of temperature biofeedback in the treatment of migraine. *Biofeedback and Self-Regulation, 7,* 435–442.

Jurish, S. E., Blanchard, E. B., Andrasik, F., Teders, S. J., Neff, D. F., & Arena, J. G. (1983). Home- versus clinic-based treatment of vascular headache. *Journal of Consulting and Clinical Psychology, 51,* 743–751.

Kaganov, J. A., Bakal, D. A., & Dunn, B. E. (1981). The differential contribution of muscle contraction and migraine symptoms to problem headache in the general population. *Headache, 21,* 157–163.

Kayan, A., & Hood, J. D. (1984). Neuro-otological manifestations of migraine. *Brain, 107,* 1123–1142.

Kewman, D., & Roberts, A. H. (1980). Skin temperature biofeedback and migraine headaches: A double-blind study. *Biofeedback and Self-Regulation, 5,* 327–345.

Kudrow, L. (1980). *Cluster headache. Mechanisms and management.* Oxford, England: Oxford University Press.

Kudrow, L., & Sutkus, B. J. (1979). MMPI pattern specificity in primary headache disorders. *Headache, 19,* 18–24.

Kuritsky, A., Toglia, U. J., & Thomas, D. (1981). Vestibular function in migraine. *Headache, 21,* 110–112.

Kuritzky, A., Ziegler, D. K., & Hassanein, R. (1981). Vertigo, motion sickness and migraine. *Headache, 21,* 227–231.

Lacroix, J. M., Clarke, M. A., Bock, J. C., Doxey, N., Wood, A., & Lavis, S. (1983). Biofeedback and relaxation in the treatment of migraine headaches: Comparative effectiveness and physiological correlates. *Journal of Neurology, Neurosurgery, and Psychiatry, 46,* 525–532.

Lake, A., Rainey, J., & Papsdorf, J. D. (1979). Biofeedback and rational-emotive therapy in the management of migraine headache. *Journal of Applied Behavior Analysis, 12,* 127–140.

Lance, J. W., (1982). *Mechanism and management of headache* (4th ed.). London: Butterworths.

Lance, J. W., Anthony, M., & Somerville, B. (1970). Comparative trial of serotonin antagonists in the management of migraine. *British Medical Journal, 2,* 327–330.

Lance, J. W., Lambert, G. A., Goadsby, P, J., & Duckworth, J. W. (1983). Brainstem influences on the cephalic circulation: Experimental data from cat and monkey of relevance to the mechanism of migraine. *Headache, 23,* 258–265.

Largen, J. W., Mathew, R. J., Dobbins, K., & Claghorn, J. L. (1981). Specific and non-specific effects of skin temperature control in migraine management. *Headache, 21,* 36–44.

Laruitzen, M., & Olesen, J. (1984). Regional cerebral blood flow during migraine attacks by Xenon-33 inhalation and emission tomography. *Brain, 107,* 447–461.

Lauritzen, M., Olsen, T. S., Lassen, N. A., & Paulson, O. B. (1983). Changes in regional cerebral blood flow during the course of classic migraine attacks. *Annals of Neurology, 13,* 633–641.

Loh, L., Nathan, P. W., Schott, G. D., & Zilkha, K. J. (1984). Acupuncture versus medical treatment for migraine and muscle tension headaches. *Journal of Neurology, Neurosurgery and Psychiatry, 47,* 333–337.

Ludvigsson, J. (1974). Propranolol used in prophylaxis of migraine in children. *Acta Neurologica Scandinavica, 50,* 109–115.

Mathew, N. T., Stubits, E., & Nigam, M. P. (1982). Transformation of episodic migraine into daily headache: Analysis of factors. *Headache, 22,* 66–68.

Medina, J. L., & Diamond, S. (1978). The role of diet in migraine. *Headache, 18,* 31–34.

Mitchell, K. R., & Mitchell, D. M. (1971). Migraine: An exploratory treatment application of programmed behaviour therapy techniques. *Journal of Psychosomatic Research, 15,* 137–157.

Mitchell, K. R., & White, R. G. (1977). Behavioral self-management: An application to the problem of migraine headaches. *Behavior Therapy, 8,* 213–221.

Moffett, A., Swash, M., & Scott, D. F. (1972). Effect of tyramine in migraine: A double-blind study. *Journal of Neurology, Neurosurgery and Psychiatry, 35,* 496–499.

Moffett, A., Swash, M., & Scott, D. F. (1974). Effect of chocolate in migraine: A double-blind study. *Journal of Neurology, Neurosurgery and Psychiatry, 37,* 445–448.

Monro, J., Brostoff, J., Carini, C., & Zilkha, K. (1980). Food Allergy in migraine. *Lancet, ii,* 1–4.

Morley, S. (1977). Migraine: A generalized vasomotor dysfunction? A critical review of evidence. *Headache, 17,* 71–74.

Morley S. (1985). An experimental investigation of some assumptions underpinning psychological treatments of migraine. *Behavior Research and Therapy, 23,* 65–74.

Mullinix, J. M., Norton, B. J., Hack, S., & Fishman, M. A. (1978). Skin temperature biofeedback and migraine. *Headache, 17,* 242–244.

Nappi, G., Facchinetti, F., Martignoni, E., Petralgia, F., Bono, G., Micieli, G., Rosaschino, C., Manzoni, G. C., & Genazzani, A. R. (1985). Plasma and CSF endorphin levels in primary and symptomatic headaches. *Headache, 25,* 141–144.

Olesen, J., Tfelt-Hansen, P., Henricksen, L., & Larsen, B. (1981). The common migraine attack may not be initiated by cerebral ischaemia. *Lancet, 2,* 438–440.

Passchier, J., van der Helm-Hylkema, H., & Orlebeke, J. F. (1984). Psychophysiological characteristics of migraine and tension headache patients. Differential effects of sex and pain state. *Headache, 24,* 131–139.

Paulley, J. W., & Haskell, D. A. L. (1975). The treatment of migraine without drugs. *Journal of Psychosomatic Research, 19,* 367–374.

Peck, D. F., & Attfield, M. E. (1981). Migraine symptoms on the Waters Headache Questionnaire: a statistical analysis. *Journal of Psychosomatic Research, 25,* 281–288.

Pikoff, H. (1984). Is the muscular model of headache still viable? A review of conflicting data. *Headache, 24,* 186–198.

Price, K. P., & Clarke, L. K. (1979). Classical conditioning of digital pulse volume in migraineurs and normal controls. *Headache, 19,* 328–332.

Price, K. P., & Tursky, B. (1976). Vascular reactivity of migraineurs and non-migraineurs: a comparison of responses to self-control procedures. *Headache, 16,* 210–217.

Raskin, N. H., & Knittle, S. C. (1976). Ice cream headache and orthostatic symptoms in patients with migraine. *Headache, 16,* 222–225.

Raskin, N. H., & Schwartz, R. K. (1980). Icepick-like pain. *Neurology, 30,* 203–205.

Sakai, F., & Meyer, J. S. (1978). Regional cerebral hemodynamics during migraine and cluster headaches measured by the ^{133}Xe inhalation method. *Headache, 18,* 122–132.

Sargent, J. D., Walters, E. D., & Green, E. E. (1973). Psychosomatic self-regulation of migraine headaches. *Seminars in Psychiatry, 5,* 415–428.

Selby, G., & Lance J. W. (1960). Observations on 500 cases of migraine and allied vascular headache. *Journal of Neurology, Neurosurgery, and Psychiatry, 23,* 23–32.

Sicuteri, F. (1967). Vasoneuroactive substances and their implication in vascular pain. *Research and clinical Studies in Migraine, 1,* 6–45.

Sicuteri, F. (1976) Migraine, a central biochemical dysnociception. *Headache, 16,* 145–159.

Silver, B. V., Blanchard, E. B., Williamson, D. A., Theobald, D. E., & Brown, D. A. (1979). Temperature biofeedback and relaxation training in the treatment of migraine headaches. *Biofeedback and Self-Regulation, 4,* 359–366.

Thompson, J. K., & Adams, H. E. (1984). Psychophysiological characteristics of headache patients. *Pain, 18,* 41–52.

Tunis, M. M. & Wolff, H. G. (1953). Studies on headache. Long-term observations of the reactivity of the cranial arteries in subjects with migraine of the vascular type. *A. M. A. Archives of Neurology and Psychiatry, 70,* 551–557.

Turin, A., & Johnson, W. G. (1976). Biofeedback therapy for migraine headaches. *Archives of General Psychiatry, 33,* 517–519.

Tyler, G. S. (1984). Toward a coding method of migraine. *Headache, 24,* 115–116.

Warner, G., & Lance, J. W. (1975). Relaxation therapy in migraine and chronic tension headache. *Medical Journal of Australia, 1,* 298–301.

Waters, W. E. (1970). Controlled clinical trial of ergotamine tartrate. *British Medical Journal, 2,* 325–327.

Waters, W. E. (1973). The epidemiological enigma of migraine. *International Journal of Epidemiology, 2,* 189–194.

Weber, R. B., & Reinmuth, O. M. (1972). The treatment of migraine with propranolol. *Neurology, 22,* 366–369.

Weeks, R., Baskin, S., Rapoport, A., Sheftell, F., & Arrowsmith, F. (1983). A comparison of MMPI personality data and frontalis electromyographic readings in migraine and combination headache patients. *Headache, 23,* 75–82.

Wolff, H. G. (1953). *Stress and disease.* Springfield, IL: Thomas.

Ziegler, D. K., Hassanein, R. S., & Couch, J. R. (1982). Headache syndromes suggested by statistical analysis of headache symptoms. *Cephalalgia, 2,* 125–134.

Ziegler, D. K., Rhodes, R. J., & Hassanein, R. S. (1978). Association of psychological measurements of anxiety and depression with headache history in a non-clinic population. *Research and clinical Studies in Headache, 6,* 123–135.

8

Thermoregulation in the Treatment of Peripheral Vascular Disorders

Trudy Block

Clinical Psychology Institute
Fort Lauderdale, FL

Glenn R. Caddy

Nova University
Fort Lauderdale, FL

INTRODUCTION

The control of peripheral temperature has been of particular interest to specialists in the behavioral medicine area, largely because of the ready applicability of the thermoregulation procedures in clinical practice. In the management of peripheral vascular conditions, including migraine headache, Raynaud's disease, and a variety of other difficulties, thermoregulation procedures are attractive to behavioral scientists because change in peripheral temperature, the index on which these procedures are based, can be measured objectively, exhibits good reliability and validity (Yates, 1980), and offers a safe indirect estimate of local blood flow (Cook, 1972; Fuller, 1977) and of autonomic arousal (Boudewyns, 1976). There are, however, a number of difficulties within the research framework upon which the thermoregulatory procedures are based, and these have mitigated against the widespread acceptance of the procedures, at least within research settings. Many of these difficulties are related to methodological deficits. Confounding of feedback with instructions, hypnosis, imagery, or autogenic phrases are frequent criticisms leveled at many research studies in this area (Blanchard & Young, 1974; Yates, 1980). The clinician, whose primary concern is to implement an effective treatment strategy, is less concerned with confounded methodologies or the issue of which variable explains the most accounted for variance. In fact, the confounds which may be of concern to the researcher are often introduced deliberately by the clinician, who, in the case of peripheral temperature training, is interested in potentiating the feedback in order to attain maximal treatment effects.

A problem that is of relevance both to the clinician and the researcher in peripheral temperature training is that of the *drift effect* (Yates, 1980). Peripheral temperature tends to drift in the direction of ambient room temperatures. In clinical as well as research settings the control of this effect is imperative and is accomplished by providing for an adequate stabilization period and baseline prior to the introduction of the training procedures (Taub & School, 1980). Another matter of concern both in research and clinical settings involves the phenomenon of *thermal lag* (defined as the interval between the occurrence of vasomotor changes, i.e., changes in blood flow, and the corresponding onset of changes in the surface temperatures). There is a linear relationship between temperature and blood flow (Cook, 1974; Surwit, Shapiro, & Feld, 1976), and, since the temperature response is subject to thermal lag, at least some researchers have turned their focus to studying the conditioning of vasomotor responses as a means of circumventing the false feedback which is likely to be given at least part of the time during the measurement of surface temperature (D. D. Montgomery, personal communication, October, 1977). The aforestated notwithstanding, Boudewyns (1976) has shown that, although temperature is not a valid predictor of blood flow during moment to moment changes following a stimulus presentation, it is a reliable measure during extended arousal and relaxation conditions. It is just such conditions which closely approximate the context in which temperature training occurs. Consequently, in addition to the more direct training of vasomotor changes, temperature training may be considered a legitimate procedure within the clinical setting. However, given the recent research focus on the training of vasomotor control rather than the control of temperature, a thorough discussion of this literature will be presented herein as well as that addressing temperature training in the treatment of peripheral vascular disorders. Before so doing, however, it would appear instructive to outline briefly the relationship between the psychophysiology of temperature and blood flow.

Psychophysiology of Temperature and Blood Flow

A close connection between blood flow and skin temperature has been noted by a number of investigators (Ackner, 1956; Cook, 1974; Plutchik, 1956; Surwit, et al., 1976). Surwit et al. (1976) state that finger temperature is linearly related to the amount of blood flow, as measured by pulse amplitude, in the finger. But, as Mittleman and Wolff (1939) note, the correlations are not perfect and depend upon other external and internal factors.

Plutchik (1956) has also found the skin temperature of the toes and fingers to be the most sensitive indicators of superficial vessel blood flow. Also of significance, however, are the findings of Fetcher, Hall and Shaub (1949), who stressed ambient temperatures as influencing the magnitudes of the correlations. Roberts, Kewman, and MacDonald (1973) measured the relationship between blood flow, pulse rate, and temperature in one subject during increasing and decreasing temperatures. Temperature decreases were accompanied by severe vasoconstriction such that blood flow was cut off almost completely. Increases of skin temperature resulted in blood flow increases and accelerated pulse rate.

As pulse amplitude is highly correlated with arteriolar tone and thus with blood flow, pulse amplitude changes have been interpreted as blood flow changes (Cook, 1974). Burton (1939) reported correlations as high as .88 between blood flow and pulse amplitude. Cook (1974) showed that localized heating was reliably accompanied by pulse amplitude increases, while cooling led to concomitant pulse amplitude decreases.

Goetz (1950) reported a close relationship between finger pulse amplitude and blood flow in the finger. He suggested pulse amplitude, recorded plethysmographically, to be useful as a direct measure of variations in the vasomotor tone of the skin's arterioles. As cutaneous vessels are innervated entirely by the sympathetic nervous system (Leukel, 1972; Plutchik, 1956), pulse amplitude is thought to be a good indicator of sympathetic responses to emotional stress (Ackner, 1956; Boudewyns, 1976; Menzies, 1937).

FACTORS AFFECTING TEMPERATURE AND VASOMOTOR CONTROL

Volitional Temperature Control

As with other biofeedback-based procedures, the volitional control of temperature has been considered to be of particular import (Shapiro & Surwit, 1976), because the patient being trained in these procedures ultimately must exercise control in his or her natural environment without the benefit of feedback, in order to alleviate the symptomatology. Examining the legitimacy and validity of volitional temperature control, some researchers have taken temperature regulation in the absence of feedback as evidence for such control. Others subjected research participants to a cold challenge following training in peripheral temperature increases, requiring their subjects to maintain increases in the face of subnormal environmental temperatures.

Stoffer, Jensen, and Nesset (1979) tested for volitional control of finger temperature using a contingent auditory feedback group, a yoked sham feedback group, and a no-feedback group. Their subjects received five sessions of training, each of which consisted of 13 minutes of feedback. After completion of training, the subjects were tested for control without feedback in a separate session held 2 days after training. During training, subjects in the contingent feedback group proved superior to subjects in the no-feedback group. However, during the test for volitional control, they exceeded both the no-feedback and the sham feedback group subjects in their ability to self-regulate temperature. Without this test, according to Stoffer et al., the erroneous assumption of no differences between contingent and sham feedback would have been made.

For some researchers (Taub, 1977; Taub & Emurian, 1976), the most convincing evidence for volitional control has been the ability of subjects to increase and decrease their skin temperatures sequentially. However, not all individuals are able to achieve such sophisticated control. Kaplan and Crawford (1979) reported a case in which a subject was consistently unable to decrease finger temperature by more than 1° F. But this subject demonstrated the ability to increase her skin temperature by as much as 17.5°F, depending upon her initial skin temperature. In an effort to convince herself of volitional control, however, this subject began to practice stopping the handwarming at an arbitrarily predetermined temperature. Once this level of control was achieved, she trained herself, not only to stop at the preselected temperature, but to maintain this temperature for a given time and then continue to another preselected point.

This individual is considered unique in autonomic conditioning research. There are some individuals who have been referred to as "temperature acrobats" (Hertzfeld & Taub, 1980). Such people are able to achieve large magnitude changes over a brief period of time without acknowledged use of cognitive strategies to aid them.

Researchers frequently report specificity of the response following learning (Taub & Emurian, 1976). Initially, the response is diffuse and occurs symmetrically. However, as control is gained, it becomes more specific to the site at which the transducer is located. Thus, increased control at the feedback locus which is uncorrelated with other monitored sites, either opposite to or unilateral but distant from the feedback site, may offer an additional means of establishing evidence for learned control.

Intervening Variables

While a number of researchers have attested to the conditionability of vasomotor responses (Snyder & Noble, 1968; Stern & Pavloski, 1974), arguments have been advanced which suggest, at least partly, the influence of intervening variables in explaining the regulation of peripheral temperature and vasomotor control. Smith (1954) remarked that, since the autonomic nervous system has no direct interaction with the external environment due to its lack of afferent functioning, it is unlikely that it is capable of learning by reinforcement principles. The argument advanced by Katkin and Murray (1968) is that observed vasomotor changes are in fact unconditioned responses to skeletal and respiratory activity. According to this view, subjects may be reinforced for skeletal, muscular, verbal, or cognitive activity, which may well serve as stimuli for autonomic nervous system responding.

Respiratory responses have most frequently been implicated as mediating vasomotor changes in conditioning experiments (Engel & Chism, 1967; Shean & Stange, 1971; Stern & Anschel, 1968). This is not surprising, as there is a physiological basis for a linkage between respiration and vasomotor changes (Ackner, 1956; Cook, 1974; Plutchik, 1956). Engel and Chism (1967) found that both increases and decreases in respiration rate decreased the average finger pulse volume. A slow rate of respiration led to immediate and sustained decreases in finger pulse volume, while a fast respiration rate reduced finger pulse volume only after 2 to 4 minutes.

With respect to finger temperature, Engel and Chism observed no moment-to-moment variation. This is consistent with the physiology of temperature, as these changes are known to take place over several minutes. These investigators nevertheless did note a monotonic decrease from 33.2°C to 33.0°C during the fast breathing condition. Respiratory changes, however, have not been consistently related to finger temperature changes (Elder, Frentz, & Lewis, 1977; Lynch, Schuri, & D'Anna, 1976).

Although the literature regarding *respiration rate* as related to vasomotor control is equivocal, the evidence for a correspondence between the *depth of respiration* and vasomotor responding is quite convincing. Plutchik (1956) noted that deep inspirations lead to a decrease in hand blood volume, which is followed by a fall in skin temperature. Deep breaths also were found to be reliably accompanied by rapid vasoconstriction, which did not adapt over six trials (Stern & Anschel, 1968).

In addition to respiration, a number of other responses have been implicated in the control of peripheral temperature and vasomotor changes. Lynch et al. (1976) investigated the effects of isometric muscle contractions on finger pulse amplitude, skin temperature, and heart rate. Although the muscle contractions occurred without gross body movements, they resulted in rapid and large magnitude changes in the dependent measures. Thus, minute movements that may elude the experimenter's notice may operate to influence vasomotor responses.

The importance of cognitive factors and their possible significance to thermo-regulation also have been examined. In a study designed to examine the effect of vivid imagery on vasomotor responses, Miller and Dworkin (1974) reported that imagery of heat on one ear and ice on the other led to differential vasodilation and vasoconstriction of the ear lobes. In studies with Raynaud's disease patients, researchers frequently cite the patients' imagery as being influential in the achievement of temperature increases (Blanchard & Haynes, 1975; Schwartz, 1973; Shapiro & Schwartz, 1972; Surwit, 1973).

Schneider (1976) explained the acquisition of finger temperature control as a function of observing the temperature via the feedback device and relating this to accompanying physiological sensations. Once recognition of this particular state occurs, the subject may learn to prolong this state and thus, modify his or her finger temperature. Cognitive processes, it would seem, represent an important factor in thermal conditioning procedures and cannot readily be dismissed.

MIGRAINE HEADACHES

The Pathophysiology of Migraine Headache

Although the specific pathophysiology of migraine headaches is not fully known, a disturbance in the cranial arteries is often implicated as the cause of what is commonly a debilitating pain (Bakal, 1975). The major forms of this psychosomatic disorder are referred to as the *classical* and the *common* migraine. The former is characterized by periods of intense intracranial and extracranial vasoconstriction. The classical migraine is also distinguished by a prodromal phase of visual, sensory, and/or motor disturbance. In the common migraine, the initial aura associated with the classical migraine is not present (Dalessio, 1972).

Dalessio describes three phases of the migraine syndrome. Initially, there is an increased lability of the blood volume components of the cephalic motor response. This is followed by vasoconstriction of the cranial vessels, with either presence or absence of prodomal symptoms. Finally, vasodilation of the extracranial arteries takes place. For both forms of migraine, the pulsating pain is produced by engorgement associated with profound vasodilation of the extracranial vasculature (Dalessio, 1972; Friedman, 1972).

Ergotamine tartrates act to produce a temporary vasoconstriction of the extracranial arteries and consequently prevent the rebound dilation. The administration of ergotamine tartrates leads to a decrease in pulse amplitude as well as a corresponding decline in reported headache intensity. The positive effect of this medication has led biofeedback researchers to employ procedures which focus on the training of constriction of the cranial arteries (Elmore & Tursky, 1981).

There are currently two psychophysiological approaches to the treatment of migraine headache, each of which focuses on a different aspect of the pattern of vasomotor activity in the syndrome. One approach is hand temperature feedback, which concentrates on symptom alleviation during the preheadache phase and views the migraine as a syndrome of sympathetic nervous system overreactivity (Elmore & Tursky, 1981). The other approach stresses vasomotor feedback. According to the former approach, migraine is the result of the dilation of cranial arteries. Temperature feedback functions to increase blood flow through vasoconstriction of the cranial arteries. Peripheral vasodilation acts to prevent or abort the headache by decreasing sympathetic vasomotor tone (Budzinski, 1973; Elmore & Tursky, 1981).

A number of authors question the necessity of temperature training in migraine alleviation. Werbach and Sandweiss (1978) assessed the common rationale which assumes that vasodilation of the cranial arteries is accompanied by peripheral vasoconstriction. Although handwarming is thought to abort migraine attacks by preventing rebound cranial vasodilation, these authors argue that there has not been a well-controlled study which demonstrates a correlation between learned handwarming and cranial vasoconstriction. Werbach and

Sandweiss also cite Price and Tursky (1976) as support for their argument, since Price and Tursky found increased rather than decreased temporal artery blood volume during voluntary digital warming.

The second psychophysiological approach to migraine therapy is based on the effects of ergotamine tartrates. Graham and Wolff (1938) noted that ingestion of this medication was associated with decreases in temporal pulse amplitude ranging from 16% to 84%. Subjective pain reduction also appeared to correspond directly to the extent of the pulse amplitude decrease. Temporal pulse amplitude feedback places its focus on the phase during which engorgement occurs, a phase which is accompanied by severe pain. The technique of temporal pulse amplitude reduction trains the subject in the voluntary constriction of the extracranial vasculature at the headache site to relieve these painful symptoms (Elmore & Turksy, 1981).

Given the aforegoing, there is little question but that the issue of temperature training efficacy versus vasomotor training efficacy, and the theoretical underpinnings of both, are of major significance in our understanding of the nature of migraine head pain and its remediation.

Temperature Training

Although some authors have questioned the relationship between temperature gain scores and reduction in migraine activity (Werbach & Sandweiss, 1978), a number of case studies and group experiments have noted an increase in hand temperature to accompany headache alleviation. A causal relationship between the magnitude of temperature change and treatment outcome may not exist. Rather, both may be a function of sympathetic relaxation accompanying the treatment procedures.

The observation by Sargent, Green, and Walters (1972) of a spontaneous 10°F increase in hand temperature, which accompanied migraine headache alleviation in a research subject, led these and other researchers to investigate hand temperature increase training as a treatment for the relief of migraine pain. Reading and Mohr (1976) taught six migraineurs to increase their hand temperature, providing visual analog feedback without any adjunctive autogenic phrases. These patients obtained mean hand temperature increases of 1.4°C by a final no-feedback period. At 1 and 2 months, follow-up sessions were conducted. The magnitude of change was .7°C, indicating considerable loss of ability to produce the hand warming response without regular practice. Despite the small changes and loss of achieved temperature gains, remarkable clinical improvements were noted. Mean headache duration per week was reduced to 5.1 hours from 23.5 hours during baseline. If handwarming was implemented at the first sign of a migraine attack, Reading and Mohr's patients were able to reduce the headache's intensity, although they could not abort it. Handwarming per se may not have been the crucial variable, as deterioration in this ability (due to lack of practice) did not effect headache improvement. Rather, the processes involved in attempting to regulate hand temperature may have influenced sympathetic nervous system relaxation and consequently led to a reduction in symptomatology.

Gainer (1978) focused on the ability to discriminate temperature increases as a factor in migraine headache reduction. He presented a case study in which skin temperature feedback alone failed to alleviate migraine activity, although the patient had gained excellent control of the response. This patient demonstrated the ability to reliably increase hand temperature by as much as 18°F. A comparison of actual and perceived temperature changes indicated correct estimation on the part of the patient only 47% of the time. When temperature discrimination training was introduced, her estimates improved to 79%, and she began to note hand temperature changes prior to headache onset. She instituted handwarming at that time. Her headache frequency dropped to zero versus three to six attacks per week prior to discrimination training. These changes were maintained throughout an 8-month follow-up. Gainer concluded that perception of early warning signs for migraines may be a prerequisite for the control of these headaches and treatment may be facilitated by the inclusion of discrimination training for certain patients.

One of the criticisms raised in respect to temperature training has involved the lack of controls for placebo effects (Blanchard & Young, 1974). In response to this criticism, Turin and Johnson (1976) investigated the placebo-expectancy component in temperature training for migraine headaches. They reasoned that, if cooling the hands proved ineffective despite the lack of positive expectations by subjects in both conditions, the placebo-expectancy effect could be ruled out. Three subjects received training in temperature cooling, and four subjects were trained in finger warming. Only two of the subjects in the cooling condition were able to achieve a temperature reduction over 10 training sessions. Clinical improvement of headache activity was evidenced by the four hand-warming subjects, while headache activity did not change or was exacerbated in the hand-cooling subjects. Once subjects in the latter group were exposed to the temperature increase condition, all participants showed significant headache improvement. The subject exposed to the lengthiest training exhibited the most dramatic improvement, with no headache activity at all after 20 weeks of training. These results attribute treatment gains to feedback for temperature increases exclusively.

Finally, Werbach and Sandweiss (1978) found an inverse relationship between hand-warming ability during the first session and reduction of migraine activity by the end of their study. They reported a total lack of correlation between temperature gain scores across sessions and treatment outcome. The ability to warm hands, they considered, was unrelated to the reduction of migraine activity.

Although the evidence is still sparse, a number of investigators (Bild & Adams, 1980; Friar & Beatty, 1976) have recently concentrated on direct vasomotor conditioning of the cranial vasculature rather than on attempting to alleviate migraine symptoms via the more indirect method of temperature training. As Keefe (1981) has pointed out, it is extremely difficult for individuals to gain voluntary control over peripheral temperature. He suggested that such training would be facilitated by providing the patient with relaxation training before instituting the temperature training phase. In cases where this procedure was applied, temperature control has been achieved fairly rapidly.

Vasomotor Training

Johnston (1977) viewed skin temperature as an unsatisfactory measure of blood flow, as it reflects changes in such flow only approximately and sluggishly, while digital pulse amplitude measured via photoelectric plethysmograph is taken as a more accurate measure. A number of investigators have focused their attention on the presumably more direct responses of vasoconstriction and vasodilation. Furthermore, questions have been raised as to the applicability of temperature training in the treatment of both migraines and Raynaud's disease (Blanchard & Young, 1974; Schwartz, 1972; Werbach & Sandweiss, 1978). These authors have implied that direct vasomotor conditioning involving the deeper vasculature in Raynaud's disease, and training for temporal vasoconstriction in migraine headache, may be a more appropriate intervention.

The first indication that vasomotor responses may be amenable to operant conditioning procurdures came from a study conducted by Lisina (cited in Razran, 1961). During an experiment to train vasodilation in the forearm to escape electric shock, a stimulus generally resulting in reflective vasoconstriction, Lisina noted a serendipitous event. Subjects were successful in acquiring the desired response only when they were able to watch their responses on the plethysmograph.

Subsequently, Snyder and Noble (1968) attempted the operant conditioning of peripheral vasoconstriction. Stern and Pavloski (1974) repeated the Snyder and Noble (1968) experiment, controlling for respiratory and muscular artifacts. Their findings supported those of Snyder and Noble, showing significant differences between the experimental and control groups. They attributed these differences to cognitive rather than somatic mediation.

Based upon findings that vasomotor control could be operantly conditioned, Friar and Beatty (1976) hypothesized that the operant control of extracranial pulse amplitude should be an effective treatment for migraine headaches. These investigators compared a group of patients trained to decrease pulse amplitude in the extracranial artery with a control group trained to decrease pulse amplitude in the index finger of the affected side. Although both groups successfully acquired the response of reducing pulse amplitude within eight sessions, only the group trained to reduce cranial artery pulse amplitude was able to achieve a reduction in migraine activity. However, it is not surprising that the group receiving feedback for finger pulse amplitude decreases did not reduce headache activity, since the effects are similar to cooling of the hands, a condition which has been shown to be related to migraine pain exacerbation (Turin & Johnson, 1976).

A number of investigators have compared EMG feedback for vasomotor changes in the treatment of migraine headache. Bild and Adams (1980) examined the effect of these types of feedback on migraine patients. They found the cephalic blood volume pulse feedback to be superior to the frontalis EMG feedback in reducing headache activity and medication intake.

Sturgis, Tollison, and Adams (1978) successfully taught two subjects to constrict the zygomatico-facial branch of the temporal artery, an artery normally dilated during migraine episodes. They employed blood volume pulse (BVP) feedback training, which was recorded as a decrease in pulse amplitude. Their subjects received 15 BVP feedback sessions. One patient was able to decrease the duration of migraines after only 4 weeks of BVP feedback training, while the second patient reported no incidents of migraine following all 15 BVP feedback sessions (see also Feuerstein & Adams, 1977).

In testing the efficacy of biofeedback for temporal pulse amplitude reduction, against increases in hand temperature with migraineurs as subjects, Elmore and Turksy (1981) found temporal pulse amplitude decrease to be a more potent treatment than handwarming. Each group of their subjects was provided with 8 training sessions of 10 trials per session, followed by one transfer of training session without feedback. These investigators also obtained data on patterns of autonomic vasomotor responding in their subjects. The temporal pulse amplitude feedback group (TPA) reduced pulse amplitude by a mean of 26% over eight training sessions. During the transfer of training session, the mean TPA group reduction was 36%. This group also obtained mean finger pulse amplitude reductions of 28% during training and 48% during transfer of training. They were able to decrease the mean hand temperature score by 1.7°C during this session. The hand temperature feedback group achieved mean pulse amplitude reductions of 23% during training. However, during the no-feedback generalization session, these subjects were only able to reduce their temporal pulse amplitude by 11%. With hand temperature feedback, this group achieved increases in finger pulse amplitude of 99% during training. There was some deterioration during the transfer of training session, when finger pulse amplitude increased by 51%. In terms of temperature changes, a 1.87°C mean increase was obtained during training and a 2.8°C increase was achieved during the test for generalization. In terms of headache activity, the group receiving feedback for vasomotor responses achieved reductions in medication intake of 53% and a decrease of 56% in headache frequency, while the hand temperature feedback group did not decrease in these clinical measures. On the contrary, the latter group experienced some increases in headache duration and severity ratings.

Compared to temperature increase training, research available to date indicates that cranial pulse amplitude reduction feedback offers a larger magnitude of change and a longer period of maintenance of migraine symptom reduction, and so, appears to be the treatment technique of choice. Developments in equipment/instrumentation, however, will be necessary in order to provide the clinician with the capacity to conveniently undertake cranial pulse amplitude training in the office environment.

RAYNAUD'S DISEASE

Pathophysiology of Raynaud's Disease

Raynaud's disease is a form of peripheral vascular disturbance caused by the tonic contraction of the smaller arteries without obvious pathological changes in their walls. It commonly involves symmetrical areas of the hands or feet causing excessive perspiration and circulatory stasis with periods of cyanosis or pallid asphyxia. The severe cases go on to dry gangrene of the phalanges. The spasm is intermittent and occurs on exposure to cold or emotional stimuli; it involves only the terminal arteries, while the main vessels continue their normal pulsations. The disease occurs most commonly in young individuals with hyperirritable nervous constitutions.

An attack of Raynaud's disease consists of three stages. At first there is constriction of the digital arteries, with complete interruption of blood flow. In this phase the skin assumes a waxy, white color. As blood begins to trickle in, the passage of blood through the capillaries is delayed and oxygen desaturation takes place. The skin's color changes to blue, a condition known as *cyanosis*. This is followed by *reactive hyperemia,* which is the vasodilation following temporary arrest of circulation, and the skin becomes pink (Shepherd & Vanhoutte, 1979).

Raynaud's disease has been described as a functional disorder of the cardiovascular system and involves an interruption of local blood flow to the digits, due to paroxysmal vasospasms (Taub & Stroebel, 1978). Raynaud himself posed sympathetic overactivity as a causal factor, while Lewis (1929) suggested a local fault in the blood vessels. Allen and Brown (1932) presented an earlier statement of the sympathetic overreactivity explanation for uncomplicated Raynaud's syndrome, while they asserted that the local fault explanation applies in advanced cases (see also Sappington, Fiorito, & Brehany, 1979; Spittel, 1972).

Vasopastic attacks are most likely to occur when ambient temperatures are in the 12°C to 15°C range. There appears to be an interaction between ambient temperature and emotional reactions. Although emotional reactions alone can trigger severe vasoconstriction in Raynaud's patients, the condition tends to be exacerbated in cold temperatures (Malmo, 1975). During an attack, these patients register digital temperatures ranging from 19°C to 24°C, while those of normals fall in the 30°C to 35°C range (Malmo, 1975).

Temperature Training

Among the currently available therapeutic choices in the treatment of Raynaud's disease, temperature biofeedback appears to be desirable with respect to side effects. There is, however, insufficient evidence that it is the treatment of choice for this condition. The relative sparsity of successfully treated patients, and an insufficient number of controlled treatment studies, prevent outcome comparisons with other treatment forms. Studies which are designed to provide rigorous controls for placebo effects, feedback type, and long-term follow-up have yet to be conducted. The behavioral treatment of Raynaud's disease primarily has consisted of training the patient to increase the temperature at the affected site. This treatment, however, has not always led to improvement in the symptomatology, and treatment gains frequently have not been maintained over time (Blanchard & Young, 1974). Because the disorder is vasomotor in origin, it has been suggested that direct training in vasodilation of the deeper vessels may produce more positive outcomes (Blanchard & Young, 1974). To date, however, training in the control of temperature has represented the primary available behavioral treatment regimen.

Emery, Schaller, and Fowler (1976) trained 12 patients by providing them with visual feedback for temperature increases in one finger. Self-reports of improvements included the ability to swim and the capacity to remain outdoors during cold temperatures without the occurrence of vasopastic attacks. One patient had been afflicted with digital ulcers that healed during the training, pointing to another potentially useful application of this technique.

In a study by Taub (1977), patients achieved mean temperature increases of 10°C. They also obtained clinically significant reductions in their symptoms, since vasopastic attacks decreased greatly even during exposure to cold environments. In addition, generalization to no-feedback situations was readily accomplished, and the response enabled these patients to reduce or abort incipient attacks voluntarily.

Treatments adjunctive to temperature feedback are also quite common in studies with Raynaud's patients. Sedlacek (1976) treated three patients with EMG and thermal feedback. He defined *control* as involving a minimum hand temperature increase of 2.8°C and the ability to maintain this temperature at 32.5°C. Sedlacek's subjects achieved these criteria by trials 9, 14, and 16, respectively.

Keefe, Surwit, and Pilon (1980) compared skin temperature feedback with autogenic training, autogenic training alone, and progressive relaxation in the treatment of primary Raynaud's disease. They used a group format in which patients assigned to the separate conditions were seen in small groups over three 1-hour sessions. Instructions appropriate to each of the above procedures were given during these sessions. In addition, all 21 patients practiced the required skills at home throughout 9 weeks of training. The results indicated equal improvement for all participants in the first 4 weeks, irrespective of treatment condition. Symptom improvement was maintained after 9 weeks of training. As the groups were not equal in vasopastic attacks during baseline, the external validity of these results is questionable, and, certainly, effects other than those due to the experimental procedures may have influenced the outcome.

The results of a study by Surwit, Pilon, and Fenton (1978) are more conclusive. Feedback plus autogenic training, compared to autogenic training alone, resulted in equal symptom improvement as well as the ability to maintain digital temperature during cold stress tests. Furthermore, there was equal improvement for patients trained in the laboratory for six biweekly sessions and those who practiced at home in addition to training during three group meetings. Subjects in both treatment groups evidenced 50% fewer vasopastic attacks relative to subjects in a waiting-for-treatment control group. The latter group received the same treatment 2 months later with similar results.

It appears that training for temperature increases is no more effective than autogenic training or relaxation in the relief of Raynaud's symptoms, and that treatments which serve to reduce sympathetic activity lead to symptom alleviation in Raynaud's disease. Certainly, Schwartz (1972) has demonstrated that Raynaud's patients appear to respond particularly well when some form of imagery or autogenic phrases are used. Although many patients afflicted with Raynaud's disease have obtained substantial temperature increases with feedback, symptom improvements have not always accompanied these changes. The speculation has been that skin surface temperature increases are not correlated with vasodilation of the deeper vessels, and intervention may be more profitable if it involves the deeper vasculature (Blanchard & Young, 1974).

For the most part, temperature training (using feedback, autogenic training, or relaxation) for the alleviation of Raynaud's symptoms has required a large number of sessions, while temperature increases have been small. Few patients have been able to produce mean changes greater than 5.5°C in magnitude, and some could not increase their temperature by more than .3°C (Blanchard & Haynes, 1975; Jacobson, Manschreck, & Silverberg, 1979; May & Weber, 1976; Peper, 1972; Sedlacek, 1976; Shapiro & Schwartz, 1972; Surwit, 1973; Surwit et al., 1978; Taub, 1977). It does not appear that digital temperature training procedures are particularly effective or cost efficient when compared to standard medical procedures in the treatment of Raynaud's disease. However, there are at least some data suggesting that vasomotor conditioning may produce superior results within briefer training periods.

Vasomotor Training

There is currently one study which suggests that vasomotor conditioning may be a more useful technique than temperature training in the treatment of Raynaud's disease. Shapiro and Schwartz (1972) provided a Raynaud's patient with feedback for digital blood volume increases, and symptom alleviation occurred within 10 sessions. This patient also remained symptom free throughout a 1½-year follow-up. This patient reported the extensive use of self-generated imagery related to warm stimuli. It is, thus, difficult to ascribe treatment gains solely to the feedback. However, the success achieved by this patient points to the necessity of conducting research examining the applicability of this biofeedback procedure to a larger number of Raynaud's patients. In addition, more studies carefully designed to isolate the influences of imagery would appear appropriate, as imagery may be a useful adjunctive tool in the facilitation of symptom improvement. Finally, comparisons of temperature training against vasomotor conditioning for Raynaud's patients may clarify questions regarding the treatment of choice.

NOVEL TREATMENT APPLICATIONS

Temperature training also has been applied in the relief of anginal pain, rheumatoid arthritis, and to increase blood flow to specific sites of injury. Although these applications have largely been reported only in anecdotal form in case studies, they warrant further investigation.

Hartman (1979) treated an angina patient who consumed excessive amounts of nitroglycerine tablets, a vasodilator substance. This patient achieved hand temperature increases ranging from 5°F to 13°F, depending upon initial temperature, up to a maximum hand temperature of 94°F. The patient was able to maintain this response for several years, and medication intake was reduced to acceptable levels. Although there were no controls for alternative explanations, further investigation appears warranted due to the direct correspondence between anginal pain and peripheral vasoconstriction. Training for hand temperature increases may be a useful technique for relief in symptomatology of angina patients, even though improvement in the condition itself does not occur.

Bird and Colborne (1980) investigated the effect of thermal feedback and relaxation in a patient with high voltage electrical burns to the left wrist. Blood flow to the area had been restricted due to the disruption of sympathetic innervation and the formation of dense gap tissue. Prior to training, the temperature of the patient's left hand remained between 77°F and 80°F, which resulted in intense pain. His pain decreased markedly when his hand temperature rose to a range of 90°F to 93°F. His physician noticed a rare regrowth of nerves, which made additional skin graft procedures unnecessary. Partial motor and sensory recovery also occurred.

In a controlled group study, Achtenberg, McGraw, and Lawlis (1981) compared biofeedback and relaxation with standard physiotherapy for rheumatoid arthritis. The biofeedback group proved consistently superior to the traditional physiotherapy group in the patient's physical functioning, as measured by a range of outcome criteria.

Finally, a group of researchers (French, Leeb, Fahrion, Law, & Jecht, 1973) investigated the reduction of sperm count through voluntary scrotal heating. Their data showed that scrotal heating can indeed be brought under volitional control and that sperm count may be dropped to subfertile levels following training. The procedure certainly points to an interesting and presumably safe method of birth control. Just how effective these procedures may be, as well as the parameters of their efficacy over time, of course, has yet to be established.

SUMMARY

The literature regarding thermoregulation and vasomotor training in the treatment of cranial and peripheral vascular disorders is both extensive and equivocal. Thus, various perspectives regarding treatment efficacy may be supported through a selective review of this literature. Although numerous studies have shown the alleviation of symptoms in migraine headache and Raynaud's disease following temperature training, others have reported few if any treatment gains, or have not linked improvement to the treatment regimen exclusively.

The finding that subjects were able to exert control over blood vessel constriction and dilation has led some researchers to focus on the direct control of the cranial vasculature in treating migraine headache. In general, these procedures have produced positive treatment outcomes on a more consistent basis than has temperature training. However, the rather sophisticated and expensive equipment that is required for vasomotor training has made this treatment strategy prohibitive to the average clinician, and its use has been primarily relegated to large research facilities.

Temperature training also has been applied in a number of other conditions, including angina, burns, and rheumatoid arthritis, with very promising results. Some investigators have also demonstrated its possible application in birth control.

Given the diverse findings in treatment evaluation studies, much additional research with respect to the pathophysiology of peripheral vascular disorders, as well as the identification of the parameters of the treatment interventions, needs to be conducted.

REFERENCES

Achtenberg, J., McGraw, P., & Lawlis, G. F. (1981). Rheumatoid Arthritis: A study of relaxation and temperature biofeedback training as an adjunctive therapy. *Biofeedback and Self-Regulation, 6,* 207–223.

Ackner, B. (1956). Emotion and the peripheral vasomotor system. *Journal of Psychosomatic Research, 1,* 3–20.

Allen, E. D., & Brown, G. E. (1932). Raynaud's disease: A clinical study of 147 cases. *Journal of the American Medical Association, 99,* 1472–1478.

Bakal, D. A. (1975). Headache: A biopsychological perspective. *Psychological Bulletin, 82,* 369–382.

Bild, R., & Adams, H. E. (1980). Modification of migraine headaches by cephalic blood volume and pulse rate and EMG biofeedback. *Journal of Consulting and Clinical Psychology, 48,* 51–57.

Bird, E. I., & Colborne, S. R. (1980). Rehabilitation of an electrical burn patient through thermal biofeedback. *Biofeedback and Self-Regulation, 5,* 283–287.

Blanchard, E. B., & Haynes, M. R. (1975). Biofeedback treatment of a case of Raynaud's disease. *Journal of Behavior Therapy and Experimental Psychiatry, 6,* 230–234.

Blanchard, E. B., & Young, L. D. (1974). Clinical applications of biofeedback training: A review of the evidence. *Archives of General Psychiatry, 30,* 573–588.

Boudewyns, P. A. (1976). A comparison of the effects of stress vs. relaxation instructions on the finger temperature response. *Behavior Therapy, 7,* 54–67.

Budzinski, T. (1973). Biofeedback procedures in the clinic. In L. Birk (Ed.), *Biofeedback: Behavioral medicine.* New York: Grune & Stratton.

Burton, A. C. (1939). The range and variability in the blood flow of the human fingers and the vasomotor regulation of body temperature. *American Journal of Physiology, 127,* 437.

Cook, M. R. (1972). The cephalic vasomotor orienting response. *Psychophysiology, 9,* 273–274.

Cook, M. R. (1974). Psychophysiology of peripheral vascular changes. In P. A. Obrist, A. H. Black, J. Brener, & L. V. DiCara (Eds.), *Cardiovascular psychophysiology.* Chicago, IL: Aldine Publishing.

Dalessio, D. J. (1972). *Wolff's headaches and other head pain.* New York: Oxford University Press.

Elder, S. T., Frentz, K. G., & Lewis, R. A. (1977). Learned self-control of surface body temperature. Abstracts of paper presented at the Eighth Annual Meeting of the Biofeedback Society of America. *Biofeedback and Self-Regulation, 2,* 279–326.

Elmore, A. M., & Tursky, B. (1981). A comparison of two psychophysiological approaches to the treatment of migraine. *Headache, 21,* 93–101.

Emery, H., Schaller, J. G., & Fowler, R. S. (1976). Biofeedback in the management of primary and secondary Raynaud's phenomenon. *Arthritis and Rheumatism, 19,* 795.

Engel, B. T., & Chism, R. A. (1967). Effect of increases and decreases in breathing rate on heart rate and finger pulse volume. *Psychophysiology, 4,* 83–89.

Fetcher, E. S., Hall, J. F., Jr., & Shaub, H. G. (1949). The skin temperature of an extremity as a measure of its blood flow. *Science, 110,* 422–423.

Feuerstein, M., & Adams, H. E. (1977). Cephalic vasomotor feedback in the modification of migraine headache. *Biofeedback and Self-Regulation, 2,* 241–254.

French, D. J., Leeb, C. S., Fahrion, S. L., Law, O. T., & Jecht, E. W. (1973). Self-induced scrotal hyperthermia in man followed by decrease in sperm output: A preliminary report. *Andrologie, 5,* 311–316.

Friar, L. R., & Beatty, J. (1976). Migraine: Management by trained control of vasoconstriction. *Journal of Consulting and Clinical Psychology, 44,* 46–53.

Friedman, A. P. (1972). Current concepts in the diagnosis and treatment of recurrent headache. *Medical Clinics of North America, 56,* 1257–1271.

Fuller, G. D. (1977). *Biofeedback: Methods and procedures in clinical practice.* San Francisco, CA: Biofeedback Press.

Gainer, J. C. (1978). Temperature discrimination training in the biofeedback treatment of migraine headache. *Journal of Behavior Therapy and Experimental Psychiatry, 9,* 185–188.

Goetz, R. H. (1950). Effects of changes in posture on peripheral circulation with special reference to skin temperature readings and plethysmogram. *Circulation, 1,* 56–75.

Graham, J. R., & Wolff, H. G. (1938). The mechanism of the migraine headache and the action of ergotamine tartrate. *Archives of Neurological Psychiatry, 39,* 737.

Hartman, C. H. (1979). Response of anginal pain to hand warming. *Biofeedback and Self-Regulation, 4,* 355–357.

Hertzfeld, G. M., & Taub, E. (1980). Effect of slide projections and tape-recorded suggestions on thermal biofeedback training. *Biofeedback and Self-Regulation, 5,* 393–405.

Jacobson, A. M., Manschreck, T. C., & Silverberg, E. (1979). Behavioral treatment for Raynaud's disease: A comparative study with long-term follow-up. *American Journal of Psychiatry, 136,* 844–846.

Johnston, D. (1977). Feedback and instructional effects in the voluntary control of digital pulse amplitude. *Biological Psychology, 5,* 159–171.

Kaplan, B. J., & Crawford, D. G. (1979). Target training: A technique for assessing self-regulation of skin temperature. *Biofeedback and Self Regulation, 4,* 87–92.

Katkin, E. S., & Murray, N. E. (1968). Instrumental conditioning of autonomically mediated behavior: Theoretical and methodological issues. *Psychological Bulletin, 70,* 52–68.

Keefe, F. J. (1981). *Thermoregulation.* Workshop presented at the Association for the Advancement of Behavior Therapy, Toronto.

Keefe, F. J., Surwit, R. S., & Pilon, R. N. (1980). Biofeedback, autogenic training, and progressive relaxation in the treatment of Raynaud's Disease: A comparative study. *Journal of Applied Behavior Analysis, 13,* 3–11.

Leukel, F. (1972). *Introduction to physiological psychology.* St. Louis, MO: C. V. Mosby Co.

Lewis, T. (1929). Experiments relating to the peripheral mechanism involved in spasmodic arrest of the circulation in the fingers, a variety of Raynaud's Disease. *Heart, 15,* 7–101.

Lynch, W. C., Schuri, U., & D'Anna, J. (1976). Effects of isometric muscle tension on vasomotor activity and heart rate. *Psychophysiology, 13,* 222–230.

Malmo, R. B. (1975). *On emotions, needs, and our archaic brain.* New York: Holt, Rinehart and Winston, Inc.

May, D. S., & Weber, C. A. (1976). Temperature feedback training for symptom reduction in primary and secondary Raynaud's Disease. *Biofeedback and Self-Regulation, 1,* 317.

Menzies, R. (1937). Conditioned vasomotor responses in human subjects. *Journal of Psychology, 4,* 75–120.

Miller, N. E., & Dworkin, B. R. (1974). Vicissitudes and opportunities. In P. A. Obrist, A. H. Black, J. Brener, & L. V. DiCara (Eds.), *Cardiovascular psychophysiology.* Chicago, IL: Aldine Publishing.

Mittleman, B., & Wolff, H. B. (1939). Affective states and skin temperature: Experimental study of subjects with "cold hands" and Raynaud's syndrome. *Psychosomatic Medicine, 1,* 271–292.

Peper, E. (1972). *Case report.* Annual meeting of the Biofeedback Research Society.

Plutchik, R. (1956). The psychophysiology of skin temperature. *Journal of General Psychology, 55,* 249–268.

Price, K. P., & Tursky, B. (1976). Vascular reactivity of migraineurs and nonmigraineurs: A comparison of responses to self-control procedures. *Headache, 16,* 210–217.

Razran, G. (1961). The observable unconscious and the inferrable conscious in current Soviet psychophysiology: Interoceptive conditioning, semantic conditioning, and the orienting reflex. *Psychological Review, 68,* 81–147.

Reading, C., & Mohr, P. D. (1976). Biofeedback control of migraine: A pilot study. *British Journal of Social and Clinical Psychology, 15,* 429–433.

Roberts, A. H., Kewman, D. G., & MacDonald H. (1973). Voluntary control of skin temperature: Unilateral changes using hypnosis and feedback. *Journal of Abnormal Psychology, 82,* 163–168.

Sappington, J. T., Fiorito, E. M., & Brehany, K. A. (1979). Biofeedback as therapy in Raynaud's Disease. *Biofeedback and Self-Regulation, 4,* 155–169.

Sargent, J. D., Green, E. E., & Walter, E. D. (1972). The use of autogenic feedback training in a pilot study of migraine and tension headaches. *Headache, 12,* 120–125.

Schneider, J. A. (1976). Finger temperature feedback procedures: Sympathetic inhibition training or placebo effect? *Psychotherapy: Theory, Research and Practice, 13,* 141–147.

Schwartz, G. E. (1973). Biofeedback as therapy, some theoretical and practical issues. *American Psychologist, 28,* 666–673.
Schwartz, G. E. (1972). Voluntary control of human cardiovascular integration and differentiation through feedback and reward. *Science, 175,* 90–93.
Sedlacek, K. (1976). EMG and thermal feedback as a treatment for Raynaud's Disease. *Biofeedback and Self-Regulation, 1,* 318.
Shapiro, D., & Schwartz, G. E. (1972). Biofeedback and visceral learning: Clinical applications. *Seminars in Psychiatry, 4,* 171–184.
Shapiro, D., & Surwit, R. S. (1976). Learned control of physiological function and disease. In H. Leitenberg (Ed.), *Handbook of behavior modification and behavior therapy.* Englewood Cliffs, NJ: Prentice-Hall.
Shean, G. D., & Stange, P. W. (1971). The effects of varied respiratory rate and volume upon finger pulse volume. *Psychophysiology, 8,* 401–405.
Shepherd, J. T., & Vanhoutte, P. M. (1979). *The human cardiovascular system: Facts and concepts.* New York: Raven Press.
Smith, K. (1954). Conditioning as an artifact. *Psychological Review, 61,* 217–225.
Snyder, C., & Noble N. (1968). Operant conditioning of vasoconstriction. *Journal of Experimental Psychology, 77,* 263–268.
Spittell, Y. N. (1972). Raynaud's phenomenon and allied vasospastic conditions. In J. F. Fairbairn, J. L. Juergens, & J. A. Spittell (Eds.), *Allen-Barker-Hines: Peripheral vascular diseases.* Philadelphia, PA: Saunders.
Stern, R. M., & Anschel, C. (1968). Deep inspiration as stimuli for responses of the autonomic nervous system. *Psychophysiology, 5,* 132–141.
Stern, R. M., & Pavloski, R. P. (1974). Operant conditioning of vasoconstriction: A verification. *Journal of Experimental Psychology, 102,* 330–332.
Stoffer, G. R., Jensen, J. S., & Nesset, B. L. (1979). Effects of contingent versus yoked temperature feedback on voluntary temperature control and cold stress tolerance. *Biofeedback and Self-Regulation, 4,* 51–61.
Sturgis, E. T., Tollison, C. D., & Adams, H. E. (1978). Modification of combined migraine: Muscle contraction headaches using BVP and EMG feedback. *Journal of Applied Behavior Analysis, 11,* 215–223.
Surwit, R. S. (1973). Biofeedback: A possible treatment for Raynaud's Disease. *Seminars in Psychiatry, 5,* 483–490.
Surwit, R. S., Pilon, R., & Fenton, C. H. (1978). Behavioral treatment of Raynaud's Disease. *Journal of Behavioral Medicine, 1,* 323–335.
Surwit, R. S., Shapiro, D., & Feld, J. L. (1976). Digital temperature autoregulation and associated cardiovascular changes. *Psychophysiology, 13,* 242–248.
Taub, E. (1977). Self-regulation of human tissue temperature. In G. E. Schwartz & J. Beatty (Eds.), *Biofeedback: Theory and research.* New York: Academic Press.
Taub, E., & Emurian, C. S. (1976). Feedback-aided self-regulation of skin temperature with a single feedback locus. *Biofeedback and Self Regulation, 1,* 147–168.
Taub, E., & School, P. J. (1980). Some methodological considerations in thermal biofeedback training. *Behavior Research Methods and Instrumentation, 10,* 617–622.

Taub, E., & Stroebel, C. F. (1978). Biofeedback in the treatment of vasoconstrictive syndromes. *Biofeedback and Self Regulation, 3,* 363–373.

Turin, A., & Johnson, W. G. (1976). Biofeedback therapy for migraine headaches. *Archives of General Psychiatry, 33,* 517–519.

Werbach, M. R., & Sandweiss, J. H. (1978). Peripheral temperatures of migraineurs undergoing relaxation training. *Headache, 18,* 211–214.

Yates, A. J. (1980). *Biofeedback and the modification of behavior.* New York: Plenum Press.

III

PSYCHODERMATOLOGY

9

The Psychophysiology of Skin Disorders

F. A. Whitlock

Cornwall, Great Britain
Formerly, University of Queensland
Australia

The term *psychosomatic* was introduced to denote diseases whose main manifestations were somatic but in whose origins psychogenic factors were considered to be playing an important role. The concept has been applied to a wide range of conditions including asthma, hypertension, peptic ulcer, and "neurodermatitis." Unfortunately, by limiting the term to a relatively small number of diseases it might be assumed that others were purely "physical" in origins and unaffected by the patient's psychological state. With respect to many dermatoses, such a proposition is manifestly incorrect. On the one hand there are conditions such as dermatitis artefacta, where the influence of the patient's mental state is the dominant aetiological factor; there are afflictions such as acne vulgaris, with which emotional disturbances are common responses to an unsightly and uncomfortable disorder; and in between lie a number of dermatoses such as lichen simplex, atopic dermatitis, and psoriasis where, whatever their fundamental causes might be, their onset and development can be markedly affected by the patient's emotional condition at the time or before the first signs of skin lesions become apparent.

In an essay of this kind it would be superfluous to review every possible variety of dermatosis for hypothetical psychological causes. It is a common failing of medicine to attribute to emotional disturbances an aetiological role when other causes remain undetected. The fundamental causes of many skin diseases remain obscure, yet time and further research ultimately may reveal the true origins of conditions such as psoriasis, vitiligo, and alopoecia areata, to name but a few, which appear to be influenced by psychological factors operating before the appearance of the skin changes. Too great a separation of the psychological from the physical may simply be a reaffirmation of Cartesian dualism, which is the very antithesis of the mind–body unity of Hippocratic medicine. Despite orthodox medical skepticism, a relationship is assumed when it is expressed in everyday language. We betray our inner feelings by blushing with shame, sweating with anxiety, and, so it is said, itching with rage.

Many dermatoses, particularly those characterized by itching and scratching, are often precipitated or aggravated by psychological tensions. Nonetheless, it has to be admitted that our understanding of these psychophysiological processes is relatively rudimentary. Dermatologists can tell us something about the pathophysiology of the conditions they treat, but few have explored their precise relationship to the patient's underlying emotional state. In this respect many patients are more royalist than the king, claiming that they are suffering from a "nerve rash" or that sudden changes in their skins have been caused by emotional shock. In most cases it is difficult to prove the causal linkage even when one shares to some degree that patient's convictions. In such examples psychological methods of treatment may be at least as beneficial as the conventional ointments and lotions whose useful placebo and protective effects help eliminate the itch–scratch cycle, with subsequent healing or amelioration of the dermatoses.

It is questionable whether the term *psychophysiological* is preferable to psychosomatic, but it has the merit of indicating the nexus of events in which psychological disturbances influence physiological states. Consequently, before examining the psychological aspects of specific dermatoses, something must be said about the underlying physiology of skin phenomena.

Itch

Although the sensation of itching is difficult to define, it is generally agreed that, when perceived, it causes scratching to obtain relief. Some itches may include components of pricking and burning, but pure itch, which can be produced experimentally by intradermal injection of histamine, is experienced as a sensation sui generis. Like other skin sensations, its perception is a psychological event that, surprisingly, has received very little attention from neurologists and experimental psychologists.

Although it is generally agreed that the itch sensation is conveyed by fine nonmedullated C-fibres, the nerves which transmit pain sensations from the skin, there is uncertainty about the nature of itch receptors in the brain. It is apparent that central, as opposed to peripheral, itching can occur (Whitlock, 1957), and recent work demonstrating that itching can be relieved by the opiate antagonist naloxone (Summerfield, 1980; Smitz, Legros, & LeMaire, 1982; Bernstein, Swift, Soltini, & Lorincz, 1982) suggests that cerebral endorphins are involved in the process of itch perception. Morphine, which relieves pain, is a well-known cause of itching. This may be due to its inhibition of cholinesterase and some possible action on cerebral endorphins, as well as its peripheral effect which releases histamine in the skin. According to Fjellner and Hagermark (1984), naloxone will not prevent histamine-induced peripheral itching, whereas it does appear to be effective in controlling central itching. The importance of this discovery lies in the support it gives to the concept of central itching, which, conceivably, could be triggered by emotional disturbances.

Vascular Changes in the Skin

In a review of flushing reactions of the skin blood vessels (Wilkins, 1983) it was observed that there are two types of vasomotor innervation—constriction and dilation—but surprisingly little was said about emotional flushing. Various diseases of the brain may be associated with flushing, for example, Parkinsonism, migraine, and diencephalic autonomic epilepsy. One might conjecture, therefore, that cerebral mechanisms exist whereby emotional, particularly facial, flushing is controlled. The neural and chemical basis for vasomotor changes in the skin has been reviewed elsewhere (Whitlock, 1976), but it is interesting to find that anxiety and depression are associated with vasomotor constriction and a fall in skin temperature (Ackner, 1956; Mittlemann & Wolff, 1943). Raynaud's disease, where peripheral vasoconstriction may be precipitated by emotional conflict, may be helped by hypnosis and biofeedback techniques designed to reduce the degree of vasoconstriction experienced by patients with this condition (Jacobson, Hackett, Surman, & Silverberg, 1973; Roberts, Kewman, & MacDonald, 1973).

Sweating

Emotional sweating is under cholinergic and adrenergic control. Thermal sweating appears to be regulated by the hypothalamus in response to changes in blood temperature, but not a great deal is known about the control of emotional sweating, although centers in the frontal lobe may be responsible.

Some Specific Dermatoses

Generalized and localized pruritus. There are patients who suffer from generalized itching with a minimum of skin lesions apart from scratch marks. Such cases, in the absence of a systemic or metabolic cause, may well be labeled as examples of psychogenic pruritus. Opinions vary on the frequency or existence of this disorder. Rothman (1960), for example, was frankly skeptical about its occurrence, arguing that it must be rare if it exists at all. On the other hand, some writers have given convincing accounts of patients with this disorder (Calnan & O'Neill, 1952; Musaph, 1964; Cairns, 1972). In some patients this localized or generalized itching may be associated with severe depression (Bien, 1933; Edwards, 1954), and appropriate treatment of the affective disorder may abolish or alleviate the skin symptoms. It must be remembered that occult causes of generalized itching such as sarcoidosis (Sharma & Balchum, 1972) and cerebral tumors (Andreev & Petkov, 1975) have to be excluded before a firm diagnosis of psychogenic itching is made. The coexistence of tension or depression is not necessarily proof of the alleged psychogenesis, as affective symptoms may well develop in response to intractable discomfort and loss of sleep. The onset of pruritus as a symptom of a cerebral disorder (King, Huff, & Jorizzo, 1982) could be regarded as partial confirmation of the existence of the phenomenon of central itching which, in some patients, is a manifestation of emotional distress. Once itching is established, the inevitable itch–scratch cycle will perpetuate the symptom. The development of conditioned scratch responses to the itch stimulus (Robertson, Jordan, & Whitlock, 1975) will protract the attack of psychogenic itching, whether or not this has developed on the basis of some generalized dermatosis. Such reflex scratching can continue during sleep, particularly during the earlier, lighter stages of sleep (Savin, Patterson, Oswald, & Adam, 1975).

Localized pruritic dermatoses. Among the more common conditions seen in dermatological practice are cases of lichen simplex and anogenital pruritus which, in many patients, will exhibit the skin changes similar to lichen simplex on other parts of the body, but now modified by circumstances of heat, moisture, and infection (Sweet, 1952). Many examples of lichen simplex originate from a minor skin lesion which becomes perpetuated by a pattern of itching and scratching. Some cases of lichen simplex and anogenital pruritus also have personal or family histories of atopy, thus rendering their skins more sensitive to minor stimuli which may be accompanied by itching. Lichen simplex patches develop on areas of skin which are easily accessible to the patient's fingers, such as the back of the neck or outer side of the thigh. Scratching of the back of the neck is a pattern of behavior commonly observed in perfectly normal individuals when experiencing some degree of emotional tension. If this state of tension also elevates skin temperature and sweating, it is understandable that patients with an inherently itchy skin will develop a persistent scratch response to the sensation, with consequent thickening (lichenification) of the affected area.

Before assuming too readily that the symptoms of anogenital pruritus are caused by psychological disturbances, it is essential that local and metabolic causes of the disorder are considered and excluded. In many patients the local conditions of heat and moisture, and the application of potentially irritating antiseptic or local anaesthetic ointments, may well perpetuate symptoms which sometimes can be the focus of repressed sexual conflicts. Macalpine (1953a), however, expressed her doubts about psychodynamic interpretations of anogenital pruritis, although it is understandable that, once the condition is well established, psychosexual problems could develop in response to the symptoms.

Abnormal Sweating

Persistent anxiety may cause a state of chronic hyperidrosis, a not unusual complaint among patients attending skin clinics (Sneddon, 1949; Davis & Bick, 1946). It is difficult to assess the frequency of excessive sweating, for, apart from its inconvenience and socially embarrassing aspects, most patients, particularly women, deal with the problem by the application of antisweat preparations as a routine cosmetic measure. According to Hurley (1982), emotional hyperhidrosis is a disorder transmitted by an autosomal dominant gene which apparently does not involve anatomical or physiological abnormalities of the sweat glands. If this is correct, these patients have little option but to fall back on local applications as palliative measures, some of which have complications of their own which can be more troublesome than the sweating they were designed to alleviate. On the other hand, psychotherapy may reduce levels of anxiety, which is the prime cause of excessive sweating. That palmar sweating is amenable to instrumental conditioning (Kuypers & Cotton, 1972) may be a pointer to the value of biofeedback techniques as a means of controlling a troublesome symptom.

Although dyshidrosis and pompholyx eruptions on the hands and feet have long been regarded as being caused by excessive sweating, predominantly of emotional origin, there is very little evidence that the condition is associated with abnormal sweat-gland activity (Shelley, 1953). Numerous theories have been formulated to account for this dermatosis, ranging from sensitivity to nickel in various foods (Fisher, 1978) to local fungal infections. No doubt the condition will be aggravated by excessive sweating of emotional origin, and Obermeyer (1955) included psychological stress among the possible causes of the condition.

Vascular Disorders of the Skin

Raynaud's disease. Raynaud's disease is characterized by recurrent, paroxysmal contractions of the small arteries and arterioles of the extremities. It is most commonly provoked by exposure to cold and the use of vibrating tools, but there is also evidence that emotional stress will precipitate attacks in those already predisposed to the disorder (Millet, Lief, & Mittlemann 1953; Mufson, 1944). Biofeedback techniques and hypnosis have been used to reduce the inherent sensitivity of the peripheral vasculature, and some authors have postulated a "Raynaud's attitude," consisting of a sense of persecution and a wish to hit back at the alleged persecutors (Gottlieb, Glaser, & Gottschalk, 1967). It is questionable whether such a psychological state is a common cause of the Raynaud phenomenon, but there is good reason for thinking that anxiety will aggravate a condition which may be helped by relaxation and hypnosis (Peters, Lundy, & Stern, 1973), the object of such exercises being to increase peripheral skin temperature and reduce levels of anxiety. Emotional tension, if present, will intensify the patient's abnormal response to cold.

Erythematous dermatitis of the face. This nonspecific dermatosis has been attributed to suppressed feelings of grief and anger (Macalpine, 1953b). The persistent redness, burning, and itching of the facial skin improved with psychotherapy, and nearly all Macalpine's patients were depressed. A variant of this condition—actinic reticuloid—was described by Ive, Magnus, Warin, and Wilson-Jones

(1969). Whereas practically all of Macalpine's patients were women, all of Ive's cases were middle-aged or elderly men. All were said to have been seriously depressed, and five of six patients attempted suicide, one with ultimate success. Apart from this report there does not appear to have been any further mention of the condition and, more importantly, the mental state of patients who are so afflicted. Nonetheless, in the light of these reports it is clearly essential that the psychological state of patients with a persistent erythematous dermatitis of the face of obscure etiology should be carefully assessed to exclude any serious degree of depression.

Rosacea. This condition presents as a persistent facial erythema with telangiectasis and papules. In some cases there is an associated ocular keratitis. The cause of the condition is unknown and, as is so often the case with conditions of obscure etiology, psychological disturbances have been invoked to explain the chronic "blush." As Twiston Davis (1951, p. 157) wrote, "The blush of rosacea may, of course, be brought about directly by indigestion, but a guilty conscience will do it equally well, and it should always be suspected." A number of authors have argued in favor of emotional disturbance being the fundamental cause of rosacea (Sneddon, 1949; Klaber & Wittkower, 1939; Hellier, 1944), but others have failed to find satisfactory evidence in support of this theory (Whitlock, 1961; Marks, 1968; Sobye, 1950). Both Whitlock and Marks reported that, in some patients, the onset of the dermatosis was preceded by an acute emotional upset, but in general their cases did not differ from controls with respect to neuroticism or other personality features. Some of Marks's patients tended to manifest more anxiety and depression, but this could have been a response to their skin disorders rather than their causes. As Sneddon has written (1982), "The obvious and successful control of the eruption by oral antibiotics achieves more than psychotherapy and sedatives."

Miscellaneous vascular disorders. Among the many dermatoses with prominent vascular changes which have been labelled as psychosomatic in origin, mention should be made of lupus erythematosus, particularly the systemic variety of the disease (SLE). There is little evidence to support such an hypothesis, although there can be no doubt that many patients with SLE can become psychotic with prominent affective symptoms (Bennett, Hughes, Bywaters, & Holt 1972). An interesting but rare condition, psychogenic purpura, caused by autoerythrocye sensitization, may be of significance in the pathogenesis of religious stigmatization (Ratnoff, 1969; Whitlock 1976; Whitlock & Hynes, 1978). Although some authorities (Critchley, 1947; Thurston,

1952) considered the phenomena of religious stigmatization to be hysterical in origin, such a diagnosis tells us very little about the actual pathogenesis of the lesions.

Specific Skin Disorders

Atopic dermatitis. According to Champion and Parish (1972), atopic dermatitis is a genetically determined disorder with an increased tendency to form IgE antibodies. Other authors (Rajka, 1975; Rechardt, 1970) have emphasized the inherent itchiness of the atopic patient's skin. Understandably, this causes scratching, which in its turn results in erosion and lichenification of the affected areas. Under the term *neurodermatitis,* an unfortunate word often taken as implying a psychological basis for the disorder, psychosomatic theorists have speculated about the nature of the underlying conflicts (Stokes, 1940; Alexander, 1952; Alexander, French, & Pollock, 1968; Musaph, 1964). Other authors (Fiske & Obermayer, 1954; Borelli, 1950) have examined personality factors, and Fiske and Obermeyer (1954, p. 263) concluded that atopic patients showed "conflictual infantile elements from the anal and phallic levels of personality development." These were manifested as sadistic, destructive, paranoid, and aggressive features with elements of masochism, insecurity, sensitivity, dependency, and marked sexual conflicts. To counter this catch-all catalogue of personality qualities, Rechardt (1970) studied patients when their skin was most troublesome and again some nine years later. Although, when younger, these patients showed a variety of emotional disturbances, by the time they were older most of these elements had disappeared. On the basis of this investigation the notion that atopic patients suffer from a fixed, disadvantageous personality pattern can hardly be sustained. There can, however, be little doubt that psychological tensions can increase the liability of these patients to itch and scratch, and that such scratching can become a conditioned response to itching, no matter how it is caused (Jordan & Whitlock, 1972).

A good deal of speculation has been focused on the concept of maternal rejection as an important factor in the genesis and perpetuation of this dermatosis. On the evidence it is not easy to accept that maternal rejection, either overt or hidden, is of primary importance in the majority of patients. No doubt an unsatisfactory mother–child relationship will increase the infant's emotional distress, with consequent aggravation of its genetically determined tendency to itch and scratch. This, in its turn, may cause an adverse maternal response, which could amount to rejection. As is so often the case with allegedly psychosomatic disorders, it is far from easy to ascertain when a psychological disturbance is the cause or the outcome of the condition under consideration. In the issue of maternal rejection the evidence will be largely retrospective and, consequently, almost impossible to validate or measure.

On balance, therefore, it must be said that the psychosomatic theories of neurodermatitis rest on somewhat shaky observations. This is not to deny that, in some patients at various stages of their lives, exacerbations of atopic dermatitis will appear to be precipitated by emotional disturbances. Should the patient come under psychological surveillance during the episode, it might too readily be assumed that emotional factors are of prime importance in the actual aetiology of the dermatosis.

Urticaria. Urticaria is an eruption of transient erythematous and oedematous swellings of the dermis and subcutaneous tissues (Champion, 1972). It is a common condition said to affect more than one-fifth of the population at some time in their lives. Although many causes have been identified, in about 70% of cases of chronic urticaria no apparent etiology can be detected. Understandably, psychological disturbances have long been considered to be important precipitants, and Champion regarded psychological factors to be relevant in 20% of patients. In a major study (Stokes, Kulchar, & Pillsbury, 1935) it was found that a "psychoneurogenous" factor, alone or in combination with other causes, was present in 83.5% of 91 patients. It was considered that the principal psychological elements were "tension make-up, neuroticism, the worry habit, shocks, family troubles and finance" (Stokes et al., 1935, p. 497). On the basis of such an over-inclusive list one might justifiably wonder how it is that most of the adult population is free from the disorder. Again, the finding by Warin and Champion (1974), that many patients with urticaria appeared to suffer from a tense, oversensitive constitution and often reported worries or emotional stress, does not clearly separate patients from those not so afflicted. Opinions on this aspect of etiology are decidedly mixed and, as usual when abnormal psychological traits are discovered, it is difficult to be certain that these existed before the eruption or have developed in response to a chronically itchy skin. Nonetheless, there is evidence that the skin's vasomotor state can be influenced by emotional changes (Graham & Wolff, 1950), and most experienced dermatologists are convinced that psychological factors are important etiological agents. On the other hand there is little evidence to support the theory that there is a specific "hives attitude" or "hives personality." Cormia (1950) found that urticaria patients were generally stable, normal individuals. Interpretation of the lesions as the equivalent of tumefaction or erection (skin erotism) (Wittkower & Russell, 1953) appears to rest more upon the preconceptions of the observers than on objectively verifiable fact.

Psoriasis. Psoriasis is yet another dermatosis whose etiology is obscure but which, as Wilkinson (1972, p. 1192) comments, "is unpredictable and capricious in its course but is usually chronic." There has been speculation about the parts played by personality and psychological disturbances in precipitating relapses and exacerbations of the disease. Obermeyer (1955), for example, considered that psoriasis patients often exhibited emotional instability and that a general spread of the eruption could follow an acutely stressful experience. Whereas itching is not a common characteristic of psoriasis, this symptom may be present in patients whose psychological states have contributed to the onset or relapse of the condition. Bolgert and Soule (1955), who found a high frequency of pruritus in their 200 cases, considered that 52.5% showed "psychasthenia," 16% anxiety, and that 1% suffered from undifferentiated psychological disturbances. Using a life-event scale, Fava, Perini, Santonastaso, and Fornasa (1980) found that the frequency of recorded incidents before the onset of an attack of psoriasis fell intermediately between their findings in cases of urticaria and patients with fungal infections. Bearing in mind the difficulty experienced by many patients and dermatologists in fixing a precise date of onset of an attack of psoriasis, it is doubtful whether a life-event questionnaire can be a reliable instrument for this kind of investigation. Another survey of 2,164 patients (Farber, Bright, & Nall, 1968) reported that 40% claimed that their attacks of psoriasis developed at times of worry, 21% found no particular relationship between psoriasis and periods of worry, and 37% were uncertain. *Worry* is a vague term given different meanings and emphasis by adults who experience worries of greater or lesser intensity at different periods of their lives. Consequently, a more precise term is required before assuming that disturbances of an individual's tranquillity are etiologically related to psoriasis. Although investigators have claimed that psoriasis patients have particular personality qualities, the weight of opinion is opposed to this hypothesis (Baughman & Sobel, 1971; Gilbert, Rodgers, & Roenigk, 1973). Seville (1977) found that the prognosis for psoriasis was better in those who were able to recount temporal relationships of stress to the onset of their dermatosis than in those who had no such recollection. When the nature of the relationship was explained, thus providing "insight," the same author (Seville, 1978) considered that the outlook for the clearing of the eruption was very much better than in those who had gained no such awareness, either because they had failed to understand the explanation, had forgotten it, or had rejected it. Nonetheless, as one writer concluded (*British Medical Journal*, 1978, p. 530), "simple psychotherapy and explanation should not replace conventional treatments. . . despite the real limitations these have." Macalpine (1954) summarized the situation when she wrote, "Because the course of psoriasis could be influenced by emotion—as is the case with most other illnesses—one should not conclude that psoriasis was a psychosomatic disorder."

Alopoecia areata. The cause of this condition, characterized by sudden patchy loss of hair on the scalp, is not known. In some cases the hair loss may involve other parts of the body, leading to a state of alopoecia totalis. Although there are many anecdotal accounts of such hair loss being preceded by some kind of emotional stress, as Rook and Dawber (1982) comment, opinions on this issue are strongly divergent. Whereas there may be some examples of alopoecia areata whose onset is significantly related to acute psychological disturbance, this is by no means a universal finding. Perini, Fornasa, Cipriani, Bettin, Zecchino, and Peserico (1984), in a well-controlled study, found an excess of both desirable and undesirable life events during the six months before the onset of episodes of alopoecia areata. This was a retrospective investigation which could not wholly eliminate the methodological difficulties which such research inevitably entails. It is not easy to obtain conclusive evidence on this issue of predisposing stress, and Macalpine (1958) considered that the case for the psychogenesis of alopoecia had not been proven. When psychological disturbance is discovered, this could be a response to rather than a cause of the hair loss. Even if one could prove a causal connection between psychological shock and the onset of the dermatosis, there is a large gap to be filled to account for its pathogenesis. That a number of autoimmune conditions are present in some patients may indicate some kind of diathesis rendering the patient more sensitive to the impact of emotional turmoil on immune mechanisms. The finding by Hoff and Riehl (1937) that alopoecia can follow hypothalamic damage certainly points to the possibility that cerebral disturbance could play a part in the pathogenesis of alopoecia areata or totalis in some instances. Unfortunately, there is no satisfactory demonstration of psychotherapy being an effective mode of treatment for a condition which undergoes spontaneous remission in a considerable number of cases.

Dermatitis artefacta and related conditions. Sneddon (1983) has reviewed the phenomena of self-inflicted dermatoses, disorders more commonly observed in younger women who present with lesions often of a bizarre shape on areas of the body readily accessible to their fingers. Sneddon and Sneddon (1975) commented on the disturbed relationships between these young patients and their overbearing mothers, likening their circumstances to those found in patients with anorexia nervosa. The prognosis was not good, as, over a period of 12 years, one-third of their cases continued to produce lesions and were still severely disabled. Although hysterical mechanisms are often mentioned as important contributions to the pathogenesis, many patients are also depressed (Fisher & Pearce, 1974). Male patients with dermatitis artefacta, more often than women, produce their lesions for personal gain, and frank psychiatric disorder is unusual. Fabisch (1980) studied 50 patients, 44 of whom were women. A variety of stresses were considered to have precipitated the disorder, and the author saw the production of these lesions as an appeal for help, a desire for self-punishment, and a means of relieving guilt and tension. In general, psychotherapy was not particularly effective, unless it was continued for several years.

A variant of dermatitis artefacta, acne excoriee, presents as itchy well-scratched papules on the face of young women. Sneddon and Sneddon (1981) regarded the condition, which could persist for up to 20 years, as a protective pattern of behavior serving to conceal emotional disturbances, often phobic states.

Most dermatologists will be familiar with patients suffering from delusions of parasitosis, insisting that their skin is infested with organisms (Lyell, 1983). Repeated scratching to remove these insects or "worms under the skin" causes excoriated lesions which may be diagnosed as examples of dermatitis artefacta. Many of these patients are deeply depressed or suffering from severe hypochondriasis, which can be caused by an underlying organic cerebral disorder, causing the skin sensations misinterpreted as due to infestation (Ladee, 1966). Hopkinson (1973) recommended pimozide as a treatment for delusions of parasitosis, but for those who are seriously depressed it may be necessary to prescribe antidepressant drugs or psychotherapy in addition to pimozide.

Under the title of "dermatological nondisease," Cotterill (1981, 1983) reported on 28 patients whose main complaints were of burning, itching, and loss of hair. Apart from scratch marks, there was no objective evidence of skin disease in these patients. All were diagnosed as examples of dysmorphophobia who often were deeply depressed. Of these 28 patients, one committed and two attempted suicide. All were female, and those with facial symptoms had a more ominous prognosis associated with psychosis and the possible risk of harming themselves.

Although the majority of artificially produced lesions of the skin do not resemble well-known dermatoses, this is not invariably the case. Millard (1984) described 13 patients (all female) who produced injuries to their skins resembling the conditions for which they were already receiving treatment. These patients were regarded as maladjusted or suffering from some kind of emotional distress.

MENTAL ILLNESS AND SKIN DISEASE

Hughes, Barraclough, Hamblin, and White (1983) recorded the responses of skin patients to the 30-item General Health Questionnaire. Thirty percent of outpatients and 60% of inpatients obtained high scores, which were particularly excessive in patients with widespread lesions of alopoecia areata of more than six months duration. These authors considered that disfigurement, stigma, and inconvenience were major causes of psychiatric symptoms in patients with acne vulgaris, eczema, and psoriasis. Two investigators (Sainsbury, 1960, Kenyon, 1962), using the Maudsley Personality Inventory, found that patients with skin diseases, allegedly psychosomatic in origin, scored higher on the neuroticism and introversion scales than patients who had sustained injuries or who were suffering from presumed non-psychosomatic complaints. Shoemaker (1963) explored the psychodynamics of 40 patients suffering from chronic urticaria and concluded that the condition was a "regressive, physiological expression of unconscious conflict when previously operating mechanisms of defense had become inadequate to bind strong affect. Anxiety is the dominant affect in this disorder." Such psychoanalytic interpretations of a condition whose etiology is obscure may not satisfy all workers, although the role of anxiety as a contributory factor may be significant. Brown (1967) examined the mental state of patients suffering from eczema. He considered that most eczema patients had vulnerable personalities and that the majority displayed some type of emotional disturbance. In 55% this could be regarded as a psychiatric illness, most often depressive and partially suppressed. Brown considered that the emotional disturbance usually preceded the onset of eczema but, taking into account the findings of Hughes et al. (1983), it could be argued that, when relatively minor psychological symptoms are revealed in skin patients, such symptoms are understandable reactions to, rather than the determining causes of, their dermatoses. It has often been asked whether psychiatric patients are more or less liable to develop skin disorders, particularly those of an allegedly allergic nature. Hebra (1866), for example, doubted whether there was any close association between skin and mental disorders, but a rather different opinion on the subject was expressed by Slorach (1953). Kidd and Meehan (1961), who surveyed 1700 long-stay psychiatric patients, found that 413 had some kind of skin disease. Of the "neurodermatoses," there were seven cases of rosacea, one alopoecia areata, one vitiligo, and a single case of atopic dermatitis. Obviously, in this context, a good deal depends on what types of skin disease are to be included. Leaving aside conditions associated with mental defect and organic brain disease, such as adenoma sebaceum in patients with tuberose sclerosis, one might conclude that the prevalence of skin disease among patients in psychiatric hospitals is very similar to that existing in the general population, providing, of course, that one omits skin eruptions caused by psychotropic drugs.

On the other hand, there appears to be general agreement that many skin patients suffer from depression (Preston, 1969; Sanborn, Sanborn, Cimbolie, & Niswander, 1972; Hughes et al., 1983). Edwards (1954) described six depressed patients, with dermatoses complicated by intense itching, whose affective states and pruritis cleared when they were treated with electroconvulsive therapy. Macalpine (1953a) reported that depressive symptoms frequently troubled patients with pruritus ani, and Greenberg (1961) considered, on the basis of five patients with severe pruritus and melancholia which responded to antidepressant treatment, that severe and persistent pruritus may be a manifestation of depression. The observation is not entirely new, for Robert Burton (1632), describing the symptoms and signs of melancholy in the body, quoted Laurentius as saying that some victims experienced a "kind of itching on the superficies of the skin like a flea biting sometimes."

This question of whether skin symptoms can replace or, in some sense, symbolize psychotic disorders was given further consideration by Gall (1970), who described 14 patients whose depressive symptoms improved or disappeared coincidentally with the onset of attacks of urticaria. On the other hand, an earlier writer (Pons, 1892) considered that some psychoses and dermatoses waxed and waned together. In contrast, it has been held that psychosis and psychosomatic disease in general can alternate with one another, although Ross (1954) and Thomas, Stern, and Lilienfield (1956) were unable to support this contention. In all probability there is no regular relationship between psychoses and psychosomatic disorder. Sometimes one appears to supplant the other; at other times they coincide. As Brosin (1952, p. 746) wrote, "The attractive theory that psychosomatic disorders . . . are a defense or barrier against psychotic patterns needs much more validation."

Treatment

Leaving aside conditions such as dermatitis artefacta and delusions of parasitosis, where the psychiatric contribution to disease is paramount, it is fairly clear that there are few dermatoses where the fundamental cause is psychological disorder. On the other hand, many conditions will be aggravated or occasionally precipitated by emotional stress, and in such circumstances some form of psychiatric intervention seems desirable. However, rather than embark on lengthy psychological explorations of their patients, many dermatologists will use conventional physical treatments supplemented in some instances with the prescribing of mild sedatives such as diazepam.

It has been shown that atopic dermatitis and other pruritic disorders can be perpetuated by a vicious circle of itching and scratching. Understandably, therefore, behavior therapists have turned their attention to conditions where biofeedback and other behavorial techniques might be valuable aids to treatment. Ratliff and Stein (1968), for example, used an aversion technique to treat a patient with a 17-year history of neurodermatitis. Six months later his skin had healed and he was free from itching and scratching. Other workers (Walton, 1960; Allen & Harris, 1966; Bar & Kuypers, 1973; Dobes, 1977) have used behavorial methods to control the scratching of patches of lichen simplex. Patients suffering from hyperidrosis and so-called dyshidrotic eczema have been taught by biofeedback methods to reduce their levels of sweating (Miller, Coger, & Dymond, 1974; Kuypers & Cotton, 1972; Duller & Gentry, 1980). Daniels (1973) employed a mixture of behavioral methods which included relaxation and light hypnosis to treat a woman with a 6-month history of headaches and urticaria. A similar blend of procedures was adopted by Waxman (1973) in the treatment of a woman with a 20-year history of psoriasis. Unfortunately, few of these studies are beyond criticism, either because the duration of follow-up was too short or because a number of independent variables such as changes in life circumstances were not sufficiently taken into account. A more sophisticated investigation by Haynes, Wilson, Jaffe, and Britton (1979) demonstrated beneficial effects of relaxation training for a small number of patients with atopic dermatitis. The degree of muscular relaxation was recorded by frontal electromyography (EMG). Although there was no uniform relationship between itching and EMG levels, there was a fairly consistent reduction in the intensity of itching in the course of each treatment session but no consistent change across sessions. At follow-up 9 to 12 months later, most of the patients reported some continued measure of improvement. Scores on the MMPI were normal for all subjects, a finding which gave no support for the belief that sufferers from atopic dermatitis also have major personality or psychological disturbances. More success is likely to be achieved when behavorial techniques are applied to break a repetitive habit of itching and scratching. If this pattern has become a conditioned response, one might expect that reciprocal inhibition or even aversion methods would have a fair chance of overcoming a self-perpetuating dermatosis. As mentioned earlier, the symptoms of Raynaud's disease may be improved by biofeedback methods of treatment. Freedman, Ianni, and Wenig (1983) reported that subjects who learned to control peripheral skin temperature and vasodilation continued to be more resistant to cold one year later. On the other hand, patients who exhibited Raynaud's *phenomenon* in association with scleroderma failed to derive any significant clinical improvement from these methods of treatment (Freedman, Ianni, & Wenig, 1984).

Light hypnosis has been used as an aid to relaxation by some behavior therapists, but one of the major topics of interest in dermatology has been the use of hypnotic suggestion for the treatment of viral warts. Does it work, or are the benefits claimed the result of chance and spontaneous remission? As might be expected, the published results offer conflict in interpretation, with some workers obtaining successful cures (Ullman & Dudek, 1960) but others (Tenzel & Taylor, 1969) reporting no obvious improvement. Surman, Gottlieb, Hackett, and Silverberg (1973) carried out a controlled trial of hypnotherapy for the removal of warts. Five months after the start of treatment, 53% of the experimental subjects had lost their warts but none of the untreated control cases had improved. The mode of action of hypnosis on warts is obscure, but, considering the viral etiology of these tumors, one might postulate some general action on the patient's immunological state. This, however, hardly explains the effect of hypnotic suggestion directed to one hand rather than to both when the "treated" side is cured with the contralateral hand remaining unchanged. Because wart charming by lay practitioners may be more successful than hypnotic suggestion by medically qualified therapists, one might conjecture that the patient's expectations make an important contribution to the outcome of the treatment. Nonetheless, there is sound evidence supporting the value of hypnosis in the treatment of other organic dermatoses such as icthyosis and the rare congenital icthyosiform erythroderma of Brocq (Mason, 1952). In addition, hypnotherapy has been used to treat a case of refractory dermatitis—possibly atopic dermatitis (Twerski & Naar, 1974). The patient improved dramatically but, unfortunately, was lost to follow-up after six months, during which time she did suffer minor relapses which responded to self-hypnosis. Probably these beneficial results were the outcome of relaxation as well as a reduction in itching and scratching.

There is experimental evidence showing that hypnosis can alter allergic skin responses, a good example being a patient sensitive to the Japanese wax tree (Ikemi & Nakagawa, 1962). Black (1969) has summarized a number of fascinating studies, carried out with his colleagues, demonstrating the effects of hypnosis on a variety of superficial vasomotor responses. It has also been claimed that blisters can be raised by hypnotic suggestion (Ullman, 1947), but earlier work on this phenomenon, mainly by German workers, has been criticized on account of methodological flaws in the experiments (Pattie, 1941; Paul, 1963). Peripheral vasomotor responses in patients with Raynaud's disease have been influenced by hypnotic suggestion (Jacobson et al., 1973), and the alteration of skin temperature by hypnotic suggestion was demonstrated by Chapman, Goodell, and Wolff (1959). The mode of action of hypnosis on vasomotor and allergic responses is not understood, but possibly an alteration of the immune response operating through the hypothalamus is one explanation (Stein, Schiavi, & Camerino, 1976; Solomon, Amkraut, & Kasper, 1974). With respect to vasomotor changes, it is likely that the general state of relaxation induced by hypnosis may be more important than any hypothetical influence of suggestion on peripheral blood vessels (Grace & Graham, 1952). Clearly, in the light of the work quoted, hypnosis as an aid to other forms of dermatological treatment needs to be examined more rigorously and with proper experimental controls.

Although most of these accounts of behavioral and hypnotic techniques stress the value of the methods used, there is also an acknowledged contribution of the benefits of ongoing psychotherapy and relaxation. Psychotherapy without the addition of behavioral methods appears to help some patients with eczema (Brown & Bettley, 1971). This was particularly evident in well-motivated patients who had suffered from some degree of emotional disturbance before the onset of their dermatoses. In the absence of these criteria, psychotherapy appeared to aggravate the patients' eczemas, a finding which clearly underlines the need to be selective in deciding which patients with persistent dermatoses might benefit from psychotherapy.

SUMMARY AND CONCLUSIONS

Although one can hardly doubt that psychological factors can influence, for better or for worse, many skin disorders, it has to be admitted that our understanding of the psychophysiological nexus whereby these changes are brought about is meager. It is an area where speculation has been rife with inadequate attention being given to strict experimental methods. Advances are most likely to come from the combined efforts of experimental psychologists, physiologists, clinicians, and immunologists, as there must be very few individuals with the ability to master and apply all these various areas of knowledge. The precise clinical observations of the dermatologist should be supported with well-designed investigations into the etiology and treatment of skin disease. After all, the skin is in many ways an ideal organ for study, as it can be seen, even if it is far from simple to disentangle the effects of both internal and external influences upon its normal functions.

REFERENCES

Ackner, B. (1956). Emotions and the peripheral vasomotor system. *Journal of Psychosomatic Research, 1,* 3–20.

Allen, K. E., & Harris, F. M. (1966). Elimination of a child's excessive scratching by training the mother in reinforcement procedure. *Behavior Research and Therapy, 4,* 79–84.

Alexander, F. (1952). *Psychosomatic medicine.* London: George Allen & Unwin.

Alexander, F., French, T. M., & Pollock, G. H. (1968). *Psychosomatic specificity* (Vol. 1, p. 11). Chicago, IL: University of Chicago Press.

Andreev, V. C., & Petkov, I. (1975). Skin manifestations associated with tumours of the brain. *British Journal of Dermatology, 92,* 675–678.

Bar, L. H. J., & Kuypers, B. R. M. (1973). Behavior therapy in dematological practice. *British Journal of Dermatology, 88,* 591–598.

Baughman, R., & Sobel, R. (1971). Psychological factors relating to psoriasis. In E. M. Farber & A. J. Cox (Eds.), *Psoriasis, Proceedings of an International Symposium.* Palo Alto, CA: Stanford University Press.

Bennett, R., Hughes, G. R. V., Bywaters, E. G. L., & Holt, P. J. L. (1972). Neuropsychiatric problems in systematic lupus erythematosus. *British Medical Journal, 4,* 342–345.

Bernstein, J. E., Swift, R. M., Soltini, K., & Lorincz, A. L. (1982). Antipruitic effect of an opiate antagonist: Naloxone hydrochloride. *Journal of Investigative Dermatology, 78,* 82–83.

Bien, E. (1933). The clinical psychogenic aspect of pruritus vulvae. *Psychoanalytical Review, 20,* 186–196.

Black, S. (1969). *Mind and body.* London: William Kimber.

Bolgert, M., & Soule, M. (1955). Etude clinique et psychosomatique de 200 cas de psoriasis. *Semaines des Hopitaux de Paris, 31,* 1251, 1267.

Borelli, S. (1950). Untersuchugen zur Psychomatik des Neurodermatites. *Hautarzt, 1,* 250–256.

British Medical Journal (1978). Psoriasis and stress [Editorial]. *British Medical Journal, 1,* 530–531.

Brosin, H. W. (1952). Prognosis in some psychosomatic diseases. *Annals of Internal Medicine, 37,* 745–750.

Brown, D. G. (1967). Emotional disturbance in eczema: a study of symptom reporting behaviour. *Journal of Psychosomatic Research, 11,* 27–40.

Brown, D. G., & Bettley, F. R. (1971). Psychiatric treatment of eczema: a controlled trial. *British Medical Journal, 2,* 729–734.

Burton, R. (1632). *The anatomy of melancholy.* Oxford: Cripps.

Cairns, R. J. (1972). The skin and nervous system. In H. H. Rook, D. S. Wilkinson, & J. G. Ebling (Eds.), *Textbook of dermatology* (2nd ed., p. 1791). Oxford, England: Blackwell.

Calnan, C. D., & O'Neill, D. (1952). Itching in tension states. *British Journal of Dermatology and Syphilis, 64,* 274–280.

Champion, R. H. (1972). Uticaria. In H. H. Rook, D. S. Wilkinson, & J. G. Ebling (Eds.), *Textbook of dermatology* (2nd ed., p. 295) Oxford, England: Blackwell.

Champion, R. H., & Parish, W. E. (1972). Atopic dermatitis. In H. H. Rook, D. S. Wilkinson, & J. G. Ebling (Eds.) *Textbook of dermatology* (2nd ed., p. 295) Oxford, England: Blackwell.

Chapman, C. F., Goodell, H. E., & Wolff, H. G. (1959). Changes in tissue vulnerability induced during hypnotic suggestion. *Journal of Psychosomatic Research, 4,* 99.

Cormia, F. E. (1950). The role of psychosomatic factors in dermatoses. *Connecticut Medical Journal, 14,* 1051–1061.

Cotterill, J. A. (1981). Dermatological non-disease: A common and potentially fatal disturbance of body image. *British Journal of Dermatology, 104,* 611–619.

Cotterill, J. A. (1983) Psychiatry and skin disease. In A. J. Rook & H. J. Maiback (Eds.), *Recent advances in dermatology* (pp. 189–212). Edinburgh, Scotland: Churchill Livingstone.

Critchley, M. (1947). Stigmatization. *Medical Annual* (p. 326). Bristol, England: Wright.

Daniels, L. K. (1973). Treatment of urticaria and severe headache by behaviour therapy. *Psychosomatics, 14,* 347–351.

Davis, D. B., & Bick, J. W. (1946). Skin reactions observed under war-time stress. *Journal of Nervous and Mental Disease, 103,* 503–508.

Dobes, R. W. (1977). Amelioration of psychosomatic dermatosis by reciprocal inhibition scratching. *Journal of Behavioural Therapy and Experimental Psychiatry, 8,* 185–187.

Duller, P., & Gentry, W. D. (1980). Use of biofeedback in treating chronic hyperidrosis: A preliminary report. *British Journal of Dermatology, 103,* 143–146.

Edwards, K. C. S. (1954). Pruritis in Melancholia. *British Medical Journal, ii,* 1527–1529.

Fabisch, W. (1980). Psychiatric aspects of dermatitis artefacta. *British Journal of Dermatology, 102,* 29–34.
Farber, E. M., Bright, R. D., & Nall, A. I. L. (1968). Psoriasis: A questionnaire survey of 2644 patients. *Archives of Dermatology, 98,* 248–257.
Fava, G. A., Perini, G. I., Santonastaso, P., & Fornasa, C. V. (1980). Life-events and psychological distress in dermatological disorders: Psoriasis, chronic urticaria and fungal infections. *British Journal of Medical Psychology, 53,* 277–282.
Fisher, A. A. (1978). Possible role of diet in pompholyx and nickel dermatitis—a critical study. *Curtis, 22,* 412–424.
Fisher, B. K., & Pearce, K. I. (1974). Neurotic excoriations: a personality evaluation. *Curtis, 14,* 251–254.
Fiske, C. E., & Obermeyer, M. E. (1954). Personality and emotional factors in chronic disseminated neurodermatitis. *Achives of Dermatology and Syphiology. 70,* 261–267.
Fjellner, B., & Hagermark, O. (1984). The influence of the opiate antagonist, Naloxone, on experimental pruritus. *Acta Dermato-Venereologica, 64,* 73–75.
Freedman, R., Ianni, P., & Wenig, P. (1983). Behavourial treatment of Raynaud's disease. *Journal Consulting and Clinical Psychology, 51,* 539–549.
Freedman, R., Ianni, P., & Wenig, P. (1984). Behavorial treatment of Raynaud's phenomenon in Scleroderma. *Journal of Behavorial Medicine, 3,* 343–353.
von Gall, H. (1970). Der Einflusz interkurrentur Hautallergien auf den Verlauf depressiver Psychosen. *Psychiatrie, Neurologie und Medizinische Psychologie (Leipzig), 22,* 259–262.
Gilbert, A. R., Rodgers, D. A., & Roenigk, H. H. (1973). Personality evaluation in psoriasis. *Cleveland Clinic Quarterly, 40,* 147–152.
Gottlieb, A. A., Glaser, G. C., & Gottschalk, L. A. (1967). Verbal and physiological responses to hypnotic suggestion of attitude. *Psychosomatic Medicine, 15,* 61–65.
Grace, W. J., & Graham, D. T. (1952). Relationship of specific attitudes and emotions to certain bodily diseases. *Psychosomatic Medicine, 14,* 243.
Graham, O. T., & Wolff, S. (1950). Pathogenesis of urticaria: Experimental study of life situations, emotions and cutaneous vascular reactions. *Journal of the American Medical Association, 143,* 1396–1402.
Greenberg, S. I. (1961). Pruritus: A symptom of depression. *Psychosomatics, 2,* 109–111.
Haynes, S. N., Wilson, C. C., Jaffe, P. G., & Britton, B. T. (1979). Biofeedback treatment of atopic dermatitis. *Biofeedback and Self-regulation, 4,* 159–209.
Hebra, F. (1866). *On diseases of the skin.* London: New Sydenham Society.
Hellier, F. F. (1944). The relation of dermatology to psychiatry. *British Medical Journal, 1,* 583–585.
Hoff, H., & Riehl, G. (1937). Zur Frage der durch Erkrankung des Zentral Nervensystem bedingten Alopecie. *Archiv fur Dermatlogie und Syphilis, 176,* 196–200.

Hopkinson, G. (1973) The psychiatric syndrome of infestation. *Psychiatria Clinica, 6,* 330–345.
Hughes, J. E., Barraclough, B. M., Hamblin, L. G., & White, J. E. (1983). Psychiatric symptoms in dermatology patients. *British Journal of Psychiatry, 143,* 51–54.
Hurley, H. J. (1982). Hyperidrosis (emotional). In S. Maddin (Ed.), *Current dermatological therapy* (p. 232). Philadelphia, PA: W. B. Saunders Company.
Ikemi, V., & Nakagawa, S. (1962). A psychosomatic study of contagious dermatitis. *Kyushu Journal of Medical Science, 13,* 335–350.
Ive, F. A., Magnus, I. A., Warin, R. P., & Wilson-Jones, E. (1969). Actinic reticuloid. *British Journal of Dermatology, 81,* 469–485.
Jacobson, A. M., Hackett, T. B., Surman, O., & Silverberg, E. L. (1973). Raynaud's phenomenon. *Journal of the American Medical Association, 225,* 739–740.
Jordan, J. M., & Whitlock, F. A. (1972). Emotions and the skin: The conditioning of scratch response in cases of atopic dermatitis. *British Journal of Dermatology, 86,* 574–585.
Kenyon, F. E. (1962). A psychiatric survey of a random sample of out-patients attending a dermatological hospital. *Journal of Psychosomatic Research, 6,* 129–135.
Kidd, C. B., & Meehan, J. C. (1961). A dermatological survey of long stay mental patients. *British Journal of Dermatology, 72,* 129–133.
King, C. A., Huff, J., & Jorizzo, J. L. (1982). Unilateral neurogenic pruritus: Paroxysmal itching associated with central nervous system lesions. *Annals of Internal Medicine, 97,* 222–223.
Klaber, A., & Wittkower, E. (1939). The pathogenesis of rosacea. *British Journal of Dermatology and Syphilis, 51,* 501–524.
Kuypers, B. R. M., & Cotton, D. W. K. (1972). Conditioning of sweating. *British Journal of Dermatology, 87,* 154–160.
Ladee, G. A. (1966). *Hypochondriacal syndromes.* Amsterdam, Holland: Elsevier.
Lyell, A. (1983). Delusions of parasitosis. *British Journal of Dermatology, 108,* 485–499.
Macalpine, I. (1953a). Pruritus ani. *Psychosomatic Medicine, 14,* 499–508.
Macalpine, I. (1953b). Psychiatric observations on facial dermatosis. *British Journal of Dermatology and Syphilis, 65,* 177–182.
Macalpine, I. (1954). A critical evaluation of psychosomatic medicine in relation to dermatology. In R. M. B. McKenna (Ed.), *Modern trends in dermatology, 2nd series.* London: Butterworth.
Macalpine, I. (1958). Is alopoecia areata psychosomatic? *British Journal of Dermatology and Syphilis, 70,* 117–131.
Marks, R. (1968). Concepts in the pathogenesis of rosacea. *British Journal of Dermatology, 80,* 170–177.
Mason, A. A. (1952). A case of congenital icthyosiform erythroderma treated by hypnosis. *British Medical Journal, II,* 422–423.
Millard, L. G. (1984). Dermatological pathomimicry: A form of patient maladjustment. *Lancet, 2,* 969–971.

Miller, R. M., Coger, R. W., & Dymond, A. M. (1974). Biofeedback skin conductance conditioning in dyshidrotic eczema. *Archives of Dermatology and Syphilis, 109,* 737–738.

Millet, J. A. P., Lief, H., & Mittlemann, B. (1953). Raynaud's disease. *Psychosomatic Medicine, 15,* 61–65.

Mittleman, B., & Wolff, H. G. (1943). Emotions and skin temperature. *Psychosomatic Medicine, 5,* 211–231.

Mufson, I. (1944). The mechanism and treatment of Raynaud's disease: a psychosomatic disturbance. *Annals of Internal Medicine, 20,* 228–238.

Musaph, H. (1964). *Itching and scratching.* Basel, Switzerland: Karger.

Obermeyer, M. E. (1955). *Psychocutaneous medicine* (p. 325). Springfield, IL: Charles C. Thomas.

Pattie, F. (1941). The production of blisters by hypnotic suggestion: A review. *Journal of Abnormal Psychology, 36,* 62–72.

Paul, G. L. (1963). The production of blisters by hypnotic suggestion: another look. *Psychosomatic Medicine, 25,* 233–244.

Perini, G. I., Fornasa, C. V., Cipriani, R., Bettin, A., Zecchino, F., & Peserico, A. (1984). Life events and alopoecia areata Psychotherapy. *Psychosomatics, 41,* 48–52.

Peters, J. E., Lundy, R. M., & Stern, R. M. (1973). Skin temperature and hypnosis. *International Journal of Clinical and Experimental Hypnosis, 21,* 205–212.

Pons, J. (1892). Sympathetic insanity. In D. Hack Tuke (Ed.), *Dictionary of psychological medicine* (p. 262). London: Churchill.

Preston, K. (1969). Depression and skin disease. *Medical Journal of Australia, i,* 326–329.

Rajka, G. (1975). *Atopic Dermatitis.* London: W. B. Saunders.

Ratliff, R. G., & Stein, N. H. (1968). Treatment of neurodermatitis by behaviour therapy: a case study. *Behaviour Research and Therapy, 6,* 397–399.

Ratnoff, O. D. (1969). Stigmata: where mind and body meet. *Medical Times, 97,* 150–163.

Rechardt, E. (1970). *An investigation in the psychosomatic aspects of prurigo Besnier.* Monographs from the Psychiatric Clinic of the Helsinki University Central Hospital, Helsinki.

Roberts, A. N., Kewman, D. G., & Macdonald, H. (1973). Voluntary control of skin temperature. *Journal of Abnormal Psychology, 82,* 163–168.

Robertson, I., Jordan, J. M., & Whitlock, F. A. (1975). Emotions and the skin II. The conditioning of scratch responses in cases of lichen simplex. *British Journal of Dermatology, 92,* 407–412.

Rook, A., & Dawber, R. (1982). *Diseases of the hair and scalp.* Oxford, England: Blackwell.

Ross, W. D. (1954). Psychosomatic disorders and psychoses. In E. Wittkower & R. A. Clehgorn (Eds.), *Recent developments in psychosomatic medicine.* London: Pitman.

Rothman, S. (1960). Pathophysiology of itch sensation. In W. Montagna (Ed.), *Advances in biology of skin, Vol. 1.* Oxford, England: Pergamon.

Sainsbury, P. (1960). Psychosomatic disorder and neurosis in out-patients attending general hospital. *Journal of Psychosomatic Research, 4,* 261–273.

Sanborn, D. E., Sanborn, C. J., Cimbolie, P., & Niswander, G. D. (1972). Suicide and stress-related dermatoses. *Diseases of the Nervous System, 33,* 391–394.

Savin, J. A., Patterson, W. D., Oswald, I., & Adam, K. (1975). Further studies of scratching during sleep. *British Journal of Dermatology, 93,* 297–302.

Seville, R. H. (1977). Psoriasis and stress. *British Journal of Dermatology, 97,* 297–302.

Seville, R. H. (1978). Psoriasis and stress II. *British Journal of Dermatology, 98,* 151–153.

Sharma, O. P., & Balchum, O. J. (1972). Alcohol-induced pain and itching by hot shower in sarcoidosis. *American review of Respiratory Disease, 106,* 763–766.

Shelley, W. B. (1953). Dyshidrosis (pompholyx). *Archives of Dermatology and Syphilology, 68,* 314–319.

Shoemaker, R. J. (1963). A search for the affective determinants of chronic urticaria. *Psychosomatics, 4,* 125–132.

Slorach, J. (1953). The skin and psychosis. In E. Wittkower & B. Russell (Eds.), *Emotional factors in skin disease.* London: Cassell.

Smitz, S., Legros, J-J., & LeMaire, M. (1982). Naloxone, itch, urticaria and angio oedema. *Annals of Internal Medicine, 97,* 788–789.

Sneddon, I. B. (1949). The mind and the skin. *British Medical Journal, I,* 472–475.

Sneddon, I. B. (1982). Rosacea and rhinophyma. In S. Maddin (Ed.), *Current dermatologic therapy* (p. 619). Philadelphia, PA: W. B. Saunders.

Sneddon, I. B. (1983). Simulated disease: Problems in diagnosis and management. *Journal of the Royal College of Physicians of London, 17,* 199–205.

Sneddon, I. B., & Sneddon, J. (1975). Self-inflicted injury: A follow-up study of 43 patients. *British Medical Journal, iii,* 527–530.

Sneddon, I. B., & Sneddon, J. (1981). Acne excoriee: A protective device. *British Journal of Dermatology, 105* (Supp. 19), 29.

Sobye, P. (1950). Rosacea, aetiology and pathogenesis. *Acta Dermato-Venereologica, 30,* 137–150.

Solomon, G. F., Amkraut, A. A., & Kasper, P. (1974). Immunity, emotions and stress. *Psychosomatics, 23,* 209–217.

Stein, M., Schiavi, R. C., & Camerino, M. (1976). Influence of brain and behaviour on the immune system. *Science, 191,* 435–440.

Stokes, J. H. (1940). The personality factor in psychoneurogenenous reactions of the skin. *Archives of Dermatology and Syphiliogy, 42,* 780–801.

Stokes, J. H., Kulchar, G. V., & Pillsbury, D. M. (1935). Effect on the skin of emotional and nervous states. Aetiologic background of urticaria with special reference to psychoneurogeneous factors. *Archives of Dermatology and Syphilogy, 31,* 470–499.

Summerfield, J. A. (1980). Naloxone modulates the perception of itch in man. *British Journal of Clinical pharmacology, 10,* 180–183.

Surman, O. S., Gottlieb, S. K., Hackett, T. B., & Silverberg, E. L. (1973). Hypnosis in the treatment of warts. *Archives of General Psychiatry, 28,* 439–441.

Sweet, R. D. (1952). On the treatment of anogenital pruritus. *Lancet, II,* 258–262.

Tenzel, J. H., & Taylor, R. L. (1969). An evaluation of hypnosis and suggestion as treatment of warts. *Psychosomatics, 10,* 252–257.

Thomas, A., Stern, M., & Lilienfield, A. (1956). Relationship of psychosis and psychosomatic disease. *Journal of Nervous and Mental Disease, 123,* 249–256.

Thurston, H. (1952). *The physical phenomena of mysticism.* London: Burns Oates.

Twerski, A. J., & Naar, R. (1974). Hypnotherapy in a case of refractory dermatitis. *American Journal of Clinical Hypnosis, 16,* 202–205.

Twiston Davis, J. H. (1951). Psychosomatic factors in dermatology. *British Journal of Physical Medicine and Industrial Hygiene, 14,* 155–160.

Ullman, M. (1947). Herpes simplex and second degree burns induced under hypnosis. *American Journal of Psychiatry, 103,* 828–830.

Ullman, M., & Dudek, S. (1960). On the psyche and warts II. Hypnotic suggestion and warts. *Psychosomatic Medicine, 22,* 68–76.

Walton, D. (1960). The application of learning theory to the treatment of a case of neurodermatitis. In H. J. Eysenck (Ed.), *Behaviour therapy and the neuroses.* Oxford, England: Pergamon.

Warin, R. P., & Champion, R. H. (1974). *Urticaria.* London: W. B. Saunders.

Waxman, D. (1973). Behavior therapy of psoriasis: A hypnoanalytic and counter-conditioning technique. *Postgraduate Medical Journal, 49,* 591–595.

Whitlock F. A. (1957). Neuropsychiatric concepts in relation to dermatology. *Transaction of the St. John's Hospital Dermatological Society, 38,* 8–12.

Whitlock, F. A. (1961). Psychosomatic aspects of rosacea. *British Journal of Dermatology, 73,* 137–148.

Whitlock, F. A. (1976). *Psychophysiological aspects of skin disease.* London: W. B. Saunders.

Whitlock, F. A., & Hynes, J. V. (1978). Religious stigmatization: A historical and psychophysiological inquiry. *Psychological Medicine, 8,* 185–202.

Wilkins, J. K. (1983). Flushing reactions. In A. J. Rook & H. I. Maiback (Eds.), *Recent advances in dermatology, No. 6.* Edinburgh, Scotland: Churchill-Livingstone.

Wilkinson, D. S. (1972). Psoriasis. In A. Rook, D. S. Wilkinson, & F. J. G. Ebling (Eds.), *Textbook of dermatology* (p. 1192). Oxford, England: Blackwell.

Wittkower, E., & Russell, B. (Eds.). (1953). *Emotional factors in skin disease.* London: Cassell.

10

The Psychological and Behavioral Basis of Dermatological Disease

John de Korte

Division of Psychodermatology,
Department of Dermatology
Academic Medical Centre
Amsterdam, The Netherlands

Herman Musaph

State University of Utrecht
Amsterdam, The Netherlands

A HISTORY OF PSYCHODERMATOLOGY

In many respects the historical development of psychodermatology corresponds with the development of psychosomatic medicine in general. It was Alexander and French who, in 1948, described seven psychosomatic diseases, one of them being neurodermatitis. For many years Alexander studied the symbolic meaning of these diseases, emphasizing the influence of psychodynamic conflicts as a psychogenic factor. Wittkower (1947) and Wittkower and Russell (1953) also concentrated on psychogenic factors. These psychoanalysts were inspired by Freudian concepts. Later on, Obermayer (1955) and Borelli (1967) wrote excellent surveys on the psyche and skin.

As psychosomatic researchers became more and more interested in psychological factors concerning the course and the treatment of disorders, within psychodermatology this led to studies on coping mechanisms in psoriasis, touching behavior in infantile eczema, and stigmatization processes in skin diseases in general. During the last few years multidisciplinary teamwork, both in research and in treatment, has become more important. Clinical practice has been enriched by psychotherapeutic approaches like group counseling and family therapy, and the patients themselves have become involved in self-helping activities. The aforementioned shift in the object of psychodermatology reflects the development of research methods and research conceptualization as well. This development may be described in three phases (Musaph, 1976).

The Anecdotal, Psychoanalytic Phase

In the 1940s and 1950s psychiatrists made detailed descriptions of emotional conflict situations being a trigger for the outburst of efflorescenties in, for instance, neurodermatitis or urticaria chronica.

A case study. A 19-year-old girl developed a skin disease characterized by vesicles over her entire body, especially the forearms. It started with pain in her hands "just as though there were splinters in them." No organic course could be found. During the interviews with the patient, she said that the vesicles appeared the day after the performance of a play in which she had a leading part as Jael, the maid servant of Maria Magdalena in ancient Jerusalem. In this play Jael, sent on an errand, is grabbed by Roman soldiers who try to rape her. This is prevented by Bar Abba, leader of the revolting Zelotes, who stabs one of the soldiers with his knife. Covered with scratches and bruises, Jael faints and then falls in love with him. Bar Abba is imprisoned. Later on, she tells Maria Magdalena about her love, and she tries to free him by telling his prison guards she is a whore and he is her only brother.

The patient said that—during the performance—it was hard to express words of love about Bar Abba, since the man who played this part was a creepy fellow, past 50, and always flirting. She also had difficulties in telling the prison guards she was a whore, especially while her parents were in the audience. They could say: "That is exactly how you really are." After the appearence of the skin disease, the mother suggested it might be a venereal disease.

In this case the play was a trigger phenomenon. From the dynamic point of view the patient had strong neurotic guilt feelings, deeply rooted in her personality, and as an endeavor to get rid of this guilt she experienced a strong need for punishment. The emotional conflict situation was actuated in the play, and the psychogenic skin disease—diagnosed as bullosia psychogenica—was to be considered as a primary expression in body language of her unbearable emotional conflict.

The many case studies published in the 1940s and 1950s have given us striking examples of the relationship between the onset of a skin disease, the presence of an emotional conflict situation, and a given personality structure. They all are rather convincing in that particular case, although the specific mechanisms in this relationship have not been described sufficiently, and the generalization of results is highly questionable. Nevertheless, these anecdotal studies have given us a better understanding of emotional factors in skin diseases. They also instigated further psychodermatological research.

The Methodological Phase

At the end of the 1950s and the beginning of the 1960s there arose strong opposition to the anecdotal approach. Psychologists wanted to purify research from biased ideology and unjustified conclusions. They pointed out that conclusions had to be drawn from material sufficient and suitable for statistical analysis, scientific evaluation, and prediction.

A good example of this new approach is a study by Baughman and Sobel (1971) on psoriasis vulgaris. Over a period of 5 years these investigators studied 252 adults who had been hospitalized for psoriasis. They used standardized personality inventories, and they came to the conclusion that there is no specific personality profile or specific emotional conflict situation appearing as a trigger phenomenon in psoriasis, "although there is a modest but statistically significant relationship between stress and psoriasis" (Baughman & Sobel, 1971, p. 603).

Another example is Brown's study, "Stress as a precipitant factor in eczema" (1972). He studied 82 cases of eczema using questionnaires and clinical interviews, with a control group of 123 outpatients of a dental hospital. He concluded that, within 12 months preceding the onset of eczema, separation experiences other than bereavement were significantly common, being admitted to by 21%, compared with 7% of the controls. Furthermore, 48% of the eczema patients admitted to having suffered from a severe shock, worry, or emotional upset within

6 months preceding the eczema onset, which is highly significant compared with 15% of the controls.

In these studies bias was largely excluded by applying a sound statistical methodology. The representative samples consisted of tens, hundreds, and sometimes thousands of patients (Farber, Bright, & Nall, 1968). The interviews were standardized, the tests were highly valid, and control groups were carefully chosen. Many hypotheses, originated in the anecdotal phase, were rejected—for instance, the hypothesis of a specific psoriasis character. Purely psychogenic skin diseases turned out to be relatively rare.

However, these studies raised questions as well. Sometimes researchers could not meet the highest methodological standards and had to restrict themselves to a sample of available patients in a clinic. In other cases, researchers became too dependent upon the self-reports of their patients. Brown (1972), for instance, described the tendency of some patients to deny emotional disturbances and to avoid subjective phenomena. And the objective Social Readjustment Rating Scale, with 40 life-events to measure life stress—as used by Baughman and Sobel (1971)—did not measure the subjective impact of these life events upon the individual patient. All in all, the methodological approach has restricted and refined the speculations of the anecdotal phase and has introduced a less subjective research method.

The Integrative Phase

In the 1970s, opposition arose to the aforementioned methodological approach. The primacy of observable behavior and statistical inference was challenged, and new tendencies in psychodermatology were outlined. Some criticism was directed towards the confinement of emotion to behavior. The great advantage is obvious: Behavior can be measured. But are we still measuring aggression in a patient suffering from itching states when we describe the Autonomous Response Pattern (ARP) of specific physiological parameters (Musaph, 1976)? Do we measure social anxiety in psoriasis when we ask a group of patients to answer 24 questions on social interactions (van der Schaar, 1976–1977)? And do we measure emotional stress in eczema by standardized questionnaires and interviews (Brown, 1972)? These are questions about the validity of this approach.

Other questions arose from the need for theoretical insight and from clinical practice. How, for instance, is a modest correlation between stress and psoriasis exacerbations to be interpreted? What are the intrapsychological mechanisms involved in the aggression regulation in psychogenic pruritus (Musaph, 1967)? What is the rationale behind the stigmatization processes in eczema? And what are the implications for clinical practice? Statistical methodology is unable to give insight into the immense diversity of human motivation.

Meanwhile new developments in psychodermatology began to occur. Contacts were made with other disciplines, such as anthropology, biology, physiology, and sociology. The result was a bombardment of information and a growing awareness that both psychoanalysts and psychologists—in their specific research objective and research methods—had isolated themselves too much from the complexity of daily dermatological practice and direct contact between the doctor and the patient. Patients themselves became more emancipated and founded patients associations, asking for more practical help and care. Psychodermatology grew from what was once called an appendix of psychoanalysis into an integrative study: the study of the relationship between somatophysiologic and psychosocial factors in the onset, course, and treatment of skin diseases.

THE PSYCHOLOGICAL SIGNIFICANCE OF THE SKIN

In order to understand the emotional life of the skin patient it is necessary to have some insight in the psychological significance of the skin. We describe the following five aspects: Perception, expression, communication, beauty, and sexuality (de Korte, 1984).

Perception. In the traditional stimulus–response model, human behavior is considered to be highly dependent on the process of perception. Thus, the skin—the largest and most fundamental sense organ—plays an important part in human behavior, especially in relation to psychological processes such as communicating, learning, and satisfying human needs.

The skin enables us to experience pain, pressure, and temperature, but also more complex sensations like itch, ache, and tickle. In general these perceptions are pseudoautomatic: One is little aware of, or selective in, skin stimuli and responses. For instance, many people scratch behind their ears without realizing either the itching or the scratching. Only when stimuli and responses become intense does awareness grow.

Expression. In many cases, reddening, sweating, growing pale, and goose skin are considered physiological expressions of emotion. From a theoretical point of view it is hard to describe the psychophysiological dynamics, but in practice many instances can be given of people reddening from shame or sweating from fear. Meerloo (1955) made a careful study of what he called *archaic skin behavior* and pointed out that the tendency to make use of skin expressions increases when the possibility of verbal expressions is limited, hampered, or considered to be undesirable. Of course, the interpretation of these physiological phenomena has to be done very carefully. Not all of them are the expression of an emotion, and even if there is an emotional equivalent, the interpretation is not self-evident. Sweating, for instance, may refer to fear, but it may also be an expression of warmth or a state of excitement.

Communication. Emotional development is largely dependent on skin contact with key figures. Especially during the first months or even the first years of life the skin is the primary organ of communication. Early deprivation of skin contact may result in a wide range of emotional and relational problems, as may be concluded from studies by Cohen (1961), Spitz (1965), and Musaph (1964). From the age of 5 onwards, skin contact decreases, largely as a result of social learning processes (Huss, 1977). In adult life skin contact is regulated, restricted, and ritualized. In Western culture there even is a taboo on touching. Nevertheless, touching remains important, although very often in an erotic or sexual context.

Beauty. To a large extent physical beauty is determined by stature, hair, and skin. Most people associate a young, sound, and tanned skin with beauty, and an old, affected, and pale skin with ugliness. In general, people invest much time and energy to approach this ideal of beauty, and some even make use of cosmetic surgery or tattoos.

The beauty of the skin is of psychological significance because of its effect on human relations. Generally speaking, a beautiful skin attracts, whereas an ugly skin easily leads to avoidance or rejection. Because of the tendency to associate an ugly skin with an ugly character, some people—especially skin patients—may suffer from stigmatization processes (halo phenomenon).

Sexuality. In essence sexuality is a dermal activity. In no other contact is the skin so deeply involved. Caressing, stroking, and kissing are only some of the activities to stimulate erotic and sexual excitement, and both male and female have their orgasm because of skin stimulation. On the one hand there is a taboo on sexuality—being associated with feelings of shame, guilt, and inferiority. On the other hand, there is a kind of surplus value: Extreme emphasis on sexuality and sexual attractiveness often reflects a need for contact, warmth, and intimacy. Some people try to compensate a lack of intimacy with sexual activities. A study by Hollender, Luborsky, and Scaramella (1969) illustrates this phenomenon. They studied 39 women with psychiatric disorders and concluded that their strong need to be held and cuddled—primarily because of lack of affective skin contact during childhood—was expressed by their desire to be held with 'adult' sexuality.

CHILD DEVELOPMENT AND SKIN CONTACT

The aforementioned significance of skin contact during early childhood has been illustrated in many studies. Bowlby (1969) put stress upon skin contact between the mother and the child in the process of attachment, which in itself is crucial for normal emotional development and intimate relationships in adulthood. Spitz (1965) studied the relationship between children with infantile eczema and their mothers, and observed a poverty of skin contact. This can be explained by repressed aggressive feelings and feelings of guilt towards these children. Only too often the mothers feel it is their fault the child has a skin disease. They may give all sorts of contents to their neurotic guilt feelings, depending on their life histories. The lack of skin contact, precisely in the phase of life when a child appears especially to need it, makes it more difficult for the child to identify with the mother, which can impede normal emotional development. An indication of the kind of relationship between a mother or a father and their child can be given by the skin contact between the key figures and the baby. In a good mother–child relationship there will be a maximum of contact between the hands of the mother and the skin of the child on her lap. The mother's hands are completely open, with the fingers slightly curved in a relaxed position. In another relationship, in which tension is typical between the mother and the baby, she will hold the baby with clenched fingers. In particular the left hand in a right-handed person, and vice versa, will show the fear of contact. We saw mothers, with unconscious aversion toward their babies, expressing this by hitting the child on their laps, pinching it and boxing it with their left hands. At the other end of the scale there is the behavior of the mother who uses her left hand to stroke, fondle, and caress the child in more or less the same way she strokes, fondles, and caresses her beloved partner.

The skin contact pattern is part of the mother's own social learning process: unconsciously she demonstrates how she has been treated by her own mother. Many mothers, still childlike themselves, have to be taught how to touch and caress a baby. However, to change their behavior, one has to combat an archaic, rigid pattern (Klaus, Kennell,

Plumb, & Zuehlke, 1970). Nevertheless, we have to promote every strategy resulting in a better skin contact between the parents and the child. This must awaken and maintain a feeling of trust, belonging, and acceptance. In this connection it is worth noting that the great advantage of breast feeding over bottle feeding is the better skin contact between the mother and the baby. And even when the mother feeds with a bottle, it is advisable to do this with a bare breast. So one should advise all young mothers to offer a bare breast when feeding, as a surface contact with the naked or nearly naked baby.

THE PSYCHOLOGICAL MEANING OF SKIN DISEASES

Psychodermatology has given us a deeper understanding of the psychological significance of skin diseases. During the anecdotal phase, for instance, much attention was paid to skin diseases considered to be a somatic expression of an emotion. Obermayer (1955) stated that patients with hyperhidrosis express their feelings of fear in excessive sweating, and that patients with rosacea express fear, shame, and guilt in the excessive redness of their skin. Borelli (1967) described feelings of the same kind in these patients, and Meerloo (1957) concluded that the presence of these skin diseases has the function of camouflage: They prevent others from observing shame and anxiety, since redness or sweating are permanently present.

Other researchers put stress upon the inability of skin patients to express their feelings. Wittkower (1947) studied acne patients and noticed that, within their families, there was a strong repression of feelings, and Musaph (1967) described the repression of aggressive feelings in patients with psychogenic pruritus. Repression of feelings may also be a patient's reaction to the skin disease itself. For instance, many patients with psoriasis or vitiligo tend to repress their emotions while they are ashamed of their skin. In general we may say that every skin patient has his own unique reactions to the disease, depending upon the objective severity of the specific skin disease, the personality structure, and the life situation. Objective severity—determined by character, size, duration, and visibility of the skin disease—is not a predominant factor in the patient's reactions. Lipowski (1983) pointed out that patients have different attitudes and different responses to the same disease. The personality structure, and the life situation of the patient, primarily determine the subjective severity of a specific skin disease. Of course, we all know this from our own experience. In clinical practice we are regularly confronted with patients having a minor skin disease and at the same time experiencing many emotional problems, and on the other hand we meet patients with severe skin diseases seemingly having no problems at all. The subjective severity is expressed by the patient's behavior or reactions. Feelings of guilt, excessive shame, and emotional armoring are especially common. Patients with excessive shame express themselves with timid or submissive behavior, or even by social isolation. And emotional armoring is often expressed by indifferent, apathetic, or even exhibitory behavior.

On a conscious level skin patients may desperately long for affectionate (skin) contact. Their reactions, however, impede this to some extent and must be seen as an unconscious protection against stress, conflict, and pain. Deprivation of skin contact may partly be compensated for by automutilation of the skin, for instance by excessive skin care, tickling, or scratching. Of course, excessive mutilation gives raise to skin diseases as well, as will be described further down. Some examples are dermatitis artefacta, trichotillomania, and cutaneous hypochondriasis. They may also negatively influence the course of the disease, as in lichen simplex, acne excorie, and pruritus anogenitalis. From this we may conclude that some skin diseases may be seen as a signal of deprivation of skin contact.

ITCHING AND SCRATCHING

Itching and scratching are fundamental phenomena in psychodermatology. They may be regarded as basic behavioral variables appearing in many patients suffering from dermatoses. In dermatology, itching is well known as a symptom of scabies, pediculosis, insect bites, urticaria, atopic dermatitis, contact dermatitis, lichen ruber planus, Morbus Duhring, and miliaria. There are also many internal diseases associated with itching states, like diabetes mellitus, nephritis, disorders of the liver, gout, disorders of the thyroid gland, food allergies, Hodgkin's disease, leukemia, and carcinomatoses. Furthermore, itching can be found in senility and during pregnancy. In fact, itching and scratching are not only well-known phenomena in medicine: They appear in every human being.

Itching is well known in situations where stories are told concerning fleas and itching states. We observed itching and scratching in students listening to explanations of psychogenic pruritus and pruritus anogenitalis. This can be explained by the mechanism of identification with the victim, well known by medical students when a patient is demonstrated.

Identification is not the only mechanism operating. There are people who feel itching in an unpleasant situation, for example, when they are verbally attacked and, as a reaction, are flabbergasted. Some people react with blushing, others with goose-skin or freezing (Todstellreflex). Some people feel itching, for instance, in their hands. Very often the explanation is clear: There is a blocking of aggressive feelings. The aggressive tendencies, forbidden by the superego, are warded off. When this happens chronically, we speak of characterological armouring. Then there is a disorder in the aggression regulation. The defense against aggressive feelings is too strong. Instead of feelings of rage, hate, or resentment, there appears an itching state.

Itching and Scratching As Derived Activities

Tinbergen (1952) defined *derived activities* as outlets through which thwarted drives can express themselves in motion. Formerly, these were called *sparking-over mechanisms*. There are innate motor patterns in fish, birds, and mammals, but not necessarily in man. Tinbergen (1952, p. 16) mentioned: "I happen to have observed that chimpanzees under certain conditions of frustration of feeding are subject to violent outbursts of scratching." In man, everybody can observe yawning; rubbing one's skin, hands, or nose; passing a hand over one's hair; pinching a part of the body; and lighting a cigarette. The person in question mostly does not know what he or she is doing, the motions being unconscious. They may be signs of embarrassment, suppressed rage, sexual excitement, or impatience. So all these examples are experienced in situations in which an emotion is thwarted off. They are derived activities.

One of these derived activities is itching, resulting in scratching. When we are confronted with psychogenic itching states, we have to ask ourselves: What is the sense of being thwarted? Why is this person unable to work through his or her emotional conflict in a more adequate way, namely, by expressing the conflict and by experiencing the corresponding emotions? Why are itching states the 'solution' to an emotional conflict situation? Psychodynamically trained psychiatrists and psychologists have related this phenomenon to a disturbance of aggression regulation. And, in fact, there are many people suffering from itching states who have difficulties with their own aggressive feelings. Generally speaking, we may say: Symptom formation in itching and scratching occurs when an anger or anxiety impulse is signalled and warded off, and the central mechanism basic to it becomes active. This may result from a neurotic personality structure. For instance, when the superego does not permit a specific emotion—like rage—to be experienced.

A case study. A 29-year-old woman consulted her general practitioner because of severe itching states over the whole body. He referred her to the dermatologist, who could not find any dermatological or internal disorder. The patient was referred to one of us, and during the first interview the patient told a remarkable story. The severe itching state had its onset during the evening her parents-in-law were visiting her. They had not seen each other for a long time, since the parents had passionately denounced the marriage of their son. They had not even joined the wedding party. After 2 years of marriage a baby was born. Friends used their utmost endeavors to persuade the grandparents to visit their grandchild. This visit was paid, apparently in harmony. Everybody did his or her best to avoid anything that could spoil the atmosphere. At the end of the evening our patient saw her parents-in-law out and closed the door behind them. At that very moment the severe itching state appeared.

It seems to us that our patient:

1. had had aggressive feelings toward her parents-in-law for years,
2. thwarted her rage feelings spasmodically,
3. had an emotional conflict situation in which contradictory feelings were present, and
4. blamed herself for being so tolerant in accepting her grandparents for her child.

In search of other neurotic mechanisms we found that the disorder in the aggression regulation had existed for many years. We had the task of helping the patient to overcome her anxiety in experiencing her aggressive feelings during psychotherapy along analytic lines. The patient's ego was strong enough to work through her conflicts. This required a corrective experience of the repressed emotion and a strengthening of the ego. Her innumerable aggressive impulses were no longer held subliminal. They became reinforced, or, when the defenses became too weak, it was necessary to experience itching states. She became able to experience the real feelings themselves. The actual conflict had provoked a slumbering conflict with infantile roots, manifested in her life history.

Itching is not always aroused in a neurotic personality structure. Normally, it may also arise in response to an external stimulus or a pathological skin condition. Furthermore, it may be caused by physiological conditions, or by normal suggestive influences, such as produced by reading this paper. Then your itching is caused by an unconscious identification mechanism with the described patients. The difference between normal and pathological itching is that the latter is fixated in time, while the former quickly disappears. When there is no dermatological explanation at all for the itching, we speak of *primary psychogenic pruritus*. As a frequent side-effect of many dermatoses it is called *secondary pruritus*.

Scratching Without Itching

It is quite possible to scratch oneself without any experience of itching. A boring speaker can provoke scratching in his audience. While waiting for a traffic light, many people put their hands to their heads and start to scratch. Very often this is a silent protest against an unwanted situation, a derived activity to overcome feelings of frustration. When itching is provoked by scratching, the itching has the function of sanctioning the scratching. Some people develop a scratching technique in which they can produce a sensation of mild pain, giving them indubitable feelings of pleasure. Such a sensation, after violent scratching, is called the *afterglow*. Some of these actions may be interpreted as masturbation equivalents, especially when scratching is done in the genital sphere. In this respect scratching is an expression of skin eroticism. Scratching without itching may be an entirely unconscious action. In our opinion right-handed people especially use the left hand to make intimate gestures, being more remote from the subject's consciousness. It may be considered as an expression of certain autoerotic and autoaggressive impulses. This means that feelings of embarrassment, anger, resentment, joy, tense expectation, sexual excitement, anxiety, and fear could be expressed in motor language.

PSYCHODERMATOLOGICAL TREATMENT

General practitioners and dermatologists familiar with the psychosomatic approach tend to be patient centered, enabling patients to discuss the emotional aspects of the skin disease and helping them overcome their psychosocial problems. In this way many patients are given a psychodermatological treatment. Nevertheless, skin patients may suffer from severe emotional and relational problems, too complicated to treat within the doctor–patient relationship.

In our department we have the opportunity to offer skin patients individual, family, or group psychotherapy. Since dermatological practice is focused on the treatment of individual patients, and since most readers will be familiar with the individual psychotherapeutic approach, we will restrict ourselves to a description of family and group psychotherapy with skin patients.

Family Therapy

Families are able to cope more or less successfully with psychosocial stress. The degree of success depends on the personalities of the family members, the kinds of relationships they have with each other, and the flexibility with which they are able to use various patterns of behavior. Within families with a restricted ability to cope with stress, these problems may become serious to such an extent that professional help is needed. For instance, when a mother with alopecia isolates herself because of feelings of shame, and the children—being neglected—develop concentration problems in school, we have an effect that runs through the family. It also happens that skin disease appears to be a symptom of more deep-seated emotional conflicts within the family. Consider, for instance, when an adolescent daughter starts to scratch excessively because of repressed erotic and sexual feelings within the family.

A case study. Two children with atopic eczema were referred to our outpatient department. The father of these children appeared to have psoriasis, and the mother was the only member of the family without a skin disease. After some time, our dermatologist noted that, in the presentation of their complaints, a different member was always in the limelight. So, when the skin of the daughter improved, the skin of the son worsened alternatively. He also noted that, somehow, the parents were bowed down by cares. Thanks to the good relationship between the dermatologist and the family, it was possible to suggest seeing the psychotherapists of the department in order to discuss their problems with their children. During the intake interview with the family, the following problems were presented:

1. Both children had sleep disturbances. They itched, scratched, and screamed during the night. Because of this the parents also slept badly, and they did not know how to react to their children.
2. The 4-year-old son also screamed and yelled during the daytime, especially when something was forbidden for him. The mother felt ashamed and, at the same time, was afraid that the father would hit the child.
3. The attention paid to the skin was time-consuming and unpleasant.

Both parents said they had to marry when the mother became pregnant. The mother experienced the marriage as a loss of face, the father as a loss of freedom.

Initially, our treatment was directive and concerned with practical problems. The partners found it hard to verbalize their feelings and experiences, and to reflect upon them. Moreover, their attitude was anxious and "wait and see." Structure and support, and quick relief from their burden, seemed appropriate. So, in order to get more sleep, it was agreed that at night the parents would alternate their care of their children. One night the father would be taking care, the other night the mother. When the son was screaming and yelling during the daytime—in order to attain an object—the parents would react consistently. A "yes" from the father would be a "yes" from the mother, and a "no" would stay a "no." Furthermore, the mother contacted the teacher of her son to discuss the family problems and to ask for support, and the father consented to not hitting the children.

These agreements, made step by step, brought relief to the parents. This enabled them to become more reflective and to discover some of their problems. They realized they behaved inconsistently towards their children, and they confronted each other with their different ideas about upbringing. We were able to ask questions about their own parents, and they were willing to reflect and to talk. One discovery had a great impact on both parents, the mother in particular. She realized that, somehow, she did not like the children sleeping better and the son seeking less attention through screaming. She became increasingly confronted with her own problems, and she felt lonelier than ever. One of the functions of their problems was discovered.

The 10 interviews we had resulted in an improvement of the family's situation. There were less sleep disturbances, less screaming during daytime, and the attention paid to the skin had become easier. Both parents, especially the mother, realized that the problems with their children had covered more deep-seated problems. We advised the parents to continue with long-term couple therapy.

In our practice we have seen many cases in which the onset, the course, or the cure of a skin disease may be influenced within the family. Therefore, we think that, in some cases, the general practitioner or dermatologist should inform himself about the family situation. Such cases include chronic skin disease in which psychosomatic aspects may play a part, cases of children with skin disease, and also when the skin disease seems to give rise to psychological stress. If problems within the family are ascertained, referral to psychotherapy has to be made very carefully to prevent defensive reactions from the patient. In the patient's mind, he or she has come for the medical treatment of a skin disease.

Family therapy may improve the course and the cure of skin diseases. It may improve the ability to cope with stress, resulting in better care of the skin. It may also resolve emotional conflicts covered by the skin disease, resulting in an improvement of the skin. In the care of our family there were weekly contacts with the dermatologist at the beginning, and 3 monthly contacts at the end. In addition, the patients experienced their skin diseases as less severe.

Group Psychotherapy

One of the advantages of group psychotherapy is that it is a very appropriate method to help patients who find it difficult to express their feelings and to reflect upon their experiences, but who are able to gain insight from the experiences of others. Sharing, identification, and interpersonal learning, for instance, are important group psychotherapeutic mechanisms. This is more important with chronic skin patients, since feelings of shame and guilt, and hampered social contacts, are common among them (de Korte & Vintura, 1986).

We organize small, open groups with skin patients who are motivated to take part in weekly sessions during a period ranging from months to several years. Within the group there is a diversity of clinical conditions, but eczema, vitiligo, psoriasis, and alopecia are common. The most important objective is to treat more deep-seated emotional conflicts in order to achieve a disidentification with the skin and an improvement of social skills. Within the therapy group many themes are discussed, such as the skin disease itself, social problems, the family situation, sexuality, and traumatic experiences. In general the development of the group process determines the themes being discussed. In this group development we distinguish four phases: orientation, exploration, integration, and termination.

In the beginning there is an orientation towards each other and towards the therapists. A central issue is the skin disease itself, and the problems everyone has in dealing with the disease. Patients talk about medical treatment, contacts with nonpatients, fear of being rejected by colleagues or acquaintances, and so on. This starts very standoffish, but very soon patients feel more free to express themselves, because they recognize their own problems in the other patients'. Experiencing and expressing pent-up emotions is an important part of the therapeutic process. The patients become more confident, and the group grows from a group of individuals—talking about *you* and *me*—towards a cohesive group—talking about *we*. This developing group cohesiveness enables the group to explore their own problems.

During the phase of exploration the patients are reflecting upon their own experiences and feelings of everyday life. They are exploring their feelings, for instance, when they are rejected by key figures like their mother, husband, or child. Gradually, this exploration becomes more and more directed towards experiences within the therapy group. With the focus on the here-and-now situation the third phase starts, the phase of integration. Patients feel the liberty of experiencing and expressing aggression, conflict, and rivalry within the group. They become more open, sincere, direct, and concerned. This long and intensive phase is of importance because of its impact upon everyday life outside the group. Patients become less concerned with their skin; they behave more easily in social situations, and they feel up to finishing group psychotherapy (de Korte, 1982).

Three out of four patients are able to finish group psychotherapy successfully: There is a disidentification with the skin and an improvement of social skills. Many patients experience an improvement of their skin as well, which probably has to do with an increased emotional stability and a lessened need to use the skin as a regulation system against psychological stress. The reverse of this phenomenon can be observed during the therapy as well: During stressful moments, patients tend to start talking about their skin. We call this "regression to the skin."

REFERENCES

Alexander, F., & French, T. M. (1948). *Studies in psychosomatic medicine.* New York: Ronald Press.

Baughman, R., & Sobel, R. (1971). Psoriasis, stress and strain. *Archives of Dermatology, 103,* 599–605.

Borelli, S. (1967). Psyche und Haut. In J. Jadassohn (Ed.), *Handbuch der Haut-und Geschlechts-Krankheiten* (Vol. 8). Berlin: Springer Verlag.

Bowlby, J. (1969). *Attachment and loss. Vol. I: Attachment.* London: The Hogarth Press.

Brown, D. G. (1972). Stress as a precipitant factor in eczema. *Journal of Psychosomatic Research, 16,* 321–327.

Cohen, S. (1961). The skin-brain barrier. *Archives of Dermatology, 83,* 106–110.

Farber, E. M., Bright, R. D., & Nall, M. L. (1968). A questionnaire survey of psoriasis. *Archives of Dermatology, 98,* 248–259.

Hollender, M. H., Luborsky, J., & Scaramella, T. J. (1969). Body contact and sexual excitement. *Archives of General Psychiatry, 20,* 188–191.

Huss, J. A. (1977). Touch with care or a caring touch? *American Journal of Occupational Therapy, 31,* 11–18.

Klaus, M. H., Kennell, J. H., Plumb, N., & Zuehlke, S. (1970). Human maternal behavior at the first contact with her young. *Pediatrics, 46,* 187–192.

de Korte, J. (1982). Psychotherapeutische Moglichkeiten bei psoriasis. *Aktuelle Dermatologie, 8,* 160–162.

de Korte, J. (1984). *The psychology of the psoriasis patient.* Essex, Holland: Amstelveen.

de Korte, J., & Vintura, L. A. (1986). Psychodermatology through the group process. In J. H. Lacey & D. A. Sturgeon (Eds.), *Proceedings of the 15th European Conference on Psychosomatic Research*. London: J. H. Libbey & Co.

Lipowski, Z. J. (1983). Psychosocial reactions to physical illness. *Canadian Medical Association Journal, 28,* 1069–1072.

Meerloo, J. A. M. (1955). Archaic behavior and the communicative act. *Psychiatric Quarterly, 29,* 60–72.

Meerloo, J. A. M. (1957). Human camouflage and identification with the environment. *Psychosomatic Medicine, 19*(2), 89–98.

Musaph, H. (1964). *Itching and scratching, psychodynamics, in dermatology.* Basel & New York: Karger.

Musaph, H. (1967). Psychogenic pruritus. *Dermatologica, 135,* 126–130.

Musaph, H. (1976). Psychodermatology. In O. W. Hill (Ed.), *Modern trends in psychosomatic medicine 3*. London: Butterworths.

Musaph, H. (1977). Skin, touch and sex. In J. Money & H. Musaph (Eds.), *Handbook of sexology*. Amsterdam, New York: Elsevier, Excerpta Medica.

Obermayer, M. E. (1955). *Psychocutaneous medicine.* Springfield, IL: C. C. Thomas.

van der Schaar, W. W. (1976–77). Psychometric investigation in 48 Dutch patients suffering from psoriasis. *Psychotherapy & Psychosomatics, 27,* 159–162.

Spitz, R. A. (1965). *The first year of life.* New York: International University Press.

Tinbergen, N. (1952). Derived activities, their causation, biological significance, origin and emancipation. *Quarterly Review of Biology, 27,* 1–32.

Wittkower, E. (1947). The psychological aspects of skin disease. *Bulletin of the Menninger Clinic, 11,* 148–168.

Wittkower, E., & Russell, B. (1953). *Emotional factors in skin diseases.* New York: Hoeber.

11

The Psychological and Behavioral Management of Psychosomatic Dermatoses

Myriam Van Moffaert

Department of Psychiatry
and
Department of Psychodermatology
University Hospital Ghent, Belgium

INTRODUCTION

A definite link between emotional factors or psychological issues on the one hand, and the genesis, onset, or precipitation of recurrent dermatoses on the other, has been previously acknowledged (Wittkower & Russell, 1953; Wittkower & Lester, 1960; Musaph, 1976; Whitlock, 1976).

Patients with psychosomatic dermatoses attribute, rightly or wrongly, their skin disorders to emotional factors: They impute an attack of alopecia areata to a psychotraumatic experience, or a recurrence of psoriasis to a particularly stressful life-event (e.g., divorce).

Physicians in general, and dermatologists in particular, are well aware of the definite role psychological factors play in the etiology and outcome of dermatoses. In their daily practice they are confronted with the secondary psychological consequences which are due to the visibility and impact of the dermatoses on the sufferer's body image and social identity.

There is an impressive body of literature on the psychogenesis of dermatoses. Many of these studies have an outstanding descriptive quality, but they are basically anecdotal. Furthermore, many of the earlier reports do not meet the methodological requirements of today. Important research papers published in the heyday of psychosomatic medicine (Alexander, 1952; Macalpine, 1958) attributed psychosomatic dermatoses to specific personality traits and specific psychological triggering conflicts and failed to make the necessary distinction between emotional causative factors and the secondary psychosocial effects of skin disorders. The anecdotal reports, which focused too narrowly on the specificity hypothesis, and the methodologically unsound early studies, have now been superseded by research articles which meet current methodological standards and which adduce statistical evidence for the quantitative correlations between life-events and a variety of skin disorders (Fava, Perini, Santonasto, & Fornasa, 1980).

Equating the psychological correlates of skin disorders with a psychological cause is still speculative (Whitlock, 1976). It is particularly the lack of insight into the exact pathophysiological pathway between stressful life experiences or personality factors and the resulting skin lesions which impedes an overall applicability of psychotherapy and behavioral treatments to dermatological disorders. More systematic research on behavioral approaches to psychodermatoses, as well as new research directions in psychoneuroimmunology and psychoneuroendocrinology should fill the present void in our knowledge (Panconesi, 1984).

Despite this present incomplete understanding of the pathophysiology of psychosomatic dermatology and of the biobehavioral pathway of dermatoses, it is generally agreed that dermatological practice needs complementary psychological and behavioral treatment techniques.

The need to integrate psychobehavioral concepts in all areas of medicine has been increasingly accepted and has resulted in a range of distinctive fields such as psychosomatic medicine, consultation-liaison psychiatry, general hospital psychiatry, and behavioral medicine. Dermatology, however, is unique in that it deals with an organ which can be readily seen and touched. Emotions are reflected directly in skin changes. The normal physiological concomitants of fear, anxiety, and shame, as well as of sexual excitation and pleasure, are visible in blushing, hair-raising, or growing pale. Aggression, frustration, or irritation may be directly expressed in itching, paresthesias, hyperhidrosis, or rash. Subjective skin symptoms, for example, pain, itching, and erythema, will differ in the intensity with which they are experienced in direct relation to emotional factors. The visibility of most dermatoses constitutes a specific problem and is bound to have a psychological impact. It elicits negative environmental responses. In Western society in particular, scars or damaged skin are objectionable. They are often, though mostly erroneously, considered contagious and may even carry the connotation of insufficient hygiene. The resulting self-depreciative feelings may reach an extent in which a complex of social fear and shame develops. A story by John Updike about a psoriasis-sufferer with a socially induced minority complex is suggestively entitled "The Leper." Apart from causing a social handicap, the visibility of dermatoses may constitute an issue in itself. Further, because the skin is the main organ of tactile interaction and its ease of accessibility has a particular impact on behavior, the impact of dermatoses on tactile communication, and consequently on bodily interactive behavior and sexual activity in particular, is immediate and crucial (Renshaw, 1980).

The skin also is a target organ for self-touching behavior. Its easy accessibility entails a variety of problems. Dermatoses which are purely organic in origin are exacerbated by habitual touching behavior. Scratching in particular brings about pathological changes in the skin and may thus aggravate a dermatosis. Because of the easy accessibility of the skin, many patients have direct access to their lesions. Touching, scratching, squeezing real or imaginary comedos, can all cause or aggravate dermatoses. Habitual skin care procedures often become part of an obsessional ritual. Prescribed skin treatment regimens can be affected by environmental stresses or by psychopathological features and result in overtreatment by the patient as part of a repetitive compulsive and potentially damaging behavior pattern. This particular feature makes dermatological disorders particularly relevant as a focus for research into the applicability of behavioral treatment techniques. The patient's behavior towards his or her lesions offers many clues for the psychological basis of skin complaints. Moreover, a large proportion of dermatoses is provoked or perpetuated by direct actions, which vary from automatic scratching and purposeless squeezing of the skin to conscious provocation of lesions on a skin site which may be symbolic of psychodynamic content. A variety of dermatoses are primarily psychological disorders which find their expression in skin symptoms (Cotterill, 1983b). Self-destructive tendencies may be expressed in trichotillomania, acné excoriée, or in factitious skin disorders. Delusions and hallucinations are frequently expressed in skin symptoms. Specific psychodermatological categories, such as delusions of infestation, dysmorphophobia, circumscript skin hypochondriasis, and the olfactory reference syndrome, have a purely psychiatric etiology and thus require a psychobehavioral approach.

Lastly, as many dermatoses have a chronic if not life-long duration, the practitioner will be compelled to deal with the psychological issues of a long-term therapeutic relationship, in which he or she will inevitably practice some form of psychological or behavioral management (Medansky & Handler, 1981).

All skin disorders, whether primarily organic or psychological in origin, may profit from a biobehavioral approach, both in terms of diagnosis and of treatment. This chapter tries to reflect the state of the art of the psychopharmacology, psychotherapy, and behavioral treatment of a variety of psychosomatic dermatoses.

PSYCHOTROPIC DRUGS IN DERMATOLOGY

A variety of psychotropic agents have been used in the treatment of psychosomatic dermatoses. The treatment with psychotropic drugs must depend on the existence of a causal link between the psychodermatological problem and a psychological factor (Crayton & Freedman, 1977).

Antipsychotics are the drugs of choice in dermatological syndromes that are rooted in psychosis, for example, delusions of infestation by insects, artifacts by self-injection of caustic concoctions, ordered by auditory hallucinations in schizophrenia.

When anxiety and/or depression are either part of the etiology or the consequence of the dermatosis, they can be reduced by anxiolytic or antidepressant drugs and so have an indirect beneficial effect on the dermatosis itself. The same indirect action may be presumed for psychotropic drugs which diminish irritability, tension or disregulation in self-aggression that lead to dermatitis artefacta (Sarti & Cossidenti, 1984).

The possible side effects of psychotropic drugs should always be evaluated. The use of benzodiazepines implies the risk of overcompliance, overconsumption, and dependency. Tricyclic antidepressants have anticholinergic side effects and may cause cardiac arrhythmias. Neuroleptics frequently have extrapyramidal side effects, occasionally leading to drug-induced dystonic reactions. The development of tardive dyskinesia is a serious, but rare, complication.

Among the vast number of reports on the drug treatment of psychophysiological skin disorders, there are only few randomly assigned, double-blind controlled clinical studies. Moreover, there is confusion over the usefulness of psychotropic drug treatment in psychodermatology. Each drug treatment has some placebo effect which is difficult to determine. The distinction between the direct cerebral effect of a psychotropic agent and its somatic effect is sometimes difficult to make; for example, beta-blocking agents in acné may act indirectly by anxiolysis through cerebral pathways or directly through reducing sebum excretion in the skin (Medansky & Handler, 1981). Psychotropic drugs act in a somatopsychic direction by their impact on the psychiatric repercussions of the somatic illness. Conversely, they have real psychosomatic effects by influencing the psychogenic factors of the psychodermatosis.

Comparative Psychotropic Drug Trials

Wittkower and Lester (1960) found that anxiety-reducing drugs were very helpful during the acute phase of any dermatosis, as adjuvants to the local dermatological treatment. They conducted a comparative study on 90 patients with varied dermatoses such as psoriasis, eczema, seborreic dermatitis, and acné vulgaris, which they treated with psychotropics exclusively. The relative efficacy of imipramine, chlorpromazine, chlordiazepoxide, meprobamate, and placebo was assessed in a double-blind non-cross-over study. In 60% of the cases a complete remission was attained. They also found that psychological symptoms tend to improve before the dermatological symptoms do, and that there is a positive correlation between the degree of improvement and the severity of the initial symptomatology. However, they found no differential effect that was a function of the type of psychotropic drug.

Neuroleptic Drugs

The efficacy of neuroleptic drugs is well documented in two different psychodermatological categories: dermatological syndromes rooted in psychotic conditions, so-called *monosymptomatic hypochondriacal psychoses* (moderate to high doses), and in pain and paresthesias (low dosage).

The main feature of monosymptomatic hypochondriacal psychosis (MHP) is a delusional belief of being diseased, despite the absence of factual evidence, which is sometimes accompanied by hallucinatory symptoms (Munro, 1983; Lyell, 1983). Among the variety of clinical forms, the most common syndromes are: the delusions of infestation, when the patient believes himself or herself to be infested with parasites or insects, and sometimes hallucinates that insects crawl over his or her skin; the delusions of dysmorphia; the olfactory reference syndrome, that is, the delusion of emitting an offensive body odor (Bishop, 1983); and the conviction of having skin cancer or a venereal disease. Exceptionally, the delusions of patients with dermal parasitosis are shared by two or even more family members or people living closely together, in a folie partagée (folie á deux, folie á trois) (Evans & Merskey, 1972).

The second indication of neuroleptics is the use of low dosages in pain and paresthesia syndromes such as glossodynia or glossopyrosis. Duke (1983) reports on the successful use of Pimozide in various conditions such as postherpetic neuralgia, neurotic excoriations, pain, and paresthesias. He suggests that the neuroleptic is useful for those conditions that defy classical dermatological management. It has only limited value in patients who suffer from severe pain alone, whereas it yields better results in patients with a combination of pain and a creeping type of paresthesia.

All neuroleptics may have both immediate and long-term side effects, mainly the iatrogenic Parkinson syndrome with extrapyramidal rigidity and the cogwheel phenomenon. Side effects such as sedation, apathy, even a more general neuroleptised syndrome (camisole chimique), are dosage bound. Dyskinesia is easily reversed by injecting an anti-Parkinson drug. Tardive dyskinesia occurs in 10% of patients treated on a chronic basis. These side effects should be accepted when psychosis is the psychodermatological indication. If, on the contrary, the neuroleptic treatment has the function of an anxiolytic, the risks of side effects may be too serious. In any case, the various risk factors have to be weighed out carefully, the nonpharmacological approaches should be given priority, and, if a tranquillizing psychotropic appears to be inevitable, benzodiazepines or anxiolytic antidepressants with sedative properties should be used. There is general agreement that the diagnostic categories of monosymptomatic delusional psychosis, delusional parasitosis, or the olfactory reference syndrome have to be treated over a sufficiently long period with a high dosage of a neuroleptic drug to get the desired effect.

There is still discussion on the diagnostic boundary between the monosymptomatic delusional psychodermatological syndromes, for which a neuroleptic drug treatment is mandatory, and the syndromes that are characterized by an overvalued idea, such as dysmorphophobia, which is rooted in the patient's personality. The importance of this phenomenological distinction is clinical: The overvalued ideas respond less favorably to neuroleptics than to insight-oriented psychotherapy. However, this point of view is challenged by Bishop (1980), who explains the overvalued ideas in terms of traumatic life experience and psychodynamics. He illustrates this with a patient with olfactory reference syndrome who complains of a persistent anal odor shortly after anal intercourse with his male friend for the first time. This hypochondriacal symptom, however, was not responsive to psychotherapy and required medication, from which the author concluded that the distinction between dysmorphophobia and monosymptomatic hypochondriasis is more of a theoretical nature than of clinical value.

A further point of discussion concerns the specificity of Pimozide in MHP. As Pimozide has specific dopamine antagonistic properties, Munro (1978) has advocated Pimozide as the drug of choice. In double-blind cross-over trials versus placebo, Pimozide was found to have a significant effect on delusions, and on pruritus.

Bourgeois and Nguyen-Lan (1986) have called the therapeutic specificity of Pimozide a myth that darkens the need for diagnostic nuances. They emphasize that the treatment should be tailored to the patient's individual needs and may include other psychotropic drugs (antidepressants), ECT, social measures, psychotherapy, or family therapy. Neuroleptic drugs other than Pimozide have been reported as equally effective if prescribed in equivalent doses—chlorpromazine 100 to 400 mg/d or trifluoroperazine 10 to 15 mg/d (Freinhar, 1984). Some of the treatment failures with Pimozide are probably not due to the inefficiency of the drug itself, but to compliance problems in these often uncooperative patients. Frithz (1979) found that, of 15 patients with delusions of infestation who had previously been treated with neuroleptics by mouth, 11 became totally symptom free after injections of depot-neuroleptics such as fluphenazine decanoate or cisflupentixole decanoate.

Various psychotropic agents (tranylcypromine, doxepin, and imipramine) have also been found to be effective in delusional-hypochondriacal dermatological syndromes, but further controlled trials are needed to elucidate this area.

Antidepressants

Depressive symptoms are not uncommon in dermatological practice. Stress-inducing life events, including loss and reactive depression, are commonly accepted as causative or precipitating factors of alopecia areata (Macalpine, 1958) and psoriasis (Fava et al., 1980). Although these dermatoses are very different on a pathophysiological level, they have in common that they are chronic and very visible diseases. It follows that many of the depressive symptoms encountered in both are a response to, rather than a cause of, the illness. Patients tend to suffer from a "leper-complex." Their self-esteem is lowered because of their appearence. They suffer from the inconvenience caused by the dermatosis itself and by the treatments, which often include occlusive dressings and the need to wear a bath cap or apply smelly ointments. They have to cope with other people's negative reactions to the unattractiveness of their skin. The efficacy of antidepressants in both conditions is doubtful, as the exact demarcation between depression as an etiological issue and as a reactive consequence is difficult to establish (Van Moffaert, 1982). Apart from the diagnosis of the dermatosis that is complicated by a depressive syndrome, one should be attentive to the diagnosis of a masked depression, also called depression sine depressione. This depressive subcategory, whose existence is not generally accepted, is characterized by somatic complaints, in this case of a dermatological nature, for which no organic explanation is found. The patient denies being depressed, but a thorough anamnesis and a probing psychiatric examination reveal different depressive symptoms, such as early awakening, anorexia, and anhedonia. The main diagnostic features lie in the course of the masking dermatological symptom, which tends to follow the diurnal pattern for depression (worse in the morning and improving later in the day).

Most antidepressant drug trials for psychosomatic skin disorders conducted between 1950 and 1970 compared tricyclic antidepressants with placebo, neuroleptics, or tranquilizers (Wittkower & Lester, 1960). Mono-amino-oxidase inhibiting antidepressants have been tried on a modest scale only, because of their potentially harmful side effects, for example, hypertensive crisis in interaction with sympathomimetic drugs, foods containing tyramine, and tricyclic antidepressants. Friedman et al. (1978) have tried Phenelzine in neurodermatitis. In a small group of 15 patients, and using diazepam as a control drug, they found the improvement with diazepam slight, while Phenelzine provided statistically significant improvements. Their working hypothesis was that change of the psychosomatic symptoms was dependent on the ultradian cycle desynchronization: Suppression of the rapid eye movement (REM) phase of the sleep–dream cycle (and its daytime counterpart of the ultradian biorhythm) seems to improve neurodermatitis (Friedman et al., 1978).

Both M.A.O.I. and tricyclic antidepressants have numerous and serious unwanted side effects: autonomic side-effects such as dry mouth, micturation difficulties, postural hypotension, and cardiovascular effects (e.g., tachycardia, changes in the E.C.G. with a risk of ventricular arrhytmias). Overdoses of tricyclic antidepressants are potentially lethal.

Second-generation antidepressants such as Mianserin, Viloxazine, and Fluvoxamine have fewer side effects and are therefore better tolerated by patients. This is important, as these are patients who have already some somatic discomfort and who will show noncompliance if the prescribed drugs have noticeable physical side effects (Sarti & Cossidenti, 1984).

Tranquilizers

Anxiety may be contributive to a dermatosis, concomitant to a skin disorder, or secondary to the skin problem. It may even be relieved by scratching (Medansky & Handler, 1981). If psychological stress, tension, anxiety, hostility, or irritation is an important factor in a dermatosis, the temporary use of anxiolytic drugs is called for. However, the prescription of an anxiolytic, in particular a benzodiazepine, can never be an isolated therapeutic answer. The patient should be introduced to alternative nonpharmacological measures to reduce anxiety as well. Furthermore, the prescription should be limited to a few weeks, covering only the acute anxiety situation, in view of the risks of dependency and overcompliance and of the possible effects of rebound of the initial anxiety symptom and the possible withdrawal effects when discontinuing the treatment. Hydroxizine hydrochloride is an antihistaminic drug which is often used by dermatologists as a tranquillizer in the treatment of urticaria (Medansky & Handler, 1981).

Novel Psychopharmacological Approaches

The possible role of cerebral endorphins in itch and pain, based on the evidence that morphine is not only analgesic but also causes pruritus, lead Bernstein et al. (1982) to use naloxone (a morphine antagonist) to treat histamine-provoked itch. They found naloxone reduced or even abolished itch. However, Fjellner and Hagermark (1984) reported that pretreatment with naloxone in 15 healthy volunteers did not influence the histamine-induced peripheral itching and cutaneous responses. The role of naloxone and other related opioid antagonists in the treatment of pruritic disorders has yet to be explicated. The role of endogenous opiate compounds (endorphins) has also been investigated in self-mutilative behavior. Richardson and Zaleski (1983) reported a reduction of self-inflicted pain behavior in an atypical Lesch-Nyhan like patient and in a Tourette's patient. These specific syndromes include self-mutilative behavior with gross psychiatric and neurologic defects or severe mental subnormality (Coppola & Rolek, 1975). It is still speculative whether or not opioid antagonists or Gaba-analogues are useful in skin self-mutilation (Primrose, 1979).

Concluding Remarks

The rational use of psychotropic drugs in psychodermatological syndromes is limited to neuroleptics in skin delusional states. The use of other psychotropic drugs in a diversity of psychophysiological skin symptoms may be promising but has not yet been supported by sufficient controlled trials.

It is noteworthy that the many reports on the use of psychotropic drugs in dermatology emphasize that the psychopharmacological treatment should always be part of an integrative approach, combining medical and psychobiobehavioral management. The need for a combined approach with diverse forms of psychotherapy is mandatory. Even when treating MHP with a neuroleptic, the need to establish a good rapport with the patient is a main treatment feature (Torch & Bishop, 1981).

PSYCHOTHERAPY IN THE MANAGEMENT OF PSYCHODERMATOSES

Dermatologists and general practitioners who pay attention to psychosocial stress factors that precede or follow skin disorders can be said to manage patients within a biopsychosocial model. They perform some rudimentary but nonetheless often effective form of psychotherapy.

Research into the application of more distinctive forms of psychotherapy in skin disorders, for example, psychoanalysis, group psychotherapy, or short-term psychotherapy, is scant and often anecdotal. As hardly any studies use adequate controls, the effectiveness of psychotherapy in the treatment of skin disorders remains hard to assess.

Analytically Oriented Psychotherapy

Although analytically oriented psychotherapy is often claimed to be largely ineffective, it has been reported as positive when combined with a supportive approach. An illustrative example is given by Koblenzer (1986), who took a patient into an insight-oriented psychotherapy once weekly after 14 years of competent but unsuccessful dermatological treatment for incapacitating and painful lesions with arthralgias. Several additional important issues in the psychotherapeutic management of dermatoses are raised in her account of the successful outcome of analytical psychotherapy. First, psychotherapy for chronical dermatological conditions may help to contain medical costs. Indeed, psychotherapy is remarkably cost effective, by limiting extensive laboratory workups, medication costs, and so on. Secondly, it puts forward a possible psychophysiological pathway of the dermatological somatization syndrome by postulating that pathways which link limbic and higher cortical centers with the hypothalamus can act as mediators. Thirdly, the combination of psychotherapy with a psychotropic regimen is mutually reinforcing, at least during the early months of psychotherapy.

The combination of psychotherapy and psychotropic drugs is also advocated by Sneddon and Sneddon (1983) in the treatment of resistant cases of acné excoriée.

In nearly 100 cases of alopecia totalis and alopecia areata, Pomey-Rey (1979) achieved outstanding results with psychotherapy, in terms of general psychological well-being, as well as concerning the remission of the hair growth disorder itself.

Many differences between the psychotherapeutic approaches to neuroses or psychosomatic diseases and psychotherapy applied to cases of dermatology have been recognized. Consoli (1984) has emphasized some particularities of the early phases of the psychotherapeutic process in dermatological patients. It appears that the patient's initial request for medical help is indistinguishable from his or her appeal for psychological help.

Rechenberger (1975) widened the scope of research from individual to interactional psychodynamics, more in particular to the fact that the resistance encountered in dermatological patients with eczema, urticaria, and psoriasis seems to go accompanied by parallel resistances in dermatologists.

The physiological etiology of psoriasis has not yet been determined, while emotional stress factors are evidently prominent in provoking relapses, so different psychotherapeutic approaches have been applied to psoriasis. Seville (1983) investigated the psychological stress events in the month preceding a relapse in patients whose psoriasis is apparently triggered by emotional stress. Psoriasis patients who have some insight in the psychodynamics of the precipitating events have a better prognosis. The author gives general directives about giving the patients a sympathetic approach and real caring, but does not inquire in the theoretical psychotherapeutic framework.

Schoenberg and Carr (1963) were the first to evaluate the efficacy of brief psychotherapy in neurodermatitis. Their approach consisted of a 12 session short-term psychotherapy focusing on reinforcement and encouragement of the expression of hostility in contemporary interpersonal conflicts. Twelve out of their 25 patients, however, did not complete the psychotherapy, while 12 out of the remaining 13 did gain a complete remission.

Psychotherapeutic treatment has also been tried in patients with skin hypochondriasis. The underlying psychodynamics are tackled in a short-term dynamic psychotherapy which focuses on the clarification of the symbolism of the choice of symptom, the decoding of the somatic symptom (Van Moffaert, 1982).

The use of these different psychotherapeutic approaches is limited to a small group of patients, because it requires either highly specialized therapists who have been trained both in dermatology and in psychotherapy or a close working association of two different specialists. On the whole it appears that the positive outcome from psychotherapy is much more dependent on nonspecific factors and on the commitment and the enthusiasm of the therapist, rather than on specific treatment variables.

The Psychotherapeutic Effect of Hospitalization

The dramatic recovery of some dermatological patients who are hospitalized but receive basically the same treatment as outpatients has been investigated by Lefebvre et al. (1980). After considering the object-relations of dermatological patients, Lefebvre et al. found that a dermatological exacerbation was linked to a threatened rupture of a narcissistic homeostasis with a key object, either an integral part of the patient's current life or a hospital staff member to whom the patient transferred his or her emotional need. In this view the therapeutic impact of the hospitalization and treatment procedures lies in permitting the recathexis of objects. Wittkower and Lester (1960) had already wondered about the often dramatic results of hospitalization. They believed that it was brought about by satisfaction of the patient's dependency needs through bed-rest, nursing, creaming and ointing, and baths. The impact of the psychodynamics of the relationship between patient and nursing team on psoriasis has been emphasized by Bosse and Hünecke (1982).

Integration of Psychotherapy in the Institutional Structure

The reported success of psychotherapeutic interventions in dermatology is more than often limited to individual cases. Specialized psychotherapeutic techniques can hardly be conducted by the practicing dermatologist and are restricted to a selected number of dermatological patients. Perhaps the most important challenge is to expand the psychotherapeutic approach into a treatment method that is integrated in the routine operation of a dermatology clinic and thus more generally available.

The structural incorporation of a psychotherapeutic dimension in a dermatology clinic varies with the availability of psychotherapists in the different settings. In some dermatological departments patients with suspected psychodermatosis are screened by a psychiatrist or a psychologist and referred to a specialized psychotherapist if necessary (Pomey-Rey, 1979). In other departments patients are offered psychotherapy by the consultation-liaison-psychiatrist or by a clinical psychologist on the premises (Van Moffaert, 1982). In still other departments staff members with a training in psychoanalysis offer psychotherapy to selected patients. Finally, there are departments that have gone as far as creating an overall psychotherapeutic climate as well as a structure in which psychotherapy is available to all patients (Rechenberger & Rechenberger, 1976).

The latter departments organize daily clinical practice on integrated psychosomatic and psychoanalytical principles. This approach is mostly inspired by heads or senior staff members who have supplemented their dermatological background with a training in psychotherapy, more in particular in psychoanalysis.

In the dermatological department under Professor J. P. Escande, at the Hopital Tarnier in Paris, the classical dermatological approach, that is, diagnosis of the lesions without discussion with the patient, has been modified considerably (Escande, 1984). The new approach involves listening to the patient in order to detect his or her general distress. The medical staff, as well as the nursing staff, have a psychoanalytical background. The gap between the somatic approach on the one hand, and the psychological treatment on the other, is bridged by their organizational integration.

Rechenberger (Rechenberger & Rechenberger, 1976) has integrated the psychotherapeutic approach in the Dermatology Clinic of the University Hospital of Düsseldorf in Germany. Her work focuses on the management of those patients who are not yet aware of a psychogenetic factor in their dermatoses, and on the effects of a disturbed mother–child relationship on specific diseases such as urticaria, psoriasis, or acné excoriée. In seminars and practical supervisions, dermatologists in training are taught how to deal with the psychosomatic components of their practice. Although dermatology in general is considered to be favorably inclined towards psychosomatic expansion of its clinical practice, research has revealed specific resistances encountered in psychodermatology. Dermatologists who have been established for a considerable number of years tend to assume that a psychosomatic dimension to their practice is time consuming and superfluous. Conversely, many of those who do accept the need for a psychosomatic approach still adhere to the fallacy that it is an innate talent that develops naturally without insight or training. It follows that dermatologists must be made aware during their formative years of an approach which will enable them to deal with the complex psychosocial issues of their practice. To train future dermatologists in general psychosomatic medicine and in the specific demands of psychodermatology, Gould and Gragg (1983) give them the opportunity to learn about the psychological aspects of their specialty by having them witness well-conducted interviews, strategic questioning, and listening techniques. At the Dermatology Department of the University of Ghent future dermatologists are trained in the general and specific aspects of psychodermatology in a series of seminars (Van Moffaert, 1986).

BEHAVIORAL STRATEGIES IN DERMATOLOGY

Many single case studies report a positive outcome of behavioral techniques in the treatment of psychodermatoses. However, there have been only few systematic behavioral intervention studies, and the applicability of behavioral techniques in psychodermatology has been insufficiently investigated (Risch & Ferguson, 1981). Yet behavioral factors have a particular impact on dermatological syndromes at different levels.

First, more than any other treatment technique, behavioral methods have a direct impact on variables that directly influence skin physiology. Indeed, hypnosis, relaxation, and so on, bring about changes in physiological parameters such as skin conductance, skin temperature, and vasomotor reactions, all of which can be decisive in the origin of skin disorders.

Secondly, the patient's gestures have a greater impact on dermatoses than on any other disease. Many functional or behaviorally determined disorders are the result of reinforced or maintained behavior. Some dermatoses (artifacts, acné excoriée, prurigo) are the direct products of patient behavior, and most dermatoses invite or even force the patient to handle his or her affected areas, which influences the course and shape of the lesions. Scratching, either induced by itch or not, squeezing, and pinching alter the skin, causing inflammation, which in its turn incites to more scratching. Excoriation caused by excessive scratching, extensive dermal tickening, lichenification, and scarring expose the organism to infection and various secondary problems. Furthermore, the application of a dermatological treatment, which often involves ointment and creams, induces the patient to manipulate his skin.

Also the daily hygienic procedures can easily become excessive and deteriorate to compulsive skin manipulation, which becomes a dermatological problem in itself.

Lastly, hospitalization in a dermatological ward has certain behavioral therapeutic effects which have not yet been sufficiently researched. It is common knowledge among dermatologists that hospitalization by itself can clear a resistant dermatosis, without any change in the dermatological treatment. It is still unclear whether this beneficial impact of hospitalization resides in the fact of being freed from the daily stress of life as an outpatient or in the regression offered to patients by the stay in hospital. Many patients point to the soothing effect they experience through the nursing procedures. The bathing, the massaging with ointments and creams, the bandaging, have all direct behavioral contents that act on many levels. On a psychodynamic level these nursing procedures reenact maternal care in early childhood. On a behavioral level the touching and massaging has a relaxing effect on the skin. All this has not yet been systematically investigated.

Behavioral Treatment Techniques

In psychodermatology diverse behavioral therapeutic strategies have been applied, either separately, mixed, or in combination with other psychological techniques. In cases where anxiety is a main causal factor, systematic desensitization can be justified. Dermatoses in which self-touching is the behavioral component are better suited for aversion techniques or token economy procedures. Hypnosis and biofeedback have already been applied to the treatment of various dermatoses. The particular combination of behavioral techniques with elements of cognitive treatment seems very promising. The association of behavioral methods with biological/cognitive techniques is a challenge for the future.

Systematic desensitization. Systematic desensitization techniques are appropriate for the treatment of dermatoses which feature anticipatory anxiety. The field of dermatology is particular in that is has to deal with all sorts of fear based on normal skin changes and especially on contagious diseases. As sexually transmitted diseases and cancer have always been the favorite targets for skin hypochondriasis, dermatologists are used to being confronted with cancerophobia and syphilophobia. These skin phobias are easily recognizable, but particularly treatment resistant. Neither psychotherapy nor psychotropics have ever yielded any spectacular results (Van Moffaert, 1982). In recent years people's fears have focused on modern scourges of sexually transmitted diseases such as herpes and AIDS, but the therapeutic strategies remain as poor as ever.

Case studies are inconclusive on the use of systematic desensitization for skin syndromes which feature anxiety and hypochondriasis. More systematic research has been done on anxiety-causing autonomic disregulations, such as excessive sweating. Bar and Kuypers (1973) have successfully treated patients with dyshidrosis with this technique. Both the skin phobia and the anticipatory anxiety, which results in neurotic fear and excessive sweating, can be tackled with systematic desensitization that breaks down the neurotic anxiety–response habit in piecemeal fashion.

Aversion therapy. Dermatological problems that are the result of persistent behavior disturbances, such as compulsive scratching and the squeezing of real or imaginary comedos, can be treated by administering an electric shock whenever the patient displays the unadaptive habit. This aversion technique proves particularly adequate for compulsive scratching. The habit of compulsive scratching often starts with a physically provoked itching, which elicits scratching to relieve the unbearable tension (itch). The relief of the itch by scratching becomes the positive reinforcer. Thus a vicious circle is created, in which the scratching persists long after the physical cause of the itch has disappeared.

Aversion therapy has been used in dermatoses ranging from neurodermatitis (Ratliff & Stein, 1968) to trichotillomania (Altman et al., 1982).

One of the possible drawbacks of aversion therapy, pointed out by Bar and Kuypers (1973), is that relapses occur as long as the compulsive behavior retains some rewarding effects. Some "booster" sessions are then indicated.

Operant techniques. This technique has been applied to syndromes as different as compulsive scratching, trichotillomania, and atopic dermatitis. In this treatment the adaptive behavior is reinforced by a reward. Unadaptive behavior is weakened or eliminated by being neglected or punished.

Although patients with neurodermatitis often display emotional problems or conflicts, their skin condition usually has a physical etiology. The persistent scratching, however, is generally the result of initial rewarding effects of this behavior (Robertson et al., 1975). The reward is double: The scratching temporarily terminates the itching feeling, and may also be reinforced by the attention the patient receives from his environment. A powerful compulsive habit develops, which perpetuates the skin problem (Walton, 1960). Operant conditioning of behavior may also improve the dermatosis. The neurodermatitis patient is rewarded for refraining from scratching for a certain amount of time. A secondary reinforcer or token can be earned according to the schedule of reinforcement and used to obtain larger rewards. If the desired behavior (not scratching) has been adopted for a longer period, an attractive reward can be given as a primary reinforcer.

Allen and Harris (1966) report the treatment of a child with persistent scratching by persuading the parents to ignore the scratching behavior and to reinforce nonscratching through rewards. Bar and Kuypers (1973) describe a 6-year-old girl who had developed a chronic neurodermatitis of the vulva by persistent (3 years) scratching after oxyuris. Here also, the parents' attitude of denying attention to the unadaptive behavior and rewarding nonscratching led to a marked improvement within a few weeks and a total extinction of the undesired habit within a few months.

Assertiveness training. This behavior technique is appropriate for patients who do not or cannot express their emotions directly and who experience extreme or considerable social fear. They often show excessive blushing, symptomatic erythema, erythrophobia, and hyperhidrosis. Patients who bottle up their emotions and who have difficulties in expressing feelings of anger or attraction tend to develop autonomic vasomotor responses, the most problematic of which is facial symptomatic erythema because of its visibility. In many cases these symptomatic autonomic vasomotor responses will entail a secondary fear of becoming red in the face (erythrophobia). Conditioning of the autonomic vasomotor responses and the erythrophobia leads to aggravation of social fear. The behavioral treatment of choice here is assertiveness training, based on Wolpe's theory of reciprocal inhibition (Risch & Ferguson, 1981).

In patients with excessive sweating during psychic stress, a similar vicious circle can be created. Fear of the hyperhidrosis develops and this "sudophobia" in itself causes the autonomous response of excessive sweating, mostly on the palms of the hand and the soles of the feet.

Assertiveness training, with or without the adjunct of systematic desensitization, is then indicated.

Biofeedback. Methodological training derived from the Schultz relaxation techniques and autohypnosis can modify physiological parameters such as skin resistance and skin temperature. Biofeedback techniques to regulate the skin temperature have two advantages: The relaxation training is quicker and controlled objectively; the temperature rises, and peripheral vasodilatation improves.

This method has been used in alopecia, pruritus vulvae, herpes, and eczema (Goldberg & Woehl, 1982). Acute anxiety produces vasoconstriction, as demonstrated by finger plethysmography. This may be reversed by relaxation, biofeedback, or hypnosis. Skin temperature regulation can be demonstrated by biofeedback. Dermatological syndromes, which include autonomic vasomotor responses or other physiological parameters such as skin conductance, can be controlled by biofeedback procedures. In dishydrotic eczema the increased epidermal hydratation is related to high skin conductivity. Training eczema patients to control relative skin conductance has been tried. The technique was described by Miller, Coger, and Dymond (1974), who applied it to cases of dyshidrotic eczema. The electronic transduction of physiological changes into auditive and visual signals teaches the patient how to modify externalized signals and alter physiological function. The effectiveness of this treatment technique could be due to the creation of marked changes in skin conductance and to lower levels of anxiety brought about by relaxation and tension reduction.

Hypnosis. Hypnotic experiments were enthusiastically used by the early researchers in psychodermatology. Hypnosis can be useful in the treatment of verrucae, the experimental production of blisters, and the investigation of vasomotor skin changes. Although eczema and psoriasis cases involving a considerable emotional factor may respond to long-term hypnotic treatment, hypnotic suggestion appears to have particularly good results in the treatment of warts (Sinclair-Gieben & Chalmers, 1959).

Specific Dermatologic Conditions and Current Treatment Strategies

In the treatment of dermatoses, behavioral and psychological techniques are substantially less strongly developed than medical intervention techniques. This is deplorable, in view of the fact that psychodermatology is particularly well suited for behavioral interventions.

There is an abundance of enthusiastic reports of positive results from behavioral treatment techniques in dermatoses that proved resistant to other forms of treatment. There are also a number of well-controlled studies that support the idea that an extension of behavioral techniques should be one of the major goals of psychodermatology.

There is no apparent consistency in the use of various behavioral techniques. It is probably too early to expect a pharmacopea with general treatment principles. We are still in the stages of trying out the possible effects of behavioral methods on those dermatological conditions that are influenced by some emotional factor: dermatoses in which the patient's mental state is the dominant factor; disorders that have no psychological etiology, but that are just natural responses to unsightly lesions; and, most frequently, dermatoses the onset or development of which is determined emotionally.

Chronic dermatoses with psychophysiological components

Atopic dermatitis (neurodermatitis). Although atopic dermatitis (also known as neurodermatitis) probably has a primary immunological cause, psychological factors certainly play a part in causing and maintaining the lesions. Emotional factors have a strong impact on the itch–scratch cycle (Faulstich et al., 1985). In 12 of the 13 patients selected and treated by Schoenberg and Carr (1963), brief psychotherapy focusing on the expression of hostility effected a remission.

The efficacy of behavioral techniques in cases of neurodermatitis is well documented. It appears that psychological methods are at least as effective as the classical medical techniques (Medansky & Handler, 1981). The behavioral procedures generally deal with the scratching behavior by selective presentation and withdrawal of the conditioned reinforcers that maintain the maladaptative scratching behavior (Jordan & Whitlock, 1972). Ratliff and Stein (1968) successfully treated one long-lasting case with a modified technique which eliminated the compulsive scratching by manipulating contingencies that are directly under the control of the therapist and the patient. However, a controlled study by Haynes et al. (1979) did not fully support the hypothesis that atopic dermatitis is amenable to intervention through behaviorally oriented treatment procedures. The patients were exposed to a fixed sequence of treatment phases, including a no-treatment baseline phase, a phase incorporating nonspecific treatment factors, and a phase involving frontal EMG feedback and relaxation instructions. Photographic analyses of the skin areas involved revealed significant remission during all phases, but no specificity in the actions of the different treatment phases could be found.

Considering that medical intervention in atopic dermatitis is merely palliative and only partially effective, and that the results of psychological and behavioral treatment are quite encouraging, there is now mixed support for the hypothesis that atopic dermatitis is amenable through behavioral treatment techniques.

Eczema. Although the specific pathophysiology of eczema is not fully known, the influence of emotional components is sufficiently acknowledged to motivate psychobehavioral treatment approaches. Most trials concerning the psychiatric treatment of eczema are uncontrolled. Brown and Bettley (1971) performed a controlled trial which suggested that brief psychiatric treatment doubled the remission chances. As they combined psychotherapy, drugs, hypnosis and relaxation, the separate actions of these treatments cannot be defined.

In infantile eczema the role of emotional factors is more obvious. Maternal or parental rejection in atopic children is crucial (Beveridge, 1974). Reports stating that about 98% of all atopic children have rejecting mothers are exaggerated, but the fact remains that atopic children are more likely to induce resentment and withdrawal in their parents, precisely because they are typically irritable. A positive attitude towards the child is extremely hard to adopt when the child displays uncontrollable bouts of scratching. By lowering the active substances in ointments and thus requiring more frequent applications, an increase of skin contact and cuddling, which is supposed to have a beneficial effect, can be integrated into the medical regimen (Brown, 1967).

Behavioral treatment concentrating on the scratching bouts, which aggravate and maintain the lesions, has had striking results. Ratliff and Stein (1968) reported a successful aversion treatment, administering a 1 mA electric shock whenever a patient with severe neurodermatitis scratched and terminating the shock as soon as the patient stopped scratching. Even simple procedures such as ignoring the scratching in order to stop the reinforcement of the scratching behavior are sometimes sufficient (Walton, 1960). In cases of dyshidrotic eczema, biofeedback procedures were found to be effective, as measured both by the marked changes in skin conductance and by lower subjective levels of anxiety (Miller et al., 1974; Miller & Coger, 1979).

Alopecia areata. Unspecific stress factors, as well as neurotic personality characteristics, have been reported as influential in attacks or relapses of alopecia areata (Puchalski & Szlendak, 1983). However, the well-controlled study by Perini et al. (1984), which recorded life events in the 6 months prior to an alopecia areata attack, did not confirm the psychogenesis of alopecia. Some authors remain confident in the effectiveness of psychoanalytical psychotherapy. In a survey of nearly 100 cases treated with psychotherapy for at least 1 year, Pomey-Rey (1979) arrived at an impressive remission rate of almost 100%. But these data are disputable in view of the fact that alopecia is a dermatosis with a high rate of spontaneous remission. Studies such as these have methodological shortcomings: The duration of follow-up is insufficiently standardized, and the possible influence of other therapeutic variables, e.g., changes in life circumstances, is not considered.

Psoriasis. Neither the significance of personality characteristics (aggression or hostility), nor the exact role of precipitating life events preceding an attack or a relapse, have been defined in psoriasis (Farber et al., 1968; Lyketsos et al., 1985; Matussek et al., 1985).

Neuroendocrinological investigations support the hypothesis that psoriatic patients perceive challenging situations as more stressful than nonpsoriatic patients (Arnetz et al., 1985). Although these pathophysiological data reinforce the commonly observed stress-induced relapses and progress of psoriatic skin disorders, there is no hard evidence for the usefulness of psychotherapeutic measures. All the same, individual and group psychotherapy have been reported as beneficial. Seville (1977, 1978, 1983) demonstrated that patients who were able to recollect emotional events preceding the psoriatic outburst and acquired insight into the psychodynamics of these precipitating events had an altogether better prognosis. Psychological interventions can help the psoriatic patient to achieve a stable and satisfying psychosocial position despite the chronic, esthetically invalidating skin disease. Group therapy with both a professional (general practitioner, psychotherapist, or dermatologist) and a psoriasis patient is likely to be most effective. It is discussed elsewhere in this volume.

Functional and/or itching dermatoses

Psychogenic pruritus. A psychobehavioral approach for patients with psychogenic pruritus has been suggested on the grounds of presumed character features such as semipermeability, the inability to manage aggressive tendencies, character armoring, and an exaggerated cleanliness and fear of disorder (Musaph, 1983). Experimental work confirms this hypothesis. There are interindividually different strategies for responding to and coping with stress, which explains why certain individuals suffer from itching in response to stress while others do not (Fjellner et al., 1985).

There is no consensus, each treatment being advocated by its own adepts, but it seems reasonable to conclude that the most opportune treatment is given by the dermatologist who helps to remove the skin lesions, administers an antipruritic drug, and shows empathic understanding of the emotional conflict situations which lead to the itch. Pruritus anogenitalis and pruritus vulvae are often particularly difficult to treat. When the itching is a concomitant of some other skin disorder, the control of the scratching habit alone may serve as an effective treatment of this skin disorder. This has been demonstrated by Dobes (1977), using a technique of reinforced inhibition in a case of resistant itching and scratching.

Behavior therapy in the treatment of urticaria can be justified by the fact that it is possible to produce wheals and to raise skin temperature by suggestion. Daniels (1973) used a combination of desensitization and covert modeling to achieve a quick symptom reduction in a patient with urticaria and migraine.

Chronic Hyperhidrosis. In chronic hyperhidrosis biofeedback has been used successfully to reduce the symptoms of excessive sweating. Duller and Gentry (1980) describe clinical improvement in 11 out of 14 adult patients. The rationale of use of biofeedback techniques in treating chronic hyperhidrosis is that it can result from anxiety and emotional stimuli and that patients can be taught behaviorally to decrease sweating.

Self-inflicted dermatoses

Dermatitis artefacta. Self-inflicted skin lesions require a combined treatment. Palliative dermatological measures such as occlusive bandages, ointments, or placebo drugs can indirectly improve the psychiatric problem by symbolizing the medical concern and care that dermatitis artefacta patients are basically craving for. In the same way, hospitalization that includes bathing and massaging by nurses can have a therapeutic value because of their symbolic meaning of care and attention. So far psychotropic drugs have only a limited role in this area. Anxiolytics, antidepressants, and neuroleptics may lessen anxiety, depression, or tension, respectively (Van Moffaert et al., 1984).

Behavioral therapies may not only be effective in stopping the self-harming behavior, but they may also be required to stop the self-mutilating habits that often persist after the psychodynamic conflicts have been resolved through psychotherapy. A supportive psychotherapeutic relationship that assesses the patient's life situation and is receptive to cathartic ventilation of anger and frustration can be established by any dermatologist who genuinely wants to help his or her patient (Fabisch, 1979).

Trichotillomania. No controlled trials have assessed the possible benefits of different therapeutic methods in the treatment of compulsive hair pulling. Trichotillomania is far less an automatic habit than is generally believed. The patient often deliberately chooses the part of the scalp which feels appropriate to be pulled and often twists or examines the hair after it has been extracted. On the grounds of the presumed psychodynamic content of hair-plucking, psychotherapy on analytic lines has been tried, with moderate results (Greenberg & Sarner, 1965).

Trichotillomania and other dermatological syndromes based on unadapted behavior often prove refractory to simple behavioral treatment. Help may be needed to detect the underlying psychopathology or the external stresses that cause the behavior. A cognitive expansion of behavioral modification techniques in trichotillomania is described by Ottens (1981). Symptom control is achieved by raising the patient's awareness of his or her hair-pulling habit and of the covert behavior that precedes the overt behavior. This technique expands a treatment that was too narrowly focused on modifying overt behavior. The cognitive component of compulsive behavior is taken as a target to produce change. Treatment procedures are built up in progressive phases: After a period in which the patient's awareness is heightened by alerting him or her for early warning postural changes which accommodate pulling, both overt and covert coping responses incompatible with hair pulling are implemented. Further, the patient is trained in covert anticipatory strategies. A last phase consists of the consolidation of the therapeutic results and optional troubleshooting.

Another procedure to reduce the hair-pulling by attention-reflection is described by Altman et al. (1982). It aims at controlling observable covarying behavior. In a case of trichotillomania in a 3-year-old, a dramatic decrease in hair-pulling was achieved when thumbsucking was penalized by application of a bad-tasting substance.

Neurotic excoriations. Neurotic excoriations are lesions that are self-inflicted by patients who cannot resist the urge to manipulate their skin. In mild cases, the habit consists of habitual, often unconscious, picking of small irregularities in the skin. In more pronounced cases, the habit becomes uncontrollable and turns into an imperative urge to dig into the skin to remove imaginary foreign bodies. Treatment is difficult, and general measures such as protection against further self-mutilation by local bandaging and antipruritic salves are recommended, combined with supportive psychotherapy (Sneddon & Sneddon, 1983). Definite directions for optimal therapy are not yet available, but Fruensgaard et al. (1979, 1980), who comprehensively reviewed the recent literature, recommend an eclectic approach, based on supportive psychotherapy.

A behavioral strategy based on the ethological correspondences between the neurotic patients' postures while compulsively inflicting lesions and the grooming activities in primates (Keehn, 1986) has been constructed by Van Moffaert (1980). It includes a behavior-substitute program conducted with a cotherapist (usually a nurse) of massages, ritual grooming sessions, and occupational therapy. In this uncontrolled study relief was gained in four of the eight patients included in the experiment.

Miscellaneous dermatological disorders

Verrucae. The occurrence of spontaneous remission in warts and the influence of emotional factors has not been explained satisfactorily. Obviously, the viral etiology may account for the connection with emotional factors and its repercussion on immunity.

Experiments in treating bilateral warts with the hypnotic suggestion that the warts would disappear on one side only are inconclusive. Surman et al. (1973) report on a group of 36 patients with bilateral warts. Untreated controls did not improve. In the 17 patients who received the hypnotic suggestion that the warts would disappear on one side only, a 53% general improvement was observed, but the side response was unselective. This suggests that hypnosis has a general effect on host response to the causative virus, but the mechanism by which hypnotic suggestion affects warts resolution is still unclear. Sinclair-Gieben and Chalmers (1959) tentatively concluded from a similar experiment that the effect of hypnosis was related to alterations in blood flow via the autonomic nervous system, and that there was evidence that capillary dilation and exudation of fluid was inhibited by hypnosis. The efficacy of hypnosis has also been demonstrated by the inhibition of the Mantoux reaction by direct suggestion under hypnosis. The problem is that there is no certainty about whether and how the depth of the hypnotic trance influences the remission of the dermatosis.

Dysmorphophobia. Dysmorphophobia is characterized by a subjective feeling of ugliness, cosmetic defect, or deformity in the appearence. In mild cases the disorder is limited to a disturbance in the "psychological" body image (Hardy, 1982). Parallels have been drawn between anorexia nervosa and dysmorphophobia in terms of the distortion of body image and the presence of an obsession phobia concerning the appearence of the body (Thomas, 1984). Although the initial diagnosis is compulsive neurosis, some cases develop delusions. One must keep in mind that an initial symptomatology of dysmorphophobia may be an ominous symptom of nascent schizophrenia (Hay, 1970). Psychotherapeutic help must be provided, especially in younger patients, in whom an in-depth personality change is still possible. Psychotherapy alone, however, rarely makes the patient abandon his or her request for incisive dermatological treatment (laser therapy, transplant) or for cosmetic surgery. Many adult dysmorphophobic patients show pronounced phobic and compulsive-obsessional symptoms (Hardy & Cotterill, 1982) and need psychotropic drug treatment. Antidepressants, tricyclic agents, or a mono-amino-oxidase inhibitor can be used. Special attention must be paid to the training in social skills, which may benefit the inhibited and socially anxious individual whose preoccupation with deformity is part of a wider deficit in social functioning (Frank, 1985). Dysmorphic delusions respond to Pimozide, but the therapeutic results are less spectacular than in other subtypes of monosymptomatic hypochondriacal psychoses, such as the delusions of infestation.

CONCLUSIONS

This survey of current work in the biobehavioral management of dermatological disorders illustrates the promising potential of psychological techniques in dermatology.

Although sufficient experimental work has been done to support the expansion of dermatology with psychological and behavioral techniques, further research is needed. Many of the trials need replication, single-case reports must be expanded to different groups of dermatological patients. The optimistic results obtained with the different behavioral approaches have not been confirmed on a long-term basis.

The study of behavioral strategies should use more sophisticated procedures to find out which dermatoses should be treated with each type of behavioral technique. Also, in the field of psychotropic drug treatment of psychodermatoses, the present empirical statements should be replaced by a rationale of the use of psychotropics. So far, experimental work makes it clear that the psychobehavioral management of dermatoses is likely to gain wider application.

REFERENCES

Alexander, F. (1952). *Psychosomatic medicine.* London: George Allen & Unwin.

Allen, K., & Harris, F. (1966). Elimination of a child's excessive scratching by training the mother in reinforcement procedures. *Behaviour Research and Therapy, 4,* 79–84.

Altman, K., Grahs, C., & Friman, P. (1982). Treatment of unobserved trichotillomania by attention-reflection and punishment of an apparent covariant. *Journal of Behaviour Therapy and Experimental Psychiatry, 13,* 337–340.

Arnetz, B. B., Fjellner, B., Eneroth, P., & Kallner, A. (1985). Stress and Psoriasis: Psychoendocrine and metabolic reactions in psoriatic patients during standardized stressor exposure. *Psychosomatic Medicine, 47,* 528–541.

Bar, L. H. J., & Kuypers, B. R. M. (1973). Behaviour therapy in dermatological practice. *British Journal of Dermatology, 88,* 591–598.

Barsky, A. J., & Klerman, G. L. (1983). Overview: Hypochondriasis, bodily complaints, and somatic styles. *The American Journal of Psychiatry, 140,* 273–283.

Bernstein, J. E., Swift, R. M., Soltani, K., & Lorincz, A. L. (1982). Antipruritic effect of an opiate antagonist, Naloxone hydrochloride. *The Journal of Investigative Dermatology, 78,* 82–83.

Beveridge, G. W. (1974). Diseases of the skin: Infantile eczema. *British Medical Journal, 1,* 154–155.

Bishop, E. R. (1980). An olfactory reference syndrome: Monosymptomatic hypochondriasis, *Journal of Clinical Psychiatry, 41,* 57–59.

Bishop, E. R. (1983). Monosymptomatic hypochondriacal syndromes in dermatology, *Journal of the American Academy of Dermatology, 9,* 152–158.

Bosse, K., & Hünecke, P. (1982). Krankheitsabhängiges Verhalten von Psoriasispatienten, Arzten und Pflegepersonal im Krankenhaus. *Akta Dermatologica, 8,* 163–166.

Bourgeois, M., & Nguyen-Lan, A. (1986). Syndrome d' Ekbom et délires d' infestation cutanée, *Annales Médico-Psychologiques, 144,* 21–39.

Brown, D. G. (1967). Emotional disturbance in eczema: A study of symptom-reporting behaviour. *Journal of Psychosomatic Research, 11,* 27–40.

Brown, D. G., & Bettley, F. R. (1971). Psychiatric treatment of eczema: A controlled trial. *British Medical Journal, 2,* 729–734.

Consoli, S. (1984). Observation au long cours d'une patiente présentant des troubles psychosomatiques et suivie en psychothérapie. *Semaine des Hopitaux de Paris, 13,* 909–915.

Coppola, R. J., & Rolek, D. F. (1975). A neuropharmacologic approach to self-mutilating behaviour. *Journal of the American Osteopathy Association, 74,* 555–557.

Cotterill, J. A. (1981a). Dermatological games. *British Journal of Dermatology, 105,* 311–320.

Cotterill, J. A. (1981b). Dermatological non-disease: A common and potentially fatal disturbance of cutaneous body image. *British Journal of Dermatology, 104,* 611–619.

Cotterill, J. A. (1983a). Biochemistry of anxiety, depression, itch and the placebo response. *Seminars in Dermatology, 2,* 171–175.

Cotterill, J. A. (1983b). Clinical features of patients with dermatologic non disease. *Seminars in Dermatology, 2,* 203–205.

Crayton, J. W., & Freedman, D. X. (1977). Psychotropic drugs in dermatologic practice. *International Journal of Dermatology, 6,* 512–519.

Daniels, L. K. (1973). Treatment of urticaria and severe headache by behaviour therapy. *Psychosomatics, 14,* 347–351.

Dobes, R. W. (1977). Amelioration of psychosomatic dermatosis by reinforced inhibition of scratching. *Journal of Behaviour Therapy and Experimental Psychiatry, 8,* 185–187.

Duke, E. E. (1983). Clinical experience with pimozide: Emphasis on its use in postherpetic neuralgia. *Journal of the American Academy of Dermatology, 8,* 845–850.

Duller, P., & Gentry, W. D. (1980). Use of biofeedback in treating chronic hyperhidrosis; a preliminary report. *British Journal of Dermatology, 103,* 143–146.

Dunbar, H. F. (1954). *Emotions and bodily change.* New York: Columbia University Press.

Escande, J. P. (1984). Organisation institutionelle d'un service hospitalier de dermatologie pour une prise en charge psychosomatique. *Semaine des Hopitaux de Paris, 3,* 916–919.

Evans, P., & Merskey, H. (1972). Shared beliefs of dermal parasitosis. *British Journal of Medical Psychology, 45,* 19–26.

Fabisch, W. (1979). Psychiatric aspects of dermatitis artefacta. *British Journal of Dermatology, 102,* 29–34.

Farber, E. M., Bright, R. D., & Nall, M. L. (1968). Psoriasis. *Archives of Dermatology, 98,* 248–259.

Faulstich, M. E., Williamson, D. A., Duchmann, E. G., Conerly, S. L., & Brantley, P. J. (1985). Psychophysiological analysis of atopic dermatitis. *Journal of Psychosomatic Research, 29,* 415–417.

Faulstich, M.E., & Williamson, D.A. (1985) An overview of atopic dermatitis: Toward a bio-behavioural integration. *Journal of Psychosomatic Research, 29,* 647–654.

Fava, G. A., Perini, G. I., Santonastaso, P., & Fornasa, C. V. (1980). Life events and psychological distress in dermatologic disorders; Psoriasis, chronic urticaria and fungal infections. *British Journal of Medical Psychology, 53,* 277–282.

Fjellner, B., & Hagermark, O. (1984). The influence of the opiate antagonist naloxone on experimental pruritus. *Acta Dermatologica Venereologica, 64,* 73–75.

Fjellner, B., Arnetz, B., Eneroth, P., & Kallner, A. (1985). Pruritus during standardized mental stress. *Acta Dermatologica Venereologica, 65,* 199–205.

Fjellner, B., & Arnetz, B. B. (1985). Psychological predictors of pruritus during mental stress. *Acta Dermatologica Venereologica, 65,* 504–508.

Frank, O. S. (1985). Dysmorphophobia. In R. N. Gain (Ed.), *Current themes in psychiatry* (pp. 257–278). Spectrum Publications.

Freinhar, J. P. (1984). Delusions of parasitosis. *Psychosomatics, 25,* 47–53.

Friedman, S., Kantor, I., Sobel, S., & Miller, R. (1978). On the treatment of neurodermatitis with a monoamime oxidase inhibitor: The chemotherapy of psychosomatic illness through A-REM suppression. *The Journal of Nervous and Mental Disease, 166,* 117–125.

Frithz, A. (1979). Delusions of infestation: Treatment by depot injections of neuroleptics. *Clinical and Experimental Dermatology, 4,* 485–488.

Fruensgaard, K., Hjortshoj, A., & Nielsen, H. (1979). Neurotic excoriations. *International Journal of Dermatology, 17,* 761–767.

Fruensgaard, K., Nielsen, H., & Hjortshoj, A. (1980). Controlled Encephalographic investigation of patients with neurotic excoriations. *Psychotherapy and Psychosomatics, 34,* 273–281.

Goldberg, S., & Woehl, M. (1982). Biofeedback en Dermatologie. *Les Nouvelles Dermatologiques, 1,* 6–9.

Gould, W. M., & Gragg, T. M. (1983). A dermatology-psychiatry liaison clinic. *Journal of the American Academy of Dermatology, 7,* 73–77.

Greenberg, H. V., & Sarner, C. A. (1965). Trichotillomania. *Archives of General Psychiatry, 12,* 482–489.

Hardy, G. E., & Cotterill, J. A. (1982). A study of depression and obsessionality in dysmorphophobic and psoriatic patients. *British Journal of Psychiatry, 140,* 19–22.

Hardy, G. E. (1982). Body image disturbance in dysmorphophobia. *British Journal of Psychiatry, 141,* 181–185.

Hay, G. G. (1970). Dysmorphophobia. *British Journal of Psychiatry, 116,* 399–406.

Haynes, S. N., Wilson, C. C., Jaffe, P. G., & Britton, B. T. (1979). Biofeedback treatment of atopic dermatitis. *Biofeedback and Self-Regulation, 4,* 195–209.

Hill, O. (1977). The psychological management of psychosomatic diseases. *British Journal of Psychiatry, 131,* 113–126.

Jordan, J. M., & Whitlock, F. A. (1972). Emotions and the skin: The conditioning of scratch responses in cases of atopic dermatitis. *British Journal of Dermatology, 86,* 574–585.

Keehn, J. D. (1986). *Animal models for psychiatry.* London: Routledge & Kegan Paul.

Koblenzer, C. S. (1983). Psychosomatic concepts in dermatology. *Archives of Dermatology, 119,* 501–512.

Koblenzer, C. S. (1985a). Psychocutaneous disease. In Demis, Dobson, & McGuire (Eds.), *Clinical dermatology.* Philadelphia, PA: Harper & Row.

Koblenzer, C. S. (1985b). The dysmorphic syndrome. *Archives of Dermatology, 121,* 780–784.

Koblenzer, C. S. (1986). Successful treatment of a chronic and disabling dermatosis by psychotherapy. *Journal of the American Academy of Dermatology, 15,* 390–393.

Lefebvre, P., Leroux, R., & Crombez, J. C. (1980). Object-relations in the dermatologic patient: A contribution to the psychoanalytic theory of psychosomatic disorder. *The Psychiatric Journal of the University of Ottawa, 5,* 17–21.

Lipowski, Z. J., Lipsitt, D. R., & Whybrow, P. C. (1977). *Psychosomatic medicine.* New York: Oxford University Press.

Lyell, A. (1983). Delusions of parasitosis. *British Journal of Dermatology, 108,* 485–499.

Lyketsos, G. C., Stratigos, J., Tawil, G., Psara, M., & Lyketsos, C. G. (1985). Hostile personality characteristics, dysthymic states and neurotic symptoms in urticaria, psoriasis and alopecia. *Psychotherapy and Psychosomatics, 44,* 122–131.

Macalpine, I. (1958). Is alopecia arcata psychosomatic? *British Journal of dermatology, 70,* 147–158.

Matussek, P., Agerer, D., & Seibt, G. (1985). Aggression in depressives and psoriatics. *Psychotherapy and Psychosomatics, 43,* 120–125.

Medansky, R. S., & Handler, R. M. (1981). Dermatopsychosomatics: Classification, physiology, and therapeutic approaches. *Journal of the American Academy of Dermatology, 5,* 125–135.

Medansky, R. S., Handler, R. M., & Medansky, D. L. (1981). Self-evaluation of acne and emotion: A pilot study. *Psychosomatics, 22,* 379–383.

Millard, L. G. (1984). Pathological pathomimicry: A form of patient maladjustment. *The Lancet, 2,* 969–971.

Miller, R. M., Coger, R. W., & Dymond, A. M. (1974). Biofeedback skin conductance conditioning in dyshidrotic eczema. *Archives of Dermatology, 109,* 737–738.

Miller, R. M., & Coger, R. W. (1979). Skin conductance conditioning with dyshidrotic eczema patients. *British Journal of Dermatology, 101,* 435–437.

Munro, A. (1978). Monosymptomatic hypochondriacal psychosis manifesting as delusions of parasitosis. *The Archives of Dermatology, 114,* 940–943.

Munro, A., & Pollock, B. (1981). Monosymptomatic psychoses which progress to schizophrenia. *Journal of Clinical Psychiatry, 42,* 474–476.

Munro, A. (1983). Delusional parasitosis: A form of monosymptomatic hypochrondriacal psychosis. *Seminars in Dermatology, 2,* 197–202.

Musaph, H. (1976). Psychodermatology. In O. W. Hill (Ed.), *Modern trends in psychosomatic medicine* (Vol. 3). London: Butterworths.

Musaph, H. (1983). Psychogenic pruritus. *Seminars in Dermatology, 2,* 217–222.

Nielsen, H., Fruensgaard, K., & Hjortshoj, A. (1980). Controlled neuropsychological investigation of patients with neurotic excoriations. *Psychotherapy and Psychosomatics, 34,* 52–61.

Ottens, A. J. (1981). Multifaceted treatment of compulsive hair pulling. *Journal of Behaviour Therapy and Experimental Psychiatry, 12,* 77–80.

Panconesi, E. (1984). The future is here; cutaneous psychoneuroimmunology as a premise. In E. Panconesi (Guest Ed.), *Stress and skin diseases: Psychosomatic dermatology.* Philadelphia, PA: J. B. Lippincott.

Perini, G. I., Fornasa, C. V., Cipriani, R., Bettin, A., Zecchino, F., & Peserico, A. (1984). Life events and alopecia areata. *Psychotherapy and Psychosomatics, 41,* 48–52.

Pomey-Rey, D. (1979). "Pour mourir guérie"?: A propos d'un cas d'acné conglobata. *Cutis, 3,* 151–157.

Pomey-Rey, D. (1979). L'écoute devant une chute de cheveux. *Cutis, 4,* 54–59.

Primrose, D. A. (1979). Treatment of self-injurious behaviour with a gaba (gamma-aminobutyric acid) analogue. *Journal of Mental Deficiency Research, 23,* 163–173.

Puchalski, Z., & Szlendak, L. (1983). Anxiety state and anxiety trait in patients with alopecia areata, rosacea and lichen ruber planus, *Zeitschrift für Hautkrankheiten, 14,* 1038–1048.

Ratliff, R. G., & Stein, N. H. (1968). Treatment of neurodermatitis by behaviour therapy: A case study. *Behavioural Research and Therapy, 6,* 397–399.

Rechenberger, I. (1975). *Tiefenpsychologisch ausgerichtete Diagnostik und Behandlung von Hautkrankheiten.* Göttingen, Germany: Vandenhoeck & Ruprecht.

Rechenberger, I. (1977). Zugang zu psychosomatischen Aspekten in der Dermatologie. *Praxis der Psychotherapie, 22,* 265–270.

Rechenberger, I., & Rechenberger, H. G. (1976). Besonderheiten eines Konsiliardienstes und einer psychosomatischen Sprechstunde in einer Universitäts-Hautklinik. *Psychotherapie, Medizinische Psychologie, 26,* 163–168.

Renshaw, D. C. (1980). Sex and the dermatologist. *International Journal of Dermatology, 19,* 469–471.

Richardson, J. S., & Zaleski, W. A. (1983). Naloxone and self-mutilation. *Biological Psychiatry, 18,* 99–101.

Risch, C., & Ferguson, J. (1981). *Behavioural treatment of skin disorders.* In J. M. Ferguson & C. B. Taylor (Eds.), *The comprehensive book of behavioural medicine, 2.* Spectrum Publications.

Robertson, I. M., Jordan, J. M., & Whitlock, F. A. (1975). Emotions and skin (II): The conditioning of scratch responses in cases of lichen simplex. *British Journal of Dermatology, 92,* 407–412.

Sarti, M. G., & Cossidenti, A. (1984). Therapy in psychosomatic dermatology. In E. Panconesi (Guest Ed.), *Stress and skin diseases: Psychosomatic dermatology.* Philadelphia, PA: Lippincott.

Savin, J. A., Patterson, W. D., Oswald, I., & Adam, C. (1975). Further studies of scratching during sleep. *British Journal of Dermatology, 93,* 297–302.

Schoenberg, B., & Carr, A. C. (1963). An investigation of criteria for brief psychotherapy of neurodermatitis. *Psychosomatic Medicine, 25,* 253–263.

Seville, R. H. (1977). Psoriasis and stress I. *British Journal of Dermatology, 97,* 297–302.

Seville, R. H. (1978). Psoriasis and stress II. *British Journal of Dermatology, 98,* 151–153.

Seville, R. H. (1983). Psoriasis, stress, insight and prognosis. *Seminars in Dermatology, 2,* 213–216.

Sinclair-Gieben, A. H. C., & Chalmers, D. (1959). Evaluation of the treatments of warts by suggestion. *Lancet, 2,* 480–482.

Sneddon, J. (1980). The psychiatrist and the dermatologist: Which ticket of admission? *Practice of Medicine, 224,* 97–99.

Sneddon, J. (1983). Patients who do not want to get better. *Seminars in Dermatology, 2,* 183–187.

Sneddon, J., & Sneddon, I. (1983). Acné excoriée: A protective device. *Clinical and Experimental Dermatology, 8,* 65–68.

Surman, O. W., Gottlieb, S. K., Hackett, T. P., & Silverberg, E. L. (1973). Hypnosis in the treatment of warts. *Archives of General Psychiatry, 28,* 439–441.

Taylor, G. J., & Doody, K. (1985). Verbal measures of alexithymia: What do they measure? *Psychotherapy and Psychosomatics, 43,* 32–37.

Thomas, C. S. (1984). Dysmorphophobia: A question of definition. *British Journal of Psychiatry, 144,* 513–516.

Torch, E. M., & Bishop, E. R. (1981). Delusions and parasitosis: Psychotherapeutic engagement. *American Journal of Psychotherapy, 35,* 101–106.

Van Moffaert, M. (1980). An eclectic approach to specific forms of dermatitis artefacta. *Proceedings of the 13th European Conference on Psychosomatic research* (pp. 217–224).

Van Moffaert, M. (1982). Psychosomatics for the practising dermatologist. *Dermatologica, 165,* 73–87.

Van Moffaert, M. (1986). Training future dermatologists in psychodermatology. *General Hospital Psychiatry, 8,* 115–118.

Van Moffaert, M., Vermander, F., & Kint, A. (1984). Dermatitis Artefacta. *International Journal of Dermatology, 24,* 236–238.

Walton, D. (1960). The application of learning theory to the treatment of a case of neurodermatitis. In H. J. Eysenck (Ed.), *Behavioural therapy and the neuroses.* London: Pergamon Press.

Whitlock, F. A. (1976). *Psychophysiological aspects of skin disease.* London: W. B. Saunders.

Wittkower, E. D., & Lester, E. (1960). Hautkrankheiten in psychosomatischer Sicht. *Acta Psychosomatica* (Documenta Geigy), *6,* 1–39.

Wittkower, E. D., & Russell, B. (1953). *Emotional factors in skin disease.* New York: Hoeber.

IV

OTHER ISSUES IN BEHAVIORAL MEDICINE

12

Behavioral Aspects of Oncology

Paul B. Jacobsen
William H. Redd

Memorial Sloan-Kettering Cancer Center and
Cornell University Medical College
New York, NY

INTRODUCTION

Recent advances in the treatment of cancer have yielded impressive gains in the observed survival rate. In the 1930s less than 1 in 5 patients with cancer was alive 5 years after diagnosis, whereas today 3 in 8 patients will survive 5 years (American Cancer Society, 1985). These gains have not been achieved without imposing great personal demands on the patient. Indeed, for some patients the side effects of treatment seem worse than the disease itself. Nausea, vomiting, loss of appetite, decreased immunity to other diseases, and fatigue are all commonly occurring side effects of conventional forms of cancer treatment. In addition to producing physical side effects, cancer treatments also give rise to behavioral side effects. The physical and psychological impact of treatment may inadvertently foster the development of aversions, phobic-like reactions, and other behavioral disorders. Besides reducing the quality of life, these behavioral side effects may also compromise health status by contributing to patient noncompliance with medical treatments.

The purpose of this chapter is to review the current status of research on the use of behavioral interventions to control physical and behavioral side effects of cancer treatment. The literature which is reviewed has been organized according to the major forms of cancer treatment. Controlling adverse reactions to chemotherapy, the topic which has received the most attention in behavioral research on oncology, is considered first. This review is followed by discussion of another well-researched topic, the use of behavioral interventions to control distress reactions to painful oncology procedures. Other forms of cancer treatment have yet to be as thoroughly investigated by behavioral researchers. There are, however, published intervention studies on the use of behavior therapies to control adverse reactions to cancer surgery, radiation therapy, hyperthermia treatment, and confinement in protective isolation. These studies are reviewed in a third section of this chapter.

Certain lines of behavioral research relevant to oncology are not considered here, since they overlap considerably with other areas of behavioral medicine. For discussion of these topics, the reader is directed to the following chapters in these volumes: Psychological Responses to Chronic Pain, Behavioral Preparation for Surgery, and Psychological and Behavioral Sequalae in Children with Chronic Disease.

ADVERSE REACTIONS TO CHEMOTHERAPY

Chemotherapy is one of the most widely prescribed methods of treating cancer. It typically involves repeated oral and intravenous administration of drugs that are toxic to the rapidly dividing cancer cells. Unfortunately, this toxic effect is not limited to neoplastic cells, but also occurs in normal cells of the bone marrow, gastrointestinal tract, reproductive system, and hair follicles. These toxic actions account for the immunosuppression, nausea, vomiting, sterility, and hair loss commonly experienced by patients during the protracted course of chemotherapy (Golden, Horwich, & Lokich, 1980).

For many patients the most noxious side effects of chemotherapy are the nausea and vomiting that may begin 1 to 2 hours after an infusion and persist for 2 to 24 hours (Frytak & Moertel, 1981). While the presence and severity of these side effects can differ greatly across patients, the factors underlying individual differences in pharmacological response are not yet completely understood. It is clear, however, that cytotoxic drugs vary considerably in emetic potential. There are certain drugs, such as cis-platinum, which tend to be associated with greater incidence and severity of posttreatment nausea and vomiting (Rozencweig, Von Hoff, Slavik, & Muggia, 1977).

In addition to posttreatment nausea and vomiting, some patients report that they also experience these reactions *before* treatment. They may become nauseated and vomit as they approach the hospital, upon seeing their doctor or oncology nurse, or as a staff member prepares for the infusion. Some patients report that even talking about chemotherapy will make them nauseated, while others state that they are nauseated the entire day before treatment. These phenomena have collectively been labeled anticipatory nausea or vomiting (ANV).

Research data suggest that the development of ANV is gradual; a longitudinal study of chemotherapy patients (Andrykowski, Redd, & Hatfield, 1985) found that, on average, anticipatory nausea occurred initially during the fifth treatment cycle. Published estimates of the prevalence of anticipatory side effects among chemotherapy patients have ranged from 18% to 57% (Andrykowski et al., 1985; Andrykowski et al., 1988; Dolgin, Katz, McGinty, & Siegel, 1985; Fetting, Wilcox, Iwata, Criswell, Bosmajian, & Sheidler, 1983; Morrow, 1982; Morrow, Arsenau, Asbury, Bennet, & Boros, 1982; Nerenz, Leventhal, & Love, 1982; Nesse, Carli, Curtis, & Kleinman, 1980; Nicholas, 1982; Scogna & Smalley, 1979; van Komen & Redd, 1985; Wilcox, Fetting, Nettesheim, & Abeloff, 1982). It should be noted that studies reporting prevalence rates have varied considerably with respect to: (a) sample size, (b) when in the course of chemotherapy treatment patients were assessed, (c) the methods by which presence or absence of ANV were assessed, and (d) the composition of samples with respect to cancer site, chemotherapy agents, and drug administration schedules. The importance of this last factor is demonstrated by the fact that, even when standardized assessment methods are used, different chemotherapy protocols have been associated with markedly different prevalence rates; for example, Andrykowski et al. (1985) found that only 20% of patients receiving fluorouracil developed anticipatory reactions, whereas 80% of patients receiving a combination of cyclophosphamide, doxorubicin, vincristine, and prednisone developed such reactions. Consequently, overall prevalence rates for chemotherapy patients are not meaningful statistics. Determining the prevalence for a specific protocol is more appropriate when attempting to identify an individual's risk of developing ANV.

Since ANV occurs prior to the administration of the cytotoxic drugs expected to produce such effects, it is presumed to have nonpharmacologic origins. This view is supported by research data which suggest that ANV arises in accord with a respondent conditioning paradigm very similar to the learned taste aversion paradigm. According to this explanation (Katz, 1982; Nesse et al., 1980; Redd & Andrykowski, 1982), ANV develops as a result of the repeated pairings of neutral stimuli (e.g., the sights, smells, and sounds of the clinic environment) with the administration of chemotherapy (unconditional stimulus) and its aftereffects (unconditional response). Through the process of conditioning, certain previously neutral stimuli become conditional stimuli such that their presence alone eventually elicit nausea and/or vomiting (conditional response). It should be noted that ANV can also be cognitively mediated; as was pointed out earlier, some patients report becoming nauseated while merely thinking about chemotherapy.

Support for the respondent learning explanation is derived from research demonstrating that patients with ANV are characterized by features that would be expected from theory and laboratory research to facilitate the acquisition of a conditional response. First, the development of ANV has consistently been associated with greater severity of the unconditional response of posttreatment nausea and vomiting (Andrykowski et al., 1985; Andrykowski et al., 1988; Dolgin et al., 1985; Fetting et al., 1983; Morrow, 1982; Nesse et al., 1980; Nicholas, 1982; van Komen & Redd, 1985; Wilcox et al., 1982). Second, greater numbers of chemotherapy treatments (i.e., more pairings of neutral clinic stimuli with posttreatment side effects) also characterizes patients with ANV (Fetting et al., 1983; Nesse et al., 1980). Third, longer infusions and the occurrence of taste sensations during infusions (factors which would reduce or bridge the interval between being in the clinic and having posttreatment side effects) also have been associated with the development of ANV (Andrykowski et al., 1985; Fetting, Wilcox, Sheidler, Donchower, Grochow, & Enterline, 1984). Finally, there are data indicating that greater anxiety or emotional distress (which has been associated with increased conditionability) also characterizes those chemotherapy patients with ANV (Altmaier, Ross, & Moore, 1982; Andrykowski et al., 1985; Nerenz et al., 1982; van Komen & Redd, 1983).

Oncologists have had only limited success with somatic treatments for relieving or eliminating the nausea and vomiting associated with chemotherapy. The commonly used antiemetic drugs (i.e., the phenothiazines) have generally not been shown to provide reliable control of chemotherapy-related nausea, and many patients complain of their strong sedative effects (Harris, 1978; Frytak & Moertel, 1981). In addition, some patients prescribed antiemetics experience marked extrapyramidal side effects such as muscle tension and rigidity. Considerable attention has recently been focused on a new antiemetic agent, metoclopramide. Preliminary results suggest that it can effectively prevent posttreatment nausea and vomiting when administered intravenously during chemotherapy infusions (Gralla, 1981). Unfortunately, metoclopramide possesses potential side effects similar to the phenothiazines (e.g., sedation, muscle tension and rigidity) which may limit its use in many cases.

Although pharmacological research has not specifically addressed ANV, clinical reports have suggested that these adverse reactions are especially resistant to treatment with antiemetics (Chang, 1981). Following the respondent conditioning conceptualization of ANV outlined above, several investigators have examined the utility of behaviorally based methods of symptom control. Five methods have been studied in experimentally designed research: hypnosis, progressive muscle relaxation, electromyographic (EMG) biofeedback, systematic desensitization, and cognitive/attentional distraction.

The efficacy of hypnosis in controlling ANV has been investigated in one study (Redd, Andresen, & Minagawa, 1982). Six women who were observed to have vomited prior to the previous three chemotherapy sessions received training in hypnosis. Training was administered by a therapist on two occasions between chemotherapy infusions. The hypnotic intervention involved suggestions for deep muscle relaxation and the introduction of relaxing imagery. Patients were encouraged to practice at home using an audiotape of one of the training sessions. Therapist-directed hypnosis was then used immediately before and during the next several chemotherapy infusions. Results indicated an immediate and complete cessation of vomiting and a reduction of self-reported nausea in the clinic whenever therapist-directed hypnosis accompanied chemotherapy. Whenever hypnosis was not used during a chemotherapy session, anticipatory nausea and vomiting returned to baseline levels.

The use of progressive muscle relaxation to control aversive side effects of chemotherapy has been investigated in two controlled studies (Burish & Lyles, 1981; Lyles, Burish, Krozely, & Oldham, 1982). In both studies, adult patients with anticipatory nausea were assessed across 5 to 10 consecutive chemotherapy treatments divided into baseline, intervention, and follow-up sessions. In one study (Burish & Lyles, 1981) 16 patients were randomly assigned for the intervention sessions to either a relaxation condition (therapist-directed progressive muscle training plus a relaxation imagery exercise immediately before and during chemotherapy) or a no-treatment control condition. The second study (Lyles et al., 1982) featured the same relaxation and no-treatment control conditions, and also included a third condition in which patients received support and encouragement from a therapist but no relaxation training (attention control condition). In the second study, 50 patients were randomly assigned to one of the three conditions. Results indicated that, compared to patients in the no-treatment control conditions, patients receiving relaxation training reported feeling less anxious, depressed, and nauseated during and after chemotherapy and showed lower pulse rates and systolic blood pressures. Nurses administering the chemotherapy also rated patients in the relaxation condition as being less anxious and nauseated during chemotherapy than the no-treatment patients. Furthermore, there were no consistent differences on dependent measures between patients in the attention and no-treatment control conditions, suggesting that the effects of relaxation training were not due simply to nonspecific intervention factors. Finally, positive results achieved during relaxation training sessions generalized to the no-intervention follow-up sessions, though the magnitude of the beneficial effects generally decreased over time.

In a related single-case study (Burish, Shartner, & Lyles, 1981), multiple muscle-site EMG biofeedback was used to augment relaxation training during drug infusions. Ten consecutive chemotherapy infusions were divided into baseline, treatment, and follow-up sessions. Results indicated that, compared to baseline sessions, the patient showed reductions in physiological arousal (EMG, pulse rate, systolic/diastolic blood pressure) and reported feeling less anxious and nauseated during biofeedback/relaxation sessions. Moreover, these changes tended to be maintained during the follow-up sessions.

Systematic desensitization has also been evaluated as a method for controlling anticipatory side effects of chemotherapy. In this research (Morrow & Morrell, 1982) the standard desensitization procedure was adapted to the treatment of ANV: A therapist conducted progressive muscle relaxation while a hierarchy of chemotherapy-related situations associated with increasing levels of nausea and/or vomiting was described. Two desensitization sessions were held between chemotherapy treatments in a setting different from where the cytotoxic drugs were administered. The study design involved random assignment of 60 patients with ANV to the desensitization condition or to one of two control conditions: no treatment or placebo treatment (two sessions of Rogerian counseling). Results indicated that, during the two chemotherapy treatments following the intervention sessions, patients in the desensitization condition reported less intense, frequent, and prolonged anticipatory nausea and vomiting than patients in the two control conditions. No significant differences were found between the placebo and no-treatment control conditions, suggesting that the therapeutic effects could not be attributed to attention and support alone.

Research on behavioral interventions for adult chemotherapy patients has focused largely on the treatment of anticipatory reactions. Among pediatric patients, there has been a greater emphasis on behavioral treatment of postchemotherapy nausea and vomiting. This difference in emphasis may reflect the fact that the safety and efficacy of antiemetic drug use with pediatric chemotherapy patients remain largely untested (Zeltzer & LeBaron, 1983). Thus, considerable interest exists in determining if behavioral interventions are an effective alternative to the unknown risks of using antiemetic medication with children.

There are two controlled studies which have used behavioral interventions to relieve postchemotherapy nausea and vomiting in pediatric patients. In one study (Zeltzer, Kellerman, Ellenberg, & Dash, 1983) a group of 12 adolescents referred because of problems with nausea and emesis underwent one to three training sessions in hypnosis before and during chemotherapy infusions. The hypnotic intervention involved the suggestion of pleasant, refreshing imagery to counteract nausea, and the use of posthypnotic suggestions for later symptom control and for easy reentry into the hypnotic state. Results indicated that reductions in the frequency and intensity of postchemotherapy emesis occurred during the hypnosis intervention period relative to the baseline period. In a second study (Zeltzer, LeBaron, & Zeltzer, 1984), 19 patients (ages 6–17 years) complaining of posttreatment nausea and vomiting were assessed across several courses of chemotherapy for which drug dosages remained unchanged. The courses were divided into baseline, intervention, and follow-up phases. After baseline assessment, patients were randomly assigned to either a hypnosis or supportive counseling intervention. In the hypnosis condition, intense use of fantasy and imagery was encouraged during drug infusion, and posthypnotic suggestions were offered aimed at improving eating and sleeping patterns at home. The supportive counseling condition consisted of distracting the child's attention through verbal means while chemotherapy was administered; the child was also instructed to remain as physically active as possible at home to avoid focusing attention on postchemotherapy side effects. Compared to baseline levels, intervention with both hypnosis and supportive counseling was associated with reductions in nausea, vomiting, and the extent to which these symptoms bothered patients. Furthermore, therapeutic gains associated with each intervention were maintained during the follow-up phase of the study. Thus, the study confirmed earlier results (Zeltzer et al., 1983) on the efficacy of hypnosis for reducing postchemotherapy nausea and vomiting. Perhaps equally important is the finding which suggested that distraction during and after chemotherapy (i.e., the supportive counseling intervention) also had therapeutic effects.

The efficacy of distraction has been further investigated in two studies that used video game playing to control adverse reactions to chemotherapy. In the first study (Kolko & Rickard-Figueroa, 1985), video games were used to treat behavioral symptoms of distress during outpatient visits for chemotherapy. Three adolescent cancer patients were studied using a single-case analysis design. Results indicated that fewer distress behaviors (e.g., crying, vomiting) were observed when the patients played video games during clinic visits. In addition, there were reductions in the number of distress symptoms experienced at home prior to chemotherapy on those days when video games were available. The second study (Redd, Jacobsen, Die-Trill, Dermatis, McEvoy, & Holland, 1987) specifically examined the effects of video game playing on nausea before and during chemotherapy. Fifteen pediatric patients (ages 9–18 years) with conditioned nausea were studied using an ABAB withdrawal design which incorporated baseline and intervention assessments within a single session. Results showed that introduction and withdrawal of the opportunity to play video games produced reductions and exacerbations, respectively, in self-reported nausea. Although video games also reduced self-reported anxiety, the effects were weaker than those for nausea. Pulse rate and systolic/diastolic blood pressure were not consistently affected, indicating that the therapeutic effects of video game playing were not associated with reductions in physiological arousal.

Researchers have speculated at length about the mechanism(s) underlying the effectiveness of behavioral interventions for controlling adverse reactions to chemotherapy (Lyles et al., 1982; Morrow & Morrell, 1982; Redd & Andrykowski, 1982). A major controversy concerns whether symptom control is achieved through distraction, relaxation, or a combination of the two factors. Intervention studies employing hypnosis, relaxation training, and desensitization cannot answer this question, since they have all confounded distraction with relaxation: Patients are typically taught to *focus attention* on the comfortable sensations produced by relaxation training or to visualize *relaxing scenes* through imagery techniques. In contrast, behavioral applications of video game playing appear to provide an opportunity to examine the effects of distraction alone. Video games are not typically experienced as relaxing; indeed, their use has been linked to patterns of physiological arousal in normal adults (Turner, Carroll, & Courtney, 1983). Consequently, results from the two studies that employed video games (Kolko & Rickard-Figueroa, 1985; Redd et al., 1987) can be interpreted as indicating that distraction alone is effective in controlling adverse reactions to chemotherapy. The finding in one of the studies (Redd et al., 1987) that reductions in nausea were not associated with decreases in physiological arousal lends further support to the view that distraction yields symptom control in the absence of relaxation. While the video game studies answer some questions, they raise others. For example, what do video games distract attention away from? In the case of conditioned nausea, does distraction yield symptom control by diverting attention away from nausea-eliciting stimuli or from the physical sensations labelled as nausea? Furthermore, the results of the video game studies do not provide an answer to the fundamental question regarding what mechanism(s) are responsible for the success of hypnosis, relaxation therapy, and desensitization in controlling adverse reactions to chemotherapy. Thus, further study is necessary before a comprehensive explanation can be provided for how behavioral procedures control nausea and vomiting in cancer chemotherapy patients.

In summary, chemotherapy-induced nausea and vomiting can give rise to anticipatory side effects of a nonpharmacologic nature. There is considerable empirical support for the view that these behavioral side effects develop via a process of respondent conditioning: through repeated pairings with posttreatment reactions, certain stimuli acquire conditional properties such that their presence alone elicits nausea and vomiting. Conditional responses to chemotherapy have been successfully treated with such behavioral interventions as hypnosis, relaxation training, EMG biofeedback, and systematic desensitization. In addition, hypnosis has been shown to partially relieve postchemotherapy nausea and vomiting in pediatric patients. Recent research suggests that distraction techniques (e.g., video game playing) are also effective in controlling adverse reactions to chemotherapy.

DISTRESS REACTIONS TO PAINFUL PROCEDURES

Another aspect of cancer treatment which can foster behavioral disorders is the repeated performance of painful medical procedures. Many treatment protocols, particularly those for leukemia, require periodic bone marrow aspirations (BMAs) and lumbar punctures (LPs). These invasive procedures are typically used in oncology for diagnostic purposes. A long needle is inserted into the iliac crest (for BMA) or the spinal column (for LP), and fluid is then withdrawn to be examined for the presence of cancerous cells. When used in conjunction with maintenance therapy for certain types of leukemia, these painful diagnostic procedures may be performed repeatedly over a 5-year period (Katz,

Kellerman, & Siegel, 1980). The procedures are usually not conducted under general anesthesia, ostensibly because of the expense and potential medical risk involved. Although local anesthesia may be used, it typically does little to relieve the acute pain caused by these procedures, especially that associated with BMA (Hilgard & LeBaron, 1984).

Because of their generally less well-developed capacities to inhibit behavioral and emotional responses, children are particularly liable to express severe pain in reaction to a BMA or LP. Physical restraint is often necessary to control reactions, such as flailing and screaming, that may prolong or make impossible the completion of the procedure. In addition to the pain associated with the procedure itself, investigators have also noted that most pediatric patients eventually display similar reactions in anticipation of procedure-related pain (Jay, Ozolins, Elliot, & Caldwell, 1983; Katz et al., 1980; LeBaron & Zeltzer, 1984). Along with these reactions immediately before pain is produced, children may also exhibit signs of anxiety (such as nausea, insomnia, and crying) hours or even days before the procedure is scheduled to occur. To better study the pain and anxiety behaviors exhibited by children immediately before and during painful oncology procedures, a number of researchers (Jay et al., 1983; Katz et al., 1980) have developed reliable observational rating scales of behavioral distress. Several factors associated with behavioral distress, as measured by these objective methods, have been identified.

Even among pediatric patients, large age differences exist in reactions to painful oncology procedures. One study (Jay et al., 1983) has shown that the level of observed distress is over five times greater in younger children (ages 2 to 6 years) than in older children (ages 7 to 12 years). Furthermore, younger children tend to display different patterns of distress; behaviors such as crying, screaming, needing restraint, and expressing pain and anxiety verbally have all been found to occur more frequently in younger children (Katz et al., 1980; LeBaron & Zeltzer, 1984). These findings probably reflect maturational differences in capacities for self-control. A second contributory factor may be the tendency for young children to misunderstand the purpose and consequences of the procedure. The younger child more often thinks that the doctor or nurse is punishing him or her for some wrong deed (Katz et al., 1980), or that he or she could die from the procedure (Jay et al., 1983; Spinetta & Maloney, 1975).

Parental anxieties also may be a factor contributing to children's distress during a painful oncology procedure. It has been shown (Jay et al., 1983) that parents' ratings of their own anxiety prior to the procedure, and their anticipation of the amount of pain their child would experience, were both highly correlated with observed distress in the treatment room. These findings are quite consistent with recent theories suggesting that a complex feedback loop exists between parent and child, with each being exquisitely sensitive to the other's emotional reactions (Bloom, 1975).

In the absence of a practical and effective pharmacologic approach, many clinicians have come to rely on behavioral interventions to control children's distress during painful oncology procedures. The efficacy of hypnosis in reducing procedure-related distress has been investigated in several controlled studies. In one study (Hilgard & LeBaron, 1982), training in hypnosis was offered to 24 pediatric patients (ages 6–19 years) reporting pain and exhibiting pain behaviors during BMA. Patients received hypnosis training during a practice session in which the procedure was rehearsed; the next BMA was then conducted under hypnosis. The hypnotic intervention featured encouragements from the therapist for intense involvement in fantasies of a distracting nature. Compared to preintervention levels, the use of hypnosis was associated with marked reductions in patients' anticipatory anxiety as rated by observers. Furthermore, both the number of observed pain behaviors and the intensity of self-reported pain decreased substantially from baseline levels when the BMA was conducted under hypnosis. Not all patients obtained relief from pain with hypnosis. Much of the variability in therapeutic response could be attributed to individual differences in susceptibility to hypnosis. Those patients who scored low on a measure of hypnotic susceptibility tended to obtain the least pain relief.

In another study (Kellerman, Zeltzer, Ellenberg, & Dash, 1983), 16 adolescents with cancer were trained to use hypnosis during BMA, LP, or injection of chemotherapeutic agents. The hypnotic intervention included a practice session in which patients received suggestions for relaxation and increased well-being and posthypnotic suggestions for reduced discomfort and greater mastery during the upcoming painful procedure. During the procedure itself, a therapist offered additional suggestions for enhanced comfort. Data for the three oncology procedures were pooled, and comparisons were made between procedures completed before and after hypnosis training. Results were consistent with earlier findings: the hypnotic intervention was associated with decreases in patients' ratings of discomfort for the periods before, during, and after a painful procedure was performed.

In a third study (Zeltzer & LeBaron, 1982) two behavioral techniques were compared for their efficacy in reducing pain and anxiety during oncology procedures. Following baseline assessment, 45 pediatric patients (ages 6–17 years) receiving repeated BMAs and LPs were randomly assigned to either a hypnotic or a nonhypnotic intervention. In the hypnotic condition, the therapist encouraged involvement in visual imagery and fantasies during a practice session and during an actual procedure session. The nonhypnotic condition featured a practice session designed to help the child control fear; during the actual procedure, the therapist provided verbal distraction and instruction in deep breathing. The findings showed that, for patients receiving BMAs, pain was reduced to a large extent by hypnosis and to a smaller but still significant extent by the nonhypnotic techniques; in contrast, anxiety was reduced only by hypnosis. For patients receiving LPs, only hypnosis relieved pain, while anxiety was reduced to a large degree by hypnosis and to a lesser degree by nonhypnotic techniques. The investigators speculated that the greater pain relief provided by hypnosis may reflect differences in the success of each intervention in distracting patients from the procedures. It is suggested that the children may have quickly lost interest in the nonhypnotic distraction techniques (e.g., counting, deep breathing) and refocused their attention on painful stimuli; in contrast, the use of creative hypnotic fantasies may have successfully distracted attention away from noxious stimulation for more extended periods of time.

Since many children are not easily engaged in hypnosis, there has been interest in determining the usefulness of other behavioral techniques for reducing distress during painful oncology procedures. An alternative approach is the use of a multicomponent intervention program based on the model of stress inoculation (Meichenbaum & Turk, 1976). The *package,* as it is referred to by its developers (Jay & Elliot, 1983), consists of five primary components: (a) the viewing of a film in which a child models good coping behavior during BMA and LP; (b) instruction in deep breathing to induce relaxation and to serve as a distraction; (c) the use of emotive imagery to inhibit anxiety and to foster mastery of pain; (d) behavioral rehearsal of the procedure to provide information, desensitize the situation, and practice coping techniques; and (e) positive reinforcement in the form of a trophy awarded for lying still during the procedure and doing the breathing exercise. In a test of the intervention's efficacy, 56 patients (ages 3–13 years) received the cognitive-behavioral package, a pharmacologic intervention (oral Valium), and minimal treatment (attention control) in a randomized order (Jay, Katz, Elliot, & Siegel, 1987). Results indicated that children exhibited less distress and reported less pain in the cognitive-behavioral condition than in the attention-control condition. The cognitive-behavioral package was effective in reducing distress in both younger and older children. No significant differences in observed distress or self-reported pain were evident between the pharmacologic and control conditions.

In summary, pediatric cancer patients who must undergo repeated painful diagnostic procedures are at risk for developing behavioral reactions characterized by severe anxiety and verbal and physical resistance. There is corroborated evidence that hypnosis is an effective means of reducing both observed distress behaviors and subjective discomfort in older children and adolescents; however, the degree of relief provided may be limited by such factors as hypnotic susceptibility. An alternative approach to controlling procedure-related distress is the use of a multicomponent package of behavioral techniques based on the model of stress inoculation. Data suggest that this package may be effective in reducing distress behavior in younger children, an age group believed less likely to benefit from hypnosis.

ADVERSE REACTIONS TO OTHER CANCER TREATMENTS

Forms of cancer treatment other than chemotherapy and painful diagnostic procedures have received much less attention from behavioral investigators. However, several preliminary studies (primarily employing single-case designs) suggest that behavioral interventions are effective in controlling adverse reactions to such treatments as cancer surgery, radiation therapy, hyperthermia treatment, and confinement in protective isolation.

Surgery

In separate single-case studies, two researchers have described how adverse side effects of surgery for cancer can be treated with the appropriate behavioral interventions. The first study (Nigl, 1979) was of a 62-year-old patient who had not eaten solid food for at least 3 years following radical oral surgery and postoperative radiation therapy for mucosal skin cancer in her oral cavity. The patient's problems with eating involved difficulties with coordination and control of tongue and jaw movements. Treatment consisted of seven training sessions in which the patient engaged in chewing movements while EMG biofeedback was provided. Over the course of treatment, the patient regained the ability to eat solid food. Follow-up assessment at 1 and 4 months indicated that the therapeutic effect was maintained. The change in eating habits was also associated with improvements in mood and self-esteem. Because of the uncontrolled nature of the study, definitive conclusions cannot be drawn; however, the dramatic nature of the results suggests that biofeedback may be useful in improving physical and psychological functioning in some patients following head and neck surgery.

The second study (Redd, 1980a) was of a 53-year-old patient who had been unable to retain solid food in the month following an esophagectomy and partial gastrectomy for carcinoma of the stomach. At the time of study, the patient's digestive system was functional and there was no tumor obstruction. Nevertheless, the patient complained of discomforting throat sensations while eating and would regurgitate all solid foods. She attributed the throat sensations to tumor recurrence, despite assurances to the contrary. Following baseline assessment, the patient was instructed in progressive muscle relaxation; she then underwent a series of desensitization sessions in which relaxation was paired with presentation of food. By the seventh day of treatment, the patient was able to retain all foods presented without gagging or regurgitating. Interspersed with desensitization sessions were control sessions in which food presentation was not paired with relaxation. Continued eating problems during control sessions suggested that desensitization was responsible for the therapeutic effect. Although her eating problems did not recur after desensitization was completed, the patient continued to complain of sensations in her throat; not until the 6-month follow-up session did the patient report she no longer believed a tumor was causing her discomfort. This study suggests that certain eating disorders in cancer patients are a result of inadvertant respondent conditioning. In the present case, the unusual throat sensation appears to have become a conditional stimulus for eliciting regurgitation, an association possibly strengthened by the patient's anxiety that the sensation represented cancer recurrence.

Radiation Therapy

The most commonly used form of radiation therapy involves directing a beam of ionizing radiation at malignant tissue in order to destroy it. However, in addition to destroying malignant tissue, radiation also affects nearby normal tissue, thereby causing a variety of adverse side effects. The specific nature of the side effects depends upon the area of the body treated. For example, when the treated areas include the digestive system, symptoms of nausea, vomiting, and loss of appetite are likely to result. In one study (Welch, 1980) approximately 79% of patients receiving radiation to the trunk reported some degree of nausea and vomiting. Antiemetic medications are of limited usefulness in controlling these radiation-induced side effects (Frytak & Moertel, 1981). Despite the evidence documenting the pervasiveness of these adverse reactions and the relative ineffectiveness of pharmacologic interventions, little behavioral research has been carried out with patients receiving radiation therapy. The need for research in this area is illustrated by a single-case study (Hamberger, 1982) in which relaxation therapy was used successfully to treat gastrointestinal side effects. The patient was a 68-year-old male who had experienced stomach pain, nausea, and vomiting during radiation treatments for bladder cancer. These symptoms continued to occur on a periodic basis once treatment was completed. While the persistence of the symptoms was consistent with known long-term physical effects of radiation therapy, baseline assessment indicated that, in the present case, gastrointestinal attacks were initiated and maintained by feelings of tension. Behavioral treatment involved training in progressive muscle relaxation; the patient then practiced using this skill while imagining specific stressful situations. Following training, the patient was directed to use feelings of tension in everyday life as cues to begin progressive muscle relaxation. The relaxation intervention resulted in the immediate cessation of gastric attacks in the first month following training. A return to baseline levels occurred during the second month when the patient failed to employ relaxation as a response to stress; however, resumption of the regular application of relaxation resulted in a reinstatement of the complete cessation of gastric attacks. Follow-up indicated that the therapeutic effects continued to be maintained after 6 months and 1 year.

Hyperthermia Treatment

Hyperthermia is an experimental cancer treatment which involves placement of a magnetrode in a specific tumor site; electrical energy is then passed through the magnetrode to destroy cancerous tissue by heating it above 42°C (Storm, Harrison, Elliot, Kaiser, Silberman, & Morton, 1981). The treatment typically produces an acute, deep aching sensation, the intensity of which is proportional to the wattage of electricity administered. In approximately one-third of patients, the pain can be so marked that watt dosage must be decreased or treatment terminated even though temperature measurements indicate that no tissue damage is occurring (Reeves, Redd, Storm, & Minagawa, 1983). In the absence of a known, effective analgesic for hyperthermia pain, a study was conducted (Reeves et al., 1983) to determine if hypnosis was useful in controlling patient discomfort. Twenty-eight patients with far-advanced cancer undergoing their first course of hyperthermia treatment were studied. Patients were stratified into groups high and low in hypnotic susceptibility and then randomly assigned to either a hypnotic condition or a no-treatment condition. Following baseline assessment during two hyperthermia treatments, the hypnosis groups received two training sessions in which they were given posthypnotic suggestions for analgesia during subsequent treatments. Results indicated that self-reported pain decreased across the next two treatments in the hypnosis group high in susceptibility, yet remained unchanged in the hypnosis group low in susceptibility and in the no-treatment control groups. These findings regarding the moderating effects of hypnotic susceptibility on pain relief are similar to those obtained with the use of hypnosis to control pain during invasive diagnostic procedures (Hilgard & LeBaron, 1982). Results such as these point to need for continued study of alternative behavioral approaches to pain control.

Confinement in Protective Isolation

As mentioned previously, cancer chemotherapy has toxic effects on both healthy and cancerous cells. Among the healthy cells sensitive to the toxic effects of chemotherapy are those located in bone marrow and blood, which are involved in the functioning of the body's immune system. Suppression of immune system functioning typically occurs as an unwanted side effect of chemotherapy. However, in patients being prepared for bone marrow transplantation, immunosuppression is deliberately induced with chemotherapy and other agents; the immune system is subsequently restored via the intravenous administration of healthy bone marrow and other blood products. During immunosuppression, the body's ability to resist disease and combat infection can be seriously compromised. In fact, infections are a leading cause of death in cancer chemotherapy patients (Kellerman, Siegel, & Rigler, 1980). To reduce the risk of life-threatening infections, cancer patients who are immunosuppressed may be isolated in a germ-free environment for periods exceeding 200 days (Kellerman, Rigler, & Siegel, 1977). While in isolation, adult patients have been noted to refuse medications; to exhibit childlike, demanding, and dependent behaviors; and to withdraw by feigning sleep or refusing to acknowledge staff presence (Kellerman et al., 1977). These reactions have been attributed to the severe restrictions protective isolation imposes on social interaction. Patients are isolated in individual rooms from which they cannot leave for the duration of their stay, and all visitors must typically wear masks, gowns, and gloves. Furthermore, the involved preparations necessary before entering a patient's room tend to discourage staff from making frequent, casual visits with such patients. In one study (Redd, 1980b), a behavioral intervention was used to control psychosomatic symptoms which had developed in two adult patients housed in protective isolation rooms. The first patient, a 24-year-old male, had developed a deep cough which continued to worsen despite the use of medication. The second patient, a 63-year-old female, developed persistent retching for which no medical cause could be identified. Baseline assessment, using audio recordings, indicated that the target symptoms (coughing, retching) dramatically increased in frequency whenever a nurse was present. The behavioral intervention involved instructing the nurses to avoid focusing discussions with patients on the targeted symptoms; nurses were also directed to leave the room immediately after completing a procedure if the targeted behavior occurred, but to remain and talk with the patient for at least 10 minutes if the symptom ceased or did not occur. Seven nurses implemented the intervention on a staggered schedule in order to provide experimental control. Results indicated that suppression of symptoms was obtained with both patients by all nurses and that each successive nurse required fewer visits to achieve symptom suppression. Follow-up assessment 2 weeks later indicated that symptoms had not returned to baseline levels. Thus, the results of the study suggested that the patients' symptoms were being positively reinforced by nursing contacts. The social deprivation associated with protective isolation provided an optimal setting for the inadvertant reinforcement of undesirable behaviors, a situation which was rectified by altering the social reinforcement contingencies.

The studies reviewed in this section describe the successful use of behavioral interventions to control adverse reactions to cancer surgery, radiation therapy, hyperthermia treatment, and confinement in protective isolation. The interventions which were applied to treatment-related problems included biofeedback, behavior modification (i.e., selective reinforcement) and various anxiety-reduction procedures (i.e., hypnosis, progressive muscle relaxation, systematic desensitization). Anxiety-reduction techniques were found to be effective against both acute pain resulting from hyperthermia treatment and persistent gastrointestinal problems arising from radiation therapy and cancer surgery. The application of EMG biofeedback involved the successful treatment of a surgery-related eating disorder. Biofeedback was used to rehabilitate chewing and swallowing movements which had been impaired by repeated oral surgical procedures. Finally, behavior modification was found to be effective when applied to psychosomatic symptoms arising in patients confined to protective isolation. Research showed that, by altering the contingencies for which patients were rewarded with social contact, the occurrence of symptoms that had no obvious medical cause could be markedly reduced.

SUMMARY

Interventions which incorporate behavioral principles are emerging as an important adjunct to modern cancer treatment, and there is growing empirical evidence that such procedures are effective against adverse reactions to a variety of oncology procedures. The domain of comprehensive cancer care must now be expanded to include the use of behavior therapy to control treatment-related symptoms of both physical and psychological origin.

Chemotherapy-related nausea is a prime example of an adverse reaction to which behavioral interventions have been successfully applied. The impetus for this research stems, in part, from the relative ineffectiveness of currently available antiemetic agents. In behavioral research, a useful distinction has been made between the nausea and vomiting which occur before versus after administration of chemotherapeutic agents. Those symptoms occurring prior to chemotherapy infusion are presumed to have nonpharmacologic origins. This view has been supported by research suggesting that anticipatory nausea and vomiting arise through a process of respondent conditioning similar to the development of learned taste aversions. Conditioned chemotherapy-related nausea and vomiting have been successfully treated in controlled studies with five different behavioral interventions: hypnosis, relaxation, EMG biofeedback, systematic desensitization, and cognitive/attentional distraction. In addition, behavioral research has shown that hypnosis is effective against posttreatment nausea and vomiting in pediatric chemotherapy patients. The mechanisms underlying the effectiveness of these procedures remain unclear. Research with video game playing to control conditioned nausea suggests that symptom control can be obtained with distraction alone; however, these findings do not rule out the possibility that different mechanisms (e.g., relaxation) may be responsible for the effectiveness of other procedures.

Another aspect of oncology where behavioral interventions have had a major impact is the control of distress reactions during painful diagnostic procedures. Clinical care of certain forms of cancer (e.g., leukemia) can require the repeated performance of bone marrow aspirations and lumbar puncture over a period of several years. Many children and adolescents eventually display distress reactions in anticipation of these procedures; in cases where these reactions include verbal and physical resistance, completion of the procedure may be prolonged or made impossible. In the absence of a practical pharmacologic method for eliminating pain and preventing distress, the efficacy of behavioral interventions has been tested. Hypnosis has been found to be effective against procedure-related distress, but its usefulness was limited by the degree of a patient's hypnotic susceptibility. A successful alternative to hypnosis was recently developed which is appropriate for use with very young children, an age group generally low in hypnotic susceptibility. The intervention is based on the model of stress inoculation and has five primary components: modeling, deep breathing exercises, emotive imagery, behavioral rehearsal, and positive reinforcement. Research on controlling children's distress during painful oncology procedures has, for the most part, been oriented toward immediate clinical needs. Theoretical issues have emerged, nonetheless, which may influence future research on the use of behavioral interventions. These issues include identifying the factors contributing to age-related differences in hypnotic susceptibility and clarifying the role of individual and familial factors in determining a child's pattern and level of distress.

Other forms of cancer treatment have yet to be as thoroughly investigated by behavioral researchers. Results, mostly of the single-case studies, suggest that behavioral interventions can be used successfully against adverse reactions to cancer surgery, radiation therapy, hyperthermia treatment, and confinement in protective isolation. The range of problems to which behavioral techniques has been applied includes acute procedure-related pain, persistent gastrointestinal symptoms, an eating disorder of physical origin, and psychosomatic symptoms for which no obvious medical cause could be identified. To control these adverse reactions, investigators have relied on the standard behavioral techniques of hypnosis, progressive muscle relaxation, biofeedback, systematic desensitization, and behavior modification. These preliminary studies illustrate how behavioral researchers are continuing to identify new applications for behavioral interventions in oncology settings.

Research in behavior aspects of oncology is a burgeoning field. More and more cancer patients are appreciating the benefits which can by yielded by the use of behavioral interventions to control treatment-related side effects. Furthermore, research in this area is likely to experience continued growth, since oncology is a rapidly changing discipline in which innovative treatments are continually subjected to rigorous experimental study. The experimental tradition in oncology provides an environment most conducive to the conduct of behavioral research. Both disciplines value the need for hypothesis testing and empirical validation in order to advance, factors which will continue to contribute to a productive interdisciplinary collaboration.

REFERENCES

Altmaier, E. M., Ross, W. E., & Moore, K. (1982). A pilot investigation of the psychologic functioning of patients with anticipatory vomiting. *Cancer, 49,* 201–204.

American Cancer Society. (1985). *Cancer facts and figures*. New York: Author.

Andrykowski, M. A., Jacobsen, P. B., Marks, E., Gorfinkle, K., Hakes, T. B., Kaufman, R. J., Currie, V. E., Holland, J. C., & Redd, W. H. (1988). Prevalence, predictors, and course of anticipatory nausea in women receiving adjuvant chemotherapy for breast cancer. *Cancer, 62,* 2607–2613.

Andrykowski, M. A., Redd, W. H., & Hatfield, A. K. (1985). Development of anticipatory nausea: A prospective analysis. *Journal of Consulting and Clinical Psychology, 53,* 447–454.

Bloom, K. (1977). Patterning of infant vocal behavior. *Journal of Experimental Child Psychology, 23,* 367–377.

Burish, T. G., & Lyles, J. N. (1981). Effectiveness of relaxation training in reducing adverse reactions to cancer chemotherapy. *Journal of Behavioral Medicine, 4,* 65–78.

Burish, T. G., Shartner, L. D., & Lyles, J. N. (1981). Effectiveness of multiple muscle-site EMG biofeedback and relaxation training in reducing the aversiveness of cancer chemotherapy. *Biofeedback and Self-Regulation, 6,* 523–535.

Chang, J. C. (1981). Nausea and vomiting in cancer patients: An expression of psychological mechanisms? *Psychosomatics, 22,* 707–709.

Dolgin, M. D., Katz, E. R., McGinty, K., & Siegel, S. E. (1985). Anticipatory reactions in pediatric cancer patients receiving chemotherapy. *Pediatrics, 75,* 547–552.

Fetting, J. H., Wilcox, P. M., Iwata, B. A., Criswell, E. L., Bosmajian, L. S., & Sheidler, V. R. (1983). Anticipatory nausea and vomiting in an ambulatory medical oncology population. *Cancer Treatment Reports, 67,* 1093–1098.

Fetting, J., Wilcox, P., Sheidler, V., Donehower, R., Grochow, L., & Enterline, J. (1984). 'Tasting' parenteral chemotherapy for breast cancer. *Proceedings of the American Society of Clinical Oncology, 3,* 74.

Frytak, S., & Moertel, L. G. (1981). Management of nausea and vomiting in the cancer patient. *Journal of the American Medical Association, 245,* 393–396.

Golden, S., Horwich, C., & Lokich, J. (1980). *Chemotherapy and you* (DHEW Publication No. NIH 77-1136). Bethesda, MD: National Institutes of Health.

Gralla, R. J. (1981). Metoclopramide: Initial clinical studies of high-dosage regimens in cisplatin-induced emesis. In D. S. Poster, J. S. Periter, & S. Bruna (Eds.), *Treatment of cancer chemotherapy-induced nausea and vomiting* (pp. 167–176). New York: Masson.

Hamberger, L. K. (1982). Reduction of generalized aversive responding in a posttreatment cancer patient: Relaxation as an active coping skill. *Journal of Behavior Therapy and Experimental Psychiatry, 13,* 229–233.

Harris, J. G. (1978). Nausea, vomiting, and cancer treatment. *Ca—A Cancer Journal for Clinicians, 28,* 194–201.

Hilgard, J. R., & LeBaron, S. (1982). Relief of anxiety & pain in children & adolescents with cancer: Quantitative measures and clinical observations. *International Journal of Clinical & Experimental Hypnosis, 30,* 417–442.

Hilgard, J. R., & LeBaron, S. (1984). *Hypnotherapy of pain in children with cancer.* Los Altos, CA: William Kaufmann.

Jay, S. M., & Elliott, C. M. (1983). Psychological intervention for pain in pediatric cancer patients. In G. B. Humphrey, B. B. Grindey, L. R. Dehmer, R. T. Acton, & T. J. Pysher (Eds.), *Adrenal & endocrine tumors in children* (pp. 123–154). Boston, MA: Martinus Nijhoff.

Jay, S. M., Elliot, C. H., Katz, E., & Siegel, S. E. (1987). Cognitive-behavioral and pharmacologic interventions for children's distress during painful medical procedures. *Journal of Consulting and Clinical Psychology, 55,* 860–865.

Jay, S. M., Ozolins, M., Elliott, C. H., & Caldwell, S. (1983). Assessment of children's distress during painful medical procedures. *Health Psychology, 2,* 133–148.

Katz, E. R. (1982). Behavioral conditioning in the development and maintenance of vomiting in cancer patients. *Psychosomatics, 23,* 650–651.

Katz, E. R., Kellerman, J., & Siegel, S. E. (1980). Behavioral distress in children with cancer undergoing medical procedures: Developmental considerations. *Journal of Consulting and Clinical Psychology, 48,* 356–365.

Kellerman, J., Rigler, D., & Siegel, S. E. (1977). The psychological effects of isolation in protected environments. *American Journal of Psychiatry, 134,* 563–565.

Kellerman, J., Siegel, S., & Rigler, D. (1980). Special treatment modalities: Laminar air flow rooms. In J. Kellerman (Ed.), *Psychological aspects of childhood cancer* (pp. 128–154). Springfield, IL: Thomas.

Kellerman, J., Zeltzer, L., Ellenberg, L., & Dash, J. (1983). Adolescents with cancer: Hypnosis for the reduction of the acute pain and anxiety associated with medical procedures. *Journal of Adolescent Health Care, 4,* 76–81.

Kolko, D. J., & Rickard-Figueroa, J. L. (1985). Effects of video games on the adverse corollaries of chemotherapy in pediatric oncology patients: A single-case analysis. *Journal of Consulting and Clinical Psychology, 53,* 223–228.

LeBaron, S., & Zeltzer, L. (1984). Assessment of acute pain and anxiety in children and adolescents by self-reports, observer reports, and a behavior checklist. *Journal of Consulting and Clinical Psychology, 52,* 729–738.

Lyles, J. N., Burish, T. G., Krozely, M. G., & Oldham, R. K. (1982). Reducing the aversiveness of cancer chemotherapy. *Journal of Consulting and Clinical Psychology, 50,* 509–524.

Meichenbaum, D., & Turk, D. (1976). The cognitive-behavioral management of anxiety, anger, and pain. In P. O. Davidson (Ed.), *The behavioral management of anxiety depression and pain* (pp. 1–34). New York: Brunner Mazel.

Morrow, G. R. (1982). Prevalence and correlates of anticipatory nausea and vomiting in chemotherapy patients. *Journal of the National Cancer Institute, 68,* 585–588.

Morrow, G. R., Arsenau, J. C., Asbury, R. F., Bennet, J. M., & Boros, L. (1982). Anticipatory nausea and vomiting with chemotherapy. *New England Journal of Medicine, 306,* 431–432.

Morrow, G. R., & Morrell, C. (1982). Behavioral treatment for the anticipatory nausea and vomiting induced by cancer chemotherapy. *New England Journal of Medicine, 307,* 1476–1480.

Nerenz, D. R., Leventhal, H., & Love, R. R. (1982). Factors contributing to emotional distress during cancer chemotherapy. *Cancer, 50,* 1020–1027.

Nesse, R. M., Carli, T., Curtis, G. C., & Kleinman, P. D. (1980). Pretreatment nausea in cancer chemotherapy: A conditioned response? *Psychosomatic Medicine, 42,* 33–36.

Nicholas, D. R. (1982). Prevalence of anticipatory nausea and emesis in cancer chemotherapy patients. *Journal of Behavioral Medicine, 5,* 461–463.

Nigl, A. J. (1979). Electromyograph training to increase oral cavity functioning in a postoperative cancer patient. *Behavior Therapy, 10,* 423–427.

Redd, W. H. (1980a). In vivo desentization in the treatment of chronic emesis following gastrointestinal surgery. *Behavior Therapy, 11,* 421–427.

Redd, W. H. (1980b). Stimulus control and extinction of psychosomatic symptoms in cancer patients in protective isolation. *Journal of Consulting and Clinical Psychology, 48,* 448–455.

Redd, W. H., Andresen, G. V., & Minagawa, R. Y. (1982). Hypnotic control of anticipatory emesis in patients receiving cancer chemotherapy. *Journal of Consulting and Clinical Psychology, 50,* 14–19.

Redd, W. H., & Andrykowski, M. A. (1982). Behavioral intervention in cancer treatment: Controlling aversive reactions to chemotherapy. *Journal of Consulting and Clinical Psychology, 30,* 1018–1029.

Redd, W. H., Jacobsen, P. B., Die-Trill, M., Dermatis, H., McEvoy, M., & Holland, J. C. (1987). Cognitive/attentional distraction in the control of conditioned nausea in pediatric cancer patients receiving chemotherapy. *Journal of Consulting and Clinical Psychology, 55,* 391–395.

Reeves, J. L., Redd, W. H., Storm, F. K., & Minagawa, R. Y. (1983). Hypnosis in the control of pain during hyperthermia treatment of cancer. *Advances in Pain Research and Therapy, 5,* 857–861.

Rozencweig, M., Von Hoff, D. D., Slavic, M., & Muggia, F. M. (1977). Cis-diamminedichloroplatinum (II): A new anticancer drug. *Annals of Internal Medicine, 86,* 803–812.

Scogna, D. M., & Smalley, R. V. (1979). Chemotherapy-induced nausea & vomiting. *American Journal of Nursing, 79,* 1502–1504.

Spinetta, J. J., & Maloney, L. J. (1975). Death anxiety in the outpatient leukemic child. *Pediatrics, 56,* 1034–1037.

Storm, F. K., Harrison, W., Elliot, R. S., Kaiser, L. R., Silberman, A. W., & Morton, D. C. (1981). Clinical radio frequency hyperthermia by magnetic loop induction. *Journal of Microwave Power, 16,* 179–184.

Turner, J. R., Carroll, D., & Courtney, H. (1983). Cardiac and metabolic responses to 'space invaders': An instance of metabolically-exaggerated cardiac adjustment? *Psychophysiology, 20,* 544–549.

van Komen, R. W., & Redd, W. H. (1985). Personality factors associated with anticipatory nausea/vomiting in patients receiving cancer chemotherapy. *Health Psychology, 4,* 189–202.

Wilcox, P. M., Fetting, J. H., Nettesheim, K. M., & Abeloff, M. D. (1982). Anticipatory vomiting in women receiving cyclophosphamide, methotrexate, and 5-FU (CMF) adjuvant chemotherapy for breast carcinoma. *Cancer Treatment Reports, 66,* 1601–1604.

Welch, D. A. (1980). Assessment of nausea and vomiting in cancer patients undergoing external beam radiotherapy. *Cancer Nursing, 3,* 365–371.

Zeltzer, L., Kellerman, J., Ellenberg, L., & Dash, J. (1983). Hypnosis for reduction of vomiting associated with chemotherapy and disease in adolescents with cancer. *Journal of Adolescent Health Care, 4,* 77–84.

Zeltzer, L., & LeBaron, S. (1982). Hypnosis and nonhypnotic techniques for reduction of pain and anxiety during painful procedures in children and adolescents with cancer. *Journal of Pediatrics, 101,* 1032–1035.

Zeltzer, L., & LeBaron, S. (1983). Behavioral intervention for children and adolescents with cancer. *Behavioral Medicine Update, 5,* 17–22.

Zeltzer, L., LeBaron, S., & Zeltzer, P. M. (1984). The effectiveness of behavioral intervention for reduction of nausea and vomiting in children and adolescents receiving chemotherapy. *Journal of Clinical Oncology, 2,* 683–690.

13

Behavioral Aspects of Diabetes*

Suzanne Bennett-Johnson

Departments of Psychiatry,
Pediatrics, and Clinical Psychology and Health Psychology
University of Florida Health Science Center
Gainesville, FL

Diabetes mellitus is characterized by insufficient insulin production by the pancreas or the insufficient use of available insulin by body tissues. Since the absorption of glucose into muscle and fat cells is governed by insulin, insufficient insulin availability or its inefficient utilization results in abnormally high levels of blood glucose or hyperglycemia which spills over into the urine (glycosuria). In fact, "sweet urine" was recognized as a classic sign of the disease many centuries ago (Bennett, 1983). In severe cases, insulin availability is nonexistent or so minimal that the body literally "starves" despite the existence of high levels of glucose in the blood. The patient feels constantly hungry, eats large quantities of food, but loses weight. The body begins to break down fat, which results in high levels of fatty acids and ketones in the blood and urine. In an attempt to rid the body of these excessive fatty

* Supported by grants R01 HD13820 and K04 HD00686 from the National Institute of Child Health and Human Development, and the National Institute of Diabetes, Digestive and Kidney Diseases.

acids, frequent urination occurs which leads to thirst and increased fluid intake. These are the classic signs of diabetes: polyuria (excessive urination), polydipsia (excessive drinking), polyphasia (excessive eating), and glycosuria ("sweet urine"). In severe, untreated cases, the build-up of fatty acids can result in ketoacidosis, coma, and ultimately death.

Although hyperglycemia is the hallmark of diabetes mellitus, there are at least two different forms of the disorder. Insulin dependent diabetes mellitus (IDDM) is characterized by complete pancreatic failure, abrupt onset of symptoms, and proneness to ketoacidosis. Daily insulin injections are necessary for survival. This form of the disorder has also been labeled Type I diabetes or juvenile diabetes, because onset typically occurs during childhood or adolescence. Patients with IDDM almost always present with the classic signs of the disease. Non-insulin-dependent diabetes (NIDDM), also known as Type II or adult-onset diabetes, can be more difficult to diagnose, since classic signs and symptoms are not always present. Patients with this form of the disorder are typically obese adults. In many cases, the disease can be managed by weight reduction and diet modification, although exogeneous insulin replacement is sometimes required. In mild NIDDM, hyperglycemia is not evident in the fasting state but becomes apparent in response to a glucose challenge. In moderate and severe cases, hyperglycemia is apparent even after an overnight fast.

IDDM is clearly the less common form of the disorder, accounting for 5%–10% of all cases of diabetes in the United States (LaPorte & Cruikshanks, 1985). Prevalence rates vary by country and ethnic group. IDDM is rare or unknown among Japanese, Indians, Chinese, Filopinos, American Indians, Eskimos, South African Negroes, and Polynesians. In caucasion populations of the United States and Western Europe, prevalence rates range from .3 to 3.5 per 1,000 persons. Incidence rates range from 7.7 to 20.0 per 100,000 persons. Although IDDM can occur at any age, the peak incidence age is 11–12 years (Zimmet, 1983).

As with IDDM, prevalence rates for NIDDM vary by geographic location and ethnic origin. In the United States, incidence rates are estimated at 32 cases per 10,000, compared to 1–2 cases per 10,000 for IDDM (LaPorte & Cruikshanks, 1985). Worldwide, lowest prevalence rates are found among Eskimos, Athabascan Indians (Alaska), and the Chinese in Singapore. The highest rates are reported for American Indians and Pacific Island populations. NIDDM used to be rare in these groups but has become prevalent with progressive modernization of life style. It has been suggested that a genetic susceptibility to NIDDM in these populations has been unmasked by environmental factors. It is noteworthy that IDDM has remained rare in these ethnic groups despite the increasing prevalence of NIDDM (Zimmett, 1983).

The etiology of diabetes is not completely understood. There appears to be a genetic component to both IDDM and NIDDM. It has been hypothesized that IDDM is an autoimmune disease in which antibodies attack the pancreas, destroying the insulin-producing beta cells (LaPorte & Cruikshanks, 1985). Factors predictive of NIDDM onset include a family history of diabetes, obesity, and increasing age (Everhart et al., 1985). Zimmet (1983) has pointed out that the decline in glucose tolerance associated with age is probably due to the expression of increasing numbers of true diabetics over time rather than a normal consequence of the aging process. The World Health Organization's Expert Committee on Diabetes Mellitus (1980) concluded that obesity is the most powerful risk factor for NIDDM, particularly in groups with a genetic predisposition for the disease. Obesity is associated with insulin resistance or a diminished sensitivity of the body to available insulin. As a consequence, both hyperglycemia and hyperinsulinemia (abnormally high levels of insulin) occur. In most cases, these effects are reversed by weight loss. Consequently, treatment of the obese patient with NIDDM involves caloric restrictions in an effort to induce and maintain sufficient weight loss. Daily exercise is considered a useful adjunct, not only as a means of inducing weight loss, but because exercise tends to increase insulin sensitivity and hence reduce hyperglycemia (Salans, Knittle, & Hirsch, 1983).

A number of complications are associated with diabetes of long duration. These include retinopathy (a leading cause of blindness), nephropathy (a common cause of kidney failure), peripheral vascular disease (associated with gangrene and limb amputations), heart disease, hypertension, and stroke. It is believed that both the onset and severity of these complications is influenced by the patient's diabetic control (Davidson, 1981). Consequently, patients are encouraged to maintain their blood glucose levels as close to normal as possible.

Normoglycemia is, in fact, the goal of all treatment programs for diabetic patients. However, the achievement of this goal is limited by both available technology and patient motivation. IDDM, which involves complete pancreatic failure, requires daily exogeneous insulin replacement. Before 1922, when insulin was discovered, youngsters with this disorder died. Today they have a more normal life expectancy. Nevertheless, daily insulin injections do not mimic normal pancreatic function. The patient must eat frequently (three meals and three snacks a day is recommended) and avoid concentrated sweets. Since this management program cannot guarantee normoglycemia, the patient must be alert for signs of abnormally low (hypoglycemia) or high blood glucose. Patients are instructed to test their urine or blood two to four times a day in order to monitor their blood glucose levels. They must know what action to take in situations of hypo- or excessive hyperglycemia. Hypoglycemia, or "insulin shock," can be particularly serious because of its relatively rapid onset and potentially dire consequences (coma and death).

Diet is important to the management of both IDDM and NIDDM. However, for the obese patient with NIDDM the goal is to restrict calorie consumption to achieve weight loss. A substantial number of patients with NIDDM are also given oral hypoglycemic agents, or in some cases, insulin injections, in order to improve metabolic control. In such cases, both the total and distribution of the patient's caloric consumption across a day must be considered so as to avoid hypoglycemic reactions. In the past, patients with diabetes were often given carbohydrate restricted diets in order to avoid hyperglycemia. Today, there is a greater emphasis on increasing complex carbohydrate consumption and reducing fat intake due to the high incidence of heart disease in this population.

Exercise is considered advantageous to patients with either IDDM or NIDDM, as it enhances the effectiveness of available insulin. However, for patients taking insulin, diet and exercise must be coordinated so as to avoid hypoglycemic reactions.

Recently, there has been a great deal of interest in the use of portable insulin pumps. These mechanical devices deliver insulin subcutaneously at a specified rate that can be changed by the patient. For example, the infusion rate is increased at meal time and decreased before exercise. For IDDM patients, these pumps offer more continuous insulin infusion that can be more easily modified in response to eating or exercise than is the case with conventional therapy which consists of one to two insulin injections per day. However, currently available pumps are technically unable to mimic the normal pancreas by releasing insulin in response to blood glucose levels. Rather, the patient estimates his or her insulin needs and selects an infusion rate based on this estimate. The patient must regularly assess his or her blood glucose concentration in order to ensure an appropriate infusion rate. Consequently, insulin pumps should be used only by highly motivated patients. The pumps are worn 24 hours a day, with the infusion site changed every 2 days. Hazards include skin infections, the development of subcutaneous nodules at the infusion site, mechanical failure, and operator error. If a pump is inadvertently left on at a high infusion rate after a meal, for example, severe hypoglycemia may result. Nocturnal hypoglycemia is an additional potential problem typically managed by frequent monitoring of blood glucose levels at 3:00 a.m.! While there is evidence that insulin delivery via a portable infusion pump leads to blood glucose levels that more closely approximate normal, insulin pumps are still considered experimental and appropriate only for highly motivated adult or adolescent patients or well-supervised children (Raskin, 1983; Schade, Santiago, Skyler, & Rizza, 1983).

The role of psychological factors in diabetes has long been recognized. In the seventeenth century, Thomas Willis (1684) stated that he believed the disease was the result of "prolonged sorrow." Two hundred years later, Maudsley (1899) commented on the importance of anxiety as a correlate of diabetes onset. Nevertheless, until the ready availability of insulin, the study of psychological factors remained minimal, particularly in the area of IDDM. All of this changed in the early twentieth century with the advent of insulin and the development of a widespread interest in psychosomatic medicine. Heavily influenced by psychoanalytic theory, research initially focused on the elucidation of a "diabetic personality" which would predispose the individual to the disease. Dunbar (1954), for example, believed the patient with diabetes had certain personality characteristics which differentiated him or her from other illness groups. These included dependence–independence conflicts, poor sexual adjustment, anxiety, depression, and paranoid suspicion. Today, it is generally accepted that there is no specific diabetic personality. In fact, diabetes per se is not typically associated with emotional or behavioral disorders. However, there is some evidence that patients in poor health have more adjustment problems than those in good diabetic control (Johnson, 1980).

While studies of the "diabetic personality" no longer dominate psychosocial research on diabetes, an interest in behavioral, emotional, and social variables as they relate to diabetes remains. In fact, there appears to be an ever increasing interest in the psychological aspects of health and illness, as is indicated by the now common use of terms such as *behavioral medicine, health psychology,* and *behavioral pediatrics*. However, the focus of research conducted under the rubric of these various terms has changed. Past studies emphasized the study of variables within the individual (e.g., personality) and the comparison of groups of patients to healthy controls. While these studies continue to be conducted, different perspectives are now emerging. Investigators are interested in psychological variables relevant to health and adjustment within an illness population. Greater recognition is given to the fact that people respond to diabetes in very different ways. Some people do extremely well, while others are constantly sick and evidence numerous adjustment problems. Since good diabetic control is believed to prevent or diminish the severity of complications in later life (Cahill, Etzwiler, & Freinkel, 1976), the importance of behavioral factors to good diabetic control is receiving increasing attention.

The remainder of this chapter will focus on what patients with diabetes know about their disease, how they manage it, and the possible impact of psychological stress in diabetes management and metabolic control. Both the descriptive and the intervention literature will be considered.

PATIENT KNOWLEDGE ABOUT DIABETES

Knowledge about diabetes is a prerequisite for successfully managing the disease; if the patient does not know what to do, he or she cannot do it. Unfortunately, one of the consistencies found in the diabetes literature is the inadequacy of patients' knowledge about their own disease (Watts, 1980). Not only do they perform poorly on tests of general information, but errors in insulin administration and glucose testing are common among children and adults (Epstein, Coburn, Becker, Drash, & Siminero, 1980; Etzwiler & Sines, 1962; Johnson et al., 1982; Watkins, Roberts, Williams, Martin, & Coyle, 1967). To complicate matters further, it appears that patients do not have a consistent knowledge base about all aspects of the disease. Two studies assessed general knowledge about diabetes as well as skill at insulin injection and urine glucose testing in an IDDM population. The patients' skill at one diabetes management task (i.e., insulin injection) was not related to their skill at the other diabetes management task (i.e., urine testing), and the patients' skill at either urine testing or insulin injection was unrelated to their general knowledge about diabetes. This suggests that knowledge of all important aspects of diabetes care must be assessed if a clear picture of the patient's understanding of this illness is desired (Harkavy, Johnson, Silverstein, Spillar, McCallum, & Rosenbloom, 1983; Johnson et al., 1982).

With childhood diabetic populations, the youngster's cognitive developmental level is an important determinant of what the patient knows about diabetes and his or her ability to accurately carry out required diabetes management tasks. Both knowledge and skill increase in age-related stages (Etzwiler, 1962; Gilbert, Johnson, Spillar, McCallum, Silverstein, & Rosenbloom, 1982; Harkavy et al., 1983; Johnson et al., 1982; Karp, Manor, & Laron, 1970; LaGreca, Follansbee, & Skyler, 1982). Studies in the United States suggest that most youngsters are capable of self-injection around 9 years of age (Gilbert et al., 1982; Harkavy et al., 1983; Johnson et al., 1982). These findings are consistent with an English study that reported the youngster's age at diagnosis was an important determinant of how quickly the patient began regularly self-injecting. Of 27 children whose diabetes was diagnosed before the age of 9, none gave their own injections immediately after diagnosis. In contrast, 18 of 27 children whose diabetes developed at 9 years or later began self-injecting as soon as their diabetes was diagnosed (Naughten, Smith, & Baum, 1982). Kohler, Hurwitz, and Milan (1982) also reported that 83% of their 9–12-year-old patients were injecting their own insulin, while only 17% of their 5–8-year-olds were doing so. While 9-year-old youngsters may be capable of self-injection, they are not usually able to accurately test their urine or blood for glucose. It is best to wait until children are 12 years of age before expecting them to perform this task independently (Harkavy et al., 1983; Johnson et al., 1982).

Because children's knowledge of diabetes is limited by their cognitive developmental level, parents necessarily play a significant role in the management of their child's disease. Nevertheless, there are few studies that have assessed parental knowledge about diabetes. Of the studies that do exist, mothers are consistently reported to know more about diabetes than any other family member. But, adolescent patients are often as knowledgeable as their mothers and more knowledgeable than their fathers (Karp et al., 1970; Garner, Thompson, & Partridge, 1969; Etzwiler & Sines, 1962; Johnson et al., 1982; Partridge, Garner, Thompson, & Cherry, 1972). These findings are congruent with the fact that mothers usually take more responsibility for the management of the child's illness than do fathers (Etzwiler & Sines, 1962).

Adequate patient (or parent) knowledge about diabetes is deemed important because of its presumed relationship to compliance or adherence. Although there is some support for the proposition that more knowledgeable patients are more adherent (Christensen, Terry, Wyatt, Pichert, & Lorenz, 1983; Hulka, Cassel, Kupper, & Burdette, 1976; Watkins, Williams, Martin, Hogan, & Anderson, 1967; Wysocki, Czyzyk, Slonska, Krolewski, & Janeczko, 1978), there have been few empirical tests of this assumption. Similarly, few studies have examined the relationship between knowledge and diabetic control; available reports offer mixed results. In adults, for example, Stone (1961) and Peyrot and McMurry (1985) found that poorer control was associated with inadequate knowledge. Their results are consistent with a recent investigation in which good dietary knowledge was associated with lower, and consequently more adequate, levels of hemoglobin Al (one index of diabetic control; McCulloch, Young, Steel, Wilson, Prescott, & Duncan, 1983). Other investigators, however, have not found hemoglobin Al values, or other indices of diabetic control, to be significantly associated with patient knowledge (Beggan, Cregan, & Drury, 1982; Hulka, Kupper, Cassel, & Mayo, 1975; Ingersoll, Orr, Herrold, & Golden, 1986; Kaplan, Chadwick, & Schimmel, 1985; Wysocki et al.,

1978). In fact, Williams, Martin, Hogan, Watkins, and Ellis (1967) reported an inverse relationship between diabetes knowledge and diabetic control; more knowledgeable patients were in poorer health. The Williams et al. (1967) finding is not an isolated one, as it has been reported in two studies focusing on youngsters with IDDM (Hamburg & Inoff, 1982; Ludvigsson, 1977). The usual explanation is that patients in poor control may receive more diabetes relevant instruction and, consequently, become more knowledgeable.

EDUCATIONAL PROGRAMS TO IMPROVE PATIENT KNOWLEDGE

Although most diabetes educational programs have not been empirically evaluated, there is little doubt that some programs do improve the knowledge of some patients. Early studies with adults indicated that formal diabetes instruction increased patient knowledge over and above routine medical care, which gave minimal time to educational issues (Bowen, Rich, & Schlotfeldt, 1961; Hassel & Medved, 1975). One of the few studies evaluating a program's effectiveness for children and parents was reported by Etzwiler and Robb (1972). Although no control groups were used, their automated "teaching machine" did enhance diabetic knowledge in all groups exposed to this procedure. These gains were maintained at a 3-month follow-up. A controlled investigation by Epstein, Figueroa, Farkas, and Beck (1981) demonstrated the effectiveness of corrective feedback as a method of improving children's accuracy at urine glucose determinations. Heston and Lazar (1980) used an instructional book and game with 7–12-year-old patients. Youngsters who received instruction learned more than control children who remained unexposed to the program. The patient's age was associated both with how much the youngster knew before participating in the program and how much he or she learned; the 7–10-year-olds were less knowledgeable than the 11–12-year-olds. The importance of patient age to learning in children was also highlighted in a study by Harkavy et al. (1983), who reported differential improvement in patient knowledge over the course of a 2-week diabetes summer camp; 12–14-year-olds seemed to learn from the experience, while 10–11-year-olds did not. Similar findings were reported by Gilbert et al. (1982), who used a peer-modeling film to teach self-injection technique. This approach was effective for 8- and 9-year-old girls, but not for younger children of either sex. These studies suggest that cognitive development level is an important determinant of what children with diabetes know about their disease as well as of their ability to learn from educational experiences presented to them. Tailoring educational programs to the developing cognitive capabilities of the child seems to be particularly important for child and adolescent IDDM populations.

Most educational programs present relatively standard information to all patients based on the assumption that people respond to diabetes in very similar ways. Recently, there has been increasing empirical evidence that patients with this disease may experience hypo- and hyperglycemic states differently, and that standard or "classic" symptoms of hypo- or hyperglycemia are *not* experienced by all or even most patients. An initial study on this topic indicated that, while youngsters said they could "tell" when their blood sugar levels were high or low by how they felt, they frequently failed to select "classic" symptoms as the basis for this determination (Eastman, Johnson, Silverstein, Spillar, & McCallum, 1938). One possible explanation for this finding is that different patients experience different symptoms when hypo- or hyperglycemic. This hypothesis was tested with a group of 26 adolescents with IDDM. Prior to each of 40 blood glucose determination, the patient identified any symptoms he or she was experiencing (e.g., headache, tired, shakey). When the data were analyzed for the group as a whole, few significant symptom–blood glucose relationships were obtained. However, when each patient's data were analyzed separately, 24 of the 26 participants had one or more symptoms that were predictive of blood glucose levels. Different patients experienced different symptoms; most of the "classic" symptoms of hypo- or hyperglycemia were not "classic" at all and, in fact, were experienced by a minority of the patients (Freund, Johnson, Rosenbloom, Alexander, & Hansen, 1986). This research, conducted with IDDM adolescents, replicated previous findings with diabetic adults (Pennebaker, Cox, Gonder-Frederick, Wunsch, Evans, & Pohl, 1981). Both studies highlight the potential importance of individual differences between patients in the experience and management of diabetes. Educational programs that assess and utilize the patient's individual response to this disease may prove more successful than those which teach only standard information to all patients.

The goal of educational programs is not to simply improve knowledge about diabetes but to enhance adherence and diabetic control. As Lane and Evans (1979) have pointed out, outcome measures of patient educational programs should include health status, adherence, use of health services, and disease adaptation measures in addition to indicators of knowledge about the disease. Unfortunately, few studies consider more than one of these outcome measures. In a 1981 review of patient education relevant to chronic disease, Mazzuca (1982) found 320 relevant articles. However, only 30 of these were controlled studies that included outcome measures relevant to both patient adherence and health status. Using a somewhat more liberal criteria for selection, articles on diabetes program instruction that included adherence *or* health status measures will be reviewed here. Almost all of these studies have been conducted with adult patients.

Uncontrolled studies have reported a decrease in hospitalization rates for diabetic patients subsequent to an educational program (Fishbein, 1985; Jacobsen, O'Rourke, & Wolf, 1983; Merrit, Hall, Kobernus, & Tanenberg, 1983). However, none of these studies evaluated change in patient knowledge, although Merritt et al. (1983) did report small improvements in other status measures (i.e., blood glucose levels and weight) subsequent to the educational intervention. Etzwiler and Robb (1972) reported an improvement in diabetes knowledge but no improvement in the metabolic control of the children and adolescents studied. Chandalia and Bagrodia (1979) reported improvements in both patient knowledge and mean blood glucose levels in their uncontrolled study of NIDDM adults seen in a nutritional counseling program.

The few available controlled investigations have consistently documented increased patient knowledge about diabetes but variable outcomes in terms of health status (Bowen et al., 1961; Karlander & Kindstedt, 1983; Korhonen et al., 1983). It appears that, when metabolic improvements do occur, they are relatively short-lived (Korhonen et al., 1983; Whitehouse, Whitehouse, Smith, & Hohl, 1979). It is probably unreasonable to assume that adequate knowledge alone will lead to adequate health in diabetic patients. Mazzuca (1982), in his review of education programs for patients with all types of chronic disease, concluded that "efforts to improve health by increasing patient knowledge alone were rarely successful" (p. 521). Patient behavior relevant to diabetes management is clearly influenced by more than knowledge about the disease; patients may know what to do but not do it. Treatment programs need to focus on other factors that may influence patient adherence behaviors. We will return to this topic later.

ADHERENCE WITH DAILY DIABETES MANAGEMENT TASKS

Noncompliance is a problem in the treatment of most serious illnesses. Diabetes is no exception. Watkins et al. (1967) published some of the first empirical data documenting the extent of this problem in adult patients. In their sample, over half of the patients studied were making insulin dosage errors, only a third were testing their urine correctly, and only 25% were judged "acceptable" in terms of meals and spacing of meals. Difficulties following dietary prescriptions are some of the most commonly reported problems in the literature (Ary, Toobert, Wilson & Glasgow, 1986; Christensen et al., 1983; Wharton, Wicking, Wills, & Martin, 1972). Children and adolescents are sometimes accused of "cheating" by underestimating the amount of sugar in their blood or urine. The prevalence of this type of behavior is not well documented, although estimates range from 6% to 50% of the population (Belmonte, Gunn, & Gonthier, 1981; Ernould, Graff, & Bourguiguon, 1982; Simonds, 1979).

Inadvertent noncompliance occurs when the patient believes he or she is adhering to recommended treatment but, through errors in knowledge or skill, is actually noncompliant. This is probably more common than "faking" urine tests or "skipping" injections. Johnson et al. (1982) found 40% of the youngsters studied made errors of this type when self-injecting insulin, and 80% made significant errors when urine testing. Frequent errors in reading urine test results were also detected by Epstein et al. (1980), who found most errors to be in one direction; urine glucose concentrations were usually underestimated by the patient.

There are numerous factors that may interfere with a patient's efforts to be compliant (e.g., inadequate knowledge, patient–physician communication, a nonsupportive family environment, complexity of the treatment regimen, etc.) All of these cannot be discussed here, and most have not been studied in this population. In fact, only recently have data become available supporting a link between barriers to compliance and compliance behaviors. LaGreca and Hanna (1983) took the interesting approach of assessing what types of factors interfered with each aspect of the treatment regimen in a sample of youngsters with diabetes. Insulin administration presented the least problem, with the fewest interference factors; "forgetting" was the only problem mentioned. In contrast, glucose testing presented the most problems with forgetting, problems in planning (i.e., schedule conflicts, traveling), and social situations (i.e., not testing because you are at a friend's house) all reported as common barriers to adherence. In fact, some type of social interference was frequently selected as a barrier to diet management and timing of meals as well. This was particularly true for patients; mothers did not seem to be as aware of the influence social situations had on their youngsters' efforts to manage diabetes. These findings are consistent with a more recent study of both children and adults with diabetes; social situations such as eating out at restaurants and inappropriate food offers by others were the most common reasons cited for dietary nonadherence (Ary et al., 1986).

When working with childhood populations, it is clear that developmental changes associated with adolescence have marked effects on patient adherence. Tattersall and Lowe (1981) have eloquently described how diabetes interferes with most of the goals of normal adolescence. Peer conformity is important, yet youngsters with this disease may feel "different" because of delayed sexual maturation and daily regimens of injections, glucose testing, and dietary constraints. Under the increased social pressure, it becomes more and more difficult to refuse "junk" food or to eat when others do not. The desire for greater independence, and the desire to be like everyone else, may make diabetes management a battleground between teenager and parent. Concerns over future employment opportunities and health complications may dampen the adolescent's hopes for the future. Until recently, few of these clinical impressions have been empirically tested. However, there is increasing evidence that, while adolescents have better knowledge and skills than younger children (Johnson et al., 1982), and are given greater responsibility for the management of their diabetes (Allen, Tennen, McGrade, Affleck, & Ratzan, 1983; Ingersoll et al., 1986; Kohler et al., 1982), they are less compliant (Allen et al., 1983; Bobrow, Avruskin, & Siller, 1985; LaGreca et al., 1982). Christensen and her colleagues (1983) studied dietary behavior in 97 patients ranging in age from infancy to 57 years of age. Preadolescent children reported the best adherence and adolescents reported the worst. Johnson, Silverstein, Rosenbloom, Carter, and Cunningham (1986) have documented more pervasive adherence problems among diabetic adolescents. Compared to their younger counterparts, the teenagers studied were less adherent with all aspects of the diabetic regimen: insulin injection, diet, exercise, and glucose testing. Ingersoll et al. (1986) have suggested that adolescent adherence problems may be the result of giving youngsters too much responsibility too early. In their study, parental participation in diabetes management was rare in families with patients 15 years of age or older. The authors argue that many of these teenagers may not be sufficiently cognitively mature to successfully manage their diabetes; patient responsibility for diabetes management should be determined by cognitive developmental level rather than by chronological age.

The deterioration in diabetic control seen in adolescent patients (Kaar, Akerblom, Huttunen, Knip, & Sakkinen, 1984; Schafer, McCaul, & Glasgow, 1986; Waller et al., 1986) is often assumed to be the result of their poor adherence. However, studies that have attempted to empirically document a link between adherence behaviors and diabetic control have yielded conflicting results. Using a nurse's rating of patients' compliance behaviors, Kaar et al. (1984) reported that adherence to a dietary regimen was associated with better diabetic control. Wing, Nowalk, Marcus, Koeske, and Finegold (1986) found that bulimic behavior in diabetic adolescents was associated with poor metabolic control, although bulimia was not more common among diabetic patients compared to healthy controls. A strong association between adherence behaviors and diabetic control was reported by Schafer, Glasgow, McCaul, and Dreher (1983) and Kaplan et al. (1985), who studied adolescents using patient self-report of diabetes regimen behaviors. However, Schafer et al. (1986) were unable to replicate their results in a second sample of adolescent patients. Simonds, Goldstein, Walker, and Rawlings (1981) were also unable to elucidate any differences between the adherence behaviors of adolescents in good and poor diabetic control. Other investigators have found parental guidance and control over diabetes management tasks to be predictive of health status in young diabetic patients but not in adolescents (Ingersoll et al., 1986; Walker et al., 1986).

Since a variety of physical changes associated with growth and sexual development occur during the adolescent years, it is possible that powerful biological factors mask behavior/health status relationships during this developmental period. Other factors may contribute to the difficulty in delineating adherence/health status relationships as well. Most notable are the variable methods of measuring adherence, most of which are without adequate psychometric documentation. Recent research by Johnson et al. (1986) suggests that 24-hour recall interviews may be one method of obtaining reliable reports of daily diabetes management behaviors. In their study of 168 IDDM children and adolescents, both the patient and primary caretaker (usually the mother) were interviewed separately about the patient's (and parent's) diabetes-relevant behaviors in the last 24 hours. Good agreement between parent and patient was obtained, although the youngest children studied (6–9 years of age) exhibited difficulty accurately recalling behaviors involving time (e.g., how long they exercised, how many minutes before a meal they took their insulin injection). The remarkable complexity of diabetes management was further highlighted by this investigation, which subjected the 13 adherence behaviors measured to a principle component factor analyses. Five independent factors emerged which, when rotated to simple structure, offered an easily interpreted solution accounting for more than 70% of the variance. While compliance or adherence is usually treated as a unitary concept, these factor analytic results suggest that diabetes management is multifaceted; adherence behaviors relevant to one component of the treatment regimen (e.g., insulin injection) are unrelated to adherence behaviors associated with different components of the treatment program (e.g., exercise). Even dietary behaviors were not always related to one another. In the patients studied, the type of food eaten was not related to how much was eaten and neither type nor amount of food consumed was related to eating frequency. Although these results need to be replicated, particularly with NIDDM populations, they suggest that the use of *compliant* or *noncompliant* as a general descriptor of the patient is inaccurate. It appears that patient behavior relevant to each treatment component must be assessed if the provider is to have an accurate perception of the patient's daily diabetes management.

IMPROVING PATIENT COMPLIANCE

There are a number of published reports suggesting that intervention programs can be successfully used to enhance patient adherence to recommended treatment. The better studies evaluate both behavioral and health status changes associated with a particular intervention plan. Most include instruction or education as part of their intervention methods to ensure that diabetes management tasks are performed accurately and to eliminate lack of knowledge as a possible source of noncompliance.

There are few large sample empirical studies of treatment programs designed for children or adolescents. Early published reports used single subject designs, focusing on a small number of children. Lowe and Lutzker (1979) and Gross (1982) demonstrated improved patient adherence subsequent to a behavioral intervention program, but related changes in health status were not monitored. Later studies have documented posttreatment changes in diabetic control as well as changes in compliance (Carney, Schechter, & Davis, 1983; Schafer, Glasgow, & McCaul, 1982). A sample of 19 youngsters were studied by Epstein and his colleagues (1981). In the context of an intensive educational program, parents were taught to use praise and points to reward children, not only for conducting urine tests, but for getting "good" results (i.e., urine glucose readings of less than 1%). While the intervention program improved youngsters' urine test results, no change in other indices of diabetic control, hemoglobin Al and serum glucose levels, occurred. However, since urine tests do not necessarily offer a reliable estimate of blood glucose concentration, improving urine test results may not always be associated with improvements in serum glucose levels. The recent development of home blood glucose monitoring techniques offer patients a direct measure of blood glucose levels, making estimates of blood glucose levels by urine glucose tests unnecessary.

Assuming that certain situations may serve as barriers to compliance, studies which teach youngsters to effectively cope with these situations seem relevant. Gross et al. (1981) used social skills training to help shy, preadolescent youngsters more effectively cope with their peers. All five youngsters studied were described as embarrassed, ashamed, or uncomfortable about their disease. Using a single subject design, the effectiveness of a training program consisting of modeling and role-playing exercises was evaluated. During and after the program, the youngsters increased eye contact and appropriate verbalizations. An in vivo follow-up assessment was conducted in which participants responded to a waiter who pressured them to order and eat ice cream in a restaurant. All of the youngsters appropriately handled the waiter, refusing the ice cream and explaining the reasons why. Follansbee, LaGreca, and Citrin (1983) also studied the effectiveness of coping skills training in adolescent diabetics facing difficult, diabetes-related social situations. Compared to untreated controls, adolescents who received the training were more assertive and less passive or aggressive. However, these gains were not maintained at a 3-month follow-up. Neither the Gross et al. (1981) nor the Follansbee et al. (1983) investigation evaluated health status changes associated with these interventions. A control group design was employed by Kaplan et al. (1985), who taught adolescents improved social skills to assist them in resisting negative peer influences. The control group spent an equal amount of time learning medical facts about diabetes. Four months after the intervention, the social skills group had better hemoglobin Al levels than the control group. Unfortunately, although improved compliance was presumed to be responsible for the social skills intervention group's better diabetic control, changes in compliance behaviors were not assessed. Interpretation of the study's findings is further hindered by slight pretreatment group differences in hemoglobin Al levels favoring the social skills intervention group.

Galatzer, Amir, Gil, Karp, and Laron (1982) have argued that intervention at the time of diagnosis may help prevent serious noncompliance problems. Diagnosis is a time of crisis, and, if psychosocial services are applied during this crisis, future psychological adjustment problems may be avoided. In their study, 107 clinic patients and families who were seen at the time of diagnosis and thereafter by a multidisciplinary team, which included a psychologist, were more compliant than a group of 116 patients who received the services of this team sometime after diagnosis. Unfortunately, patients were not randomly assigned to the two treatment conditions, and no health status comparisons between groups were made.

Possibly because there are more patients with NIDDM, intervention studies aimed at adults with diabetes have typically employed larger samples of patients and have utilized comparison groups rather than single subject designs. As might be expected, most have been aimed at weight reduction. Earlier studies documented improved glycemic control in patients who lost weight (Bistrain et al., 1976; Doar, Thompson, Wilde, & Sewell, 1975; Olefsky, Reaven, & Farquhar, 1974). More recent treatment studies have replicated these effects (Rabkin, Boyko, Wilson, Streja, 1983; Wing, Epstein, Noralk, Koeske, & Hagg, 1985). It appears that intervention programs that involve the patient on a regular basis and are aimed at modifying behavior are more effective than routine diabetes education (Mazzuca et al., 1986; Wing et al., 1985). However, it is not entirely clear what are the critical components to these programs' success (Rabkin et al., 1983; Wing, Nowalk, Epstein, & Koeske, 1986). Although few studies provide sufficient follow-up data, maintenance of treatment gains appears particularly problematic. Wing et al. (1985) compared a behavior modification weight control program to nutrition education and standard care control groups. At the end of the 16-week treatment program, the behavior modification group had lost more weight. But at a 16-month follow-up, most of the patients' initial weight loss had been regained; the treatment and control groups were no longer discernibly different. Mazzuca et al.'s (1986) report is the only other published intervention study that included follow-up assessments 1 year or more postintervention. In their study, treated subjects were more compliant and in better diabetic control 1 year posttreatment than control subjects who were given routine care. Unfortunately, the investigators did not evaluate adherence and health status immediately following treatment, so it is not possible to ascertain whether treatment gains were maintained or declined over the follow-up period. The samples studied were very large (over 500 patients participated), making slight differences between treatment and control groups statistically significant but of questionable clinical significance. Clearly, both the induction and maintenance of therapeutic change are topics in need of further study. Whether including significant others in the treatment program would enhance the maintenance of treatment gains remains to be seen. Webb et al. (1982), for example, included a family member in their treatment program for adult IDDM patients. Although the study is methodologically weak, as no control groups were used, the authors report that patients' *relatives* lost weight, apparently as a consequence of participating in the treatment program. Perhaps engaging family members in the treatment process would offer sufficient social support for patients to maintain gains made during treatment.

THE IMPACT OF PSYCHOLOGICAL STRESS ON DIABETES

Psychological stress has been an important theoretical construct used to explain both disease onset and course. Onset theories presume that the individual is constitutionally "at-risk," but that some trauma or stress actually precipitates the disease onset. Mirsky (1948) is representative of this view: "The susceptible individual is born with a limited capacity in the efficiency of one or more regularly mechanisms but he succumbs only after exposure to a sufficiently intense or prolonged appropriate stress" (pp. 187–188). However, the search for such precipitating stressful events has been entirely retrospective in nature. Adult diabetics or parents of children with IDDM are asked about events occurring prior to disease onset. Controlled studies employ retrospective interviews with diabetic patients (or their parents) and a comparison group. Stein and Charles (1971), for example, reviewed the charts of a group of primarily lower-class patients with either IDDM or NIDDM and noted any evidence of parental loss through death, separation, or divorce. The charts of a comparison group of patients with heritable blood diseases were also reviewed. The authors reported parental losses in 45% of the patients with diabetes as compared to 16% of the controls. However, many of these losses occurred 6 to 10 years prior to any symptomatology. Further, the study's findings presume equally reliable and valid recording of family and parental information in both the diabetic and blood disease groups as well as unbiased data collection on the part of the authors, who apparently expected to find greater parental loss among patients with diabetes. A more recent controlled comparison of 13 patients with IDDM (and their siblings and neighborhood controls) also reported more stressful and more severe events prior to the diagnosis of the disease (Robinson & Fuller, 1985). However, other researchers have not been able to find much support for stress as an etiological component to diabetes onset (Bruch, 1948; Geiger, Barta, & Hubay, 1973; Koch & Molnar, 1974; Koski, 1969; Kovacs, Feinberg, Paulauskas, Finkelstein, Pollock, & Crouse-Novak, 1985). In fact, several investigators have reported that patients or parents of children with diabetes often attempt to explain the disease by pointing to some upsetting event occurring prior to its onset rather than to other factors such as heredity. Such explanations are frequently of questionable validity (Bruch, 1948; Frankel, 1975; Laron, Karp, & Frankel, 1972).

Although emotional stress may be an important precipitating factor in the onset of diabetes, retrospective studies can never adequately address this issue, since the data are so colored by the interpretation of the patient and family of why the disease developed. Prospective studies of individuals at risk would be more helpful. Unfortunately, the incidence of diabetes even in relatives of patients with the disease is too low to make prospective studies feasible. The recent identification of islet-cell autoantibodies as a possible predictor of diabetes onset (LaPorte & Cruikshanks, 1985) may make such prospective studies possible. However, it is important to recognize that stress/disease onset relationships are probably more complex than initially suggested. Stress may be more or less important, depending upon the biological predisposition of the patient. In some cases, even normal stress may be an important precipitating variable. Since stress involves the individual's reactions and ability to cope, other psychological characteristics of the patient may be as important as the stress per se. If diabetes is a disorder of the immune system, quite the reverse hypothesis could be postulated: Stress could actually prevent or decrease the likelihood of diabetes onset! In the animal literature, there is actually some support for this rather counterintuitive proposal (Huang, Plaut, Taylor, & Warehein, 1981).

While there may be some controversy over whether psychological stress is involved in the etiology of diabetes, there is general agreement that stress may influence the metabolic control of patients with the disease. In one study, adult patients were asked whether or not psychological stress affected their diabetes control; the majority perception was that stress was very influential (Cox, Taylor, Nowacek, Holley-Wilcox, Pohl, & Guthrow, 1984).

Theoretically, stress should have a significant effect on diabetic control through the effects of the stress hormones, epinephrine and norepinephrine. These catecholamines, when produced in sufficient amounts, may induce both hyperglycemia and excess ketone body production. Catecholamines antagonize the peripheral metabolic effects of insulin and stimulate glycogenolysis and gluconeogenesis by the liver, all of which should result in increased blood glucose levels in the diabetic patient. Catecholamines also encourage mobilization of free fatty acids, which are converted by the liver to ketone bodies. As mentioned previously, excessive ketone production may lead to diabetic ketoacidosis (Tarnow & Silverman, 1981–82).

One of the earliest demonstrations of stress effects in diabetes was a case report by Hinkle and Wolf (1949) describing a 15-year-old girl with a repeated history of diabetic ketoacidosis. The youngster's relationship with her mother was extremely poor, with numerous episodes of violent altercations. In a diary, the patient recorded these daily stressful events and her urine ketone test results, demonstrating a striking relationship between the two.

Subsequent studies attempted to manipulate stress using a stress interview, hypnotically induced stress, or shock. Blood glucose and ketones, urine glucose and ketones, and urine volume were usually monitored before, during, and after the stress induction. In most of these studies, adults or older adolescents participated. Increases in blood ketones and urine volumes were the changes most consistently associated with stress. Variability or even decreases in blood glucose were also reported. Urine glucose measures appeared to be least sensitive to the stress manipulations (Hinkle, Conger, & Wolf, 1950; Hinkle & Wolf, 1952; Vandenbergh, Sussman, & Titus, 1966; Vandenbergh, Sussman, & Vaughan, 1967). This early work made an important contribution. However, much of it was case-study oriented (although nondiabetic comparison subjects were sometimes used), lacked statistical tests of significance, and, most importantly, did not carefully measure the participants' experience of stress by self-report and by psychophysiological indices. The stress manipulation used may have been experienced as more or less stressful by different subjects, introducing substantial variability into what appeared to be a well-controlled experiment. It is interesting that this type of stress-induction methodology has not been consistently used to study stress effects in diabetic youngsters or adults since this early series of papers.

Rather, investigators have turned to the assessment of more naturally occurring stress. Weil, Sussman, and Crain (1967) reported increased urine glucose in 9–12-year-olds attending a summer camp for youngsters with diabetes when the campers were exposed to a competitive, compared to a noncompetitive, atmosphere. This study suffers from numerous methodological flaws (e.g., possible order effects, lack of measures of stress), but represents an initial attempt to study possible stress effects in the natural environment.

The more common approach has been to assess the relationship between life stress, as indicated by life events checklists, and health status in patients with this disease. Bedell, Giordani, Amour, Tavormina, and Boll (1977) studied chronically ill youngsters attending a 3-week residential summer camp. Approximately 40% of the participants had diabetes. Campers who had a high incidence of precamp life stress had significantly more illness episodes during their camp stay than campers with low life stress. Using the same measure of life stress (Coddington's Social Readjustment Rating Questionnaire, 1972), Chase and Jackson (1981) reported increased life stress was associated with poorer diabetic control in 15–18-year-old patients.

Other evidence supportive of a relationship between undesirable life events and changes in a patient's metabolic condition can be found in investigations of adults with the disease (Bradley, 1979; Grant, Kyle, Teichman, & Mendels, 1974). However, research of this type presents a number of problems. While there appears to be some evidence that negative life stress is associated with poorer health status, findings are not always consistent from study to study, and the strength of the relationship between stress and health is usually weak. Life event checklists have some of the same problems that standard stress induction procedures present. Different patients may experience various life events differently, and a particular patient's stressful experiences may be entirely absent from the checklist. Further, major life events are only one type of stress and are probably not representative of the daily hassles one experiences in living.

Cox et al. (1984) evaluated the relationship between daily hassles or irritations and diabetic control in a sample of 59 adult IDDM patients; a low but significant association was found between daily hassles and hemoglobin Al levels ($r = .25$). Barglow and his colleagues studied the influence of stress related to childbearing in a sample of 39 pregnant IDDM women (Barglow, Hatcher, Berndt, & Phelps, 1985). Although psychological stress was not related to hemoglobin Al levels, it was related to preparandial blood glucose measures and urine ketone test results. As expected, higher stress was associated with higher blood glucose and ketone levels. The authors argue that it may be important to monitor several different indices of diabetic control if stress/health status relationship in diabetes are to be understood.

Other investigators have emphasized the need to consider the patient's coping response as a possible moderating influence on stress/metabolic control relationships. Brand, Johnson, and Johnson (1986) found an association between undesirable life experiences prior to a summer camp and metabolic control during the child's camp stay, but only for youngsters with an internal locus of control. Those children who perceived themselves as having control over life experiences were in worse metabolic condition when faced with stress. Delamater and colleagues also reported that the way the patient copes with stress seemed to be more important than the stress itself (Delamater, Kurtz, Bubb, White, & Santiago, 1987). In this study no significant differences were found between adolescents in good and poor control in reported hassles or daily stress and irritations. However, those in poor control used more avoidance and wishful thinking than those in good control. These findings are consistent with those reported by Peyrot and McMurry (1985), who evaluated 20 IDDM adults; poor control was associated with both an internal locus of control and coping strategies involving denial, although the authors did not assess the influences of stress per se in this investigation.

Although stress and/or certain kinds of coping strategies seem to be associated with poorer metabolic control, the causal mechanism is not entirely clear. Stress is usually presumed to have a direct effect on diabetic control through the effects of the stress hormones, as described previously. However, other mechanisms are possible. Stress, for example, could influence adherence which, in turn, could influence metabolic control. Since most studies are correlational, the direction of relationships between stress and diabetic control is also unknown. Although it is presumed that stress causes poor metabolic control (either directly through the stress hormones or indirectly through its effects on compliance), the reverse could also be true: Poor metabolic control could make the patient feel more stressed. Delameter et al. (1987), for example, categorized stresses described by diabetic adolescents into the following types: interpersonal-parent, interpersonal-peer, diabetes-related, academic, and miscellaneous. Diabetes-related stress was the most frequently mentioned stress among youngsters in poor control; this category of stress was rarely mentioned by youngsters in good or fair metabolic control. Clearly, the youngster's health status may be contributing to the patient's psychological stress as well as being its consequence. An earlier study by Mazze, Lucido, and Shamoon (1983) addressed this issue in an even more provocative manner. Eighty-four adolescent and adult patients with IDDM were followed over 36 weeks. Psychological and metabolic control measures were taken at entry, at 18 weeks, and at 36 weeks. Change in metabolic control was consistently associated with change in patient reported anxiety and depression; that is when patients' diabetic control improved, they felt less anxious and less depressed. Since the intervention used in the study was aimed at improving metabolic control, the direction of the psychological/health status relationship was presumed to be one in which improved diabetic control lead to improved patient affect. However, as with all correlational studies, it is possible that the increased attention given to patients studied led to an improved psychological state (i.e., less anxiety and depression) which, in turn, led to improved metabolic control. Stress/health status relationships in diabetes are an important area for future scientific inquiry, provided that the complexity of this issue is recognized.

STRESS MANAGEMENT FOR PATIENTS WITH DIABETES

Despite the fact that stress/metabolic relationships in diabetes are not completely understood, there has been an increasing interest in intervention programs to teach patients to cope with stress. EMG biofeedback relaxation was used in two case reports of young adult women with IDDM. In both cases, biofeedback was associated with hypoglycemia and reduced insulin requirements. One of the women was in poor diabetic control and experiencing significant stress. The other was in stable control, and no mention was made of stress-related difficulties. The procedure seemed to help the more stressed patient, whose health status was in jeopardy. In contrast, the treatment appeared to be detrimental to the patient whose diabetes was non-problematic before beginning biofeedback training (Fowler, Budzynski, & Vandenbergh, 1976; Seeburg & DeBoer, 1980). As Turkat (1982) has pointed out, it seems inappropriate to use intervention programs aimed at stress-reduction in patients with no apparent stress-related problems. Additional support for the blood glucose reduction effects of relaxation training comes from a study by Surwit and Feinglos (1984). Poorly controlled NIDDM adult patients were taught progressive relaxation and given EMG biofeedback training in a carefully controlled hospital environment. Compared to untrained controls, those patients involved in the relaxation training showed lower blood glucose after eating and an improved response to the glucose tolerance test. A subsequent report by these authors suggested that a decrease in plasma cortisol appeared to be the mechanism underlying the treatment effect (Surwit & Feinglos, 1984). Cortisol is a potent hyperglycemic hormone even in nondiabetic man. Its influence is further potentiated in diabetic patients who have insufficient insulin reserve (Schade & Eaton, 1983). Lammers, Naliboff, and Straatmeyer (1984) offer another description of relaxation training used with four male adult diabetics currently experiencing stress in their lives. Unlike in the Surwit and Feinglos (1984) study, patients were treated as outpatients and treatment effectiveness was evaluated by frequent blood glucose monitoring by the patient at home. Relaxation training appeared to improve diabetic control only for the two patients with the higher blood glucose values at baseline. However, the mechanism of this treatment effect was unclear, as both successfully treated subjects did *not* describe less anxiety and tension during the treatment (compared to baseline) periods.

Stress-reduction programs of this type have not been empirically evaluated with children or adolescents with diabetes. While this is expected to change, the prevailing treatment approach has been family therapy based on the work of Salvadore Minuchin and Lester Baker and colleagues. In the 1970s they introduced the notion of the *psychosomatic family*. Such families are (a) enmeshed to such an extent that individual identities and roles are unclear, (b) overprotective of all family members, (c) rigid in maintaining the status quo, and (d) lacking in conflict resolution. The child's illness plays an important role in the family's attempts to avoid conflict. However, family conflict necessarily occurs, leading to emotional or physiological arousal, described as the *turn on* phase. A return to normal levels of physiological responding (the *turn off* phase) is handicapped by the family's attempts to avoid conflict (Baker, Minuchin, Milman, Leibman, & Todd, 1975; Minuchin, Rosman, & Baker, 1978). The child with diabetes living in such a family may become overaroused, leading to metabolic derangements. These derangements continue because of the family's inability to resolve conflict, seriously jeopardizing the child's health.

To test their model, Minuchin and Baker induced stress in several young diabetic patients during a family interview. Both the patient and the family members' physiological responding was monitored before, during, and after stress was induced. A number of youngsters showed an increase in arousal and free fatty acid production that did not turn off once the interview was terminated (Baker et al., 1975; Minuchin et al., 1978). Research findings by Anderson, Miller, Auslander, and Santiago (1981) offer additional support for this model. Compared to youngsters in poor diabetic control, those in good control had parents who encouraged greater independence and direct expression of feelings within the context of a relatively cohesive, conflict-free environment.

Family therapy is usually initiated when a youngster's problems seem to be the product of dysfunctional family interactions. In Minuchin and Baker's model, the child's diabetes has encouraged overinvolvement by one parent, usually the mother. Less maternal attention is directed at other family members, placing strain on the marital relationship and resulting in hostility by siblings toward the patient. However, these resentments are not openly expressed because the patient is not to be "upset." The parents' focus on the child's problems permits them to avoid their own marital conflicts. Consequently, the child's problems are reinforced. The goal of family therapy is to identify and change these maladaptive interactions. Usually, efforts are initially directed at alleviating the patient's symptoms so as to decrease the family's use of the child's illness as a means of avoiding or detouring family conflict. This gives the family the opportunity to identify family patterns that seem to exacerbate the child's illness. Finally these maladaptive interactions are replaced by more appropriate communication patterns (Leibman, Minuchin, & Baker, 1974).

While Minuchin and Baker's psychosomatic family has a great deal of popular appeal, its limited empirical foundation should be recognized. It is unclear how many children with unstable diabetes come from psychosomatic families. Little is known about how physiologically reactive psychosomatic diabetic youngsters are to most any stress, including family conflict. Certainly, a family's attempts to avoid conflict might develop in response to a child's somatic reactivity rather than being its unique cause. Although the authors report that their family therapy approach has been successful with a number of difficult-to-manage patients, controlled investigations have not been conducted.

METHODOLOGICAL ISSUES

Throughout this review a number of methodological issues have surfaced. The most significant of these will be highlighted here.

Measurement

Perhaps first and foremost is the need for reliable and valid measures. Typically, investigators develop a test of diabetes knowledge, ask the patient about adherence behaviors, or ask physicians to rate the patient's compliance or diabetic control. Different investigators use different measures, and concern for the psychometric properties of any of the measures used has been generally absent. Fortunately, this situation is changing. There are now available measures of patient knowledge about diabetes and skill at various treatment tasks, with reported reliability and validity data (Johnson et al., 1982; Gilbert et al., 1982; Harkavy et al., 1983; Hess & Davis, 1983; Dunn, Bryson, Hoskins, Alford, Handelsman, & Turtle, 1984). However, more work needs to be done. The development of adequate methods of assessing compliance or adherence behaviors is a particularly important area in need of investigator time and attention. Recent research by Johnson et al (1986), utilizing a 24-hour recall interview methodology, shows promise in this regard.

The measurement of health or diabetic control also needs careful consideration, as there is no one generally accepted measure of diabetic control. Glycosolated hemoglobin probably comes the closest to be ideal, single measure of diabetic control. However, many physicians would not be comfortable using this as the sole index of control and continue to monitor urine or serum sugar levels as well as urine ketones, triglycerides, and cholesterol. Consequently, different studies use different measures of diabetic control. Some select one or two biochemical indices, such as glycosolated hemoglobin or urine sugar/

ketone levels. Others ask the physician to rate the patient's control on an arbitrary scale. Although this permits the physician to incorporate both clinical and laboratory information in the selection of a control rating, until recently the reliability of such ratings was not assessed. A study by Spevack and colleagues suggests that physicians can reliably rate patients' level of diabetic control when they are given only laboratory or patient conducted test results. Reliability was reduced when physicians were provided with other information about the patient (e.g., age, sex, socioeconomic background, school attendance), as would be typically the case in a clinic setting (Spevack, Johnson, Harkavy, Silverstein, Shuster, Rosenbloom, & Malone, 1987). The study's findings suggest that physicians may be able to reliably incorporate several different indicators of metabolic control into a single diabetic control rating. However, they will be most reliable if the information presented to them is limited to purely physiologic indicators of metabolic status.

Construct Independence

Not only must reliable and valid measures of the constructs selected for study be developed, but the method of measuring these constructs must be kept independent. Often the physician or health provider is asked to rate the patient's compliance and diabetic control. This introduces the possibility of spurious relationships between variables. Physicians may believe that well-controlled youngsters are usually compliant and that poorly-controlled patients are noncompliant. A significant correlation between compliance ratings and diabetic control ratings may reflect physician beliefs rather than actual health–behavior relationships.

A related problem is the lack of clear differentiation between constructs. For example, a number of investigators include compliance behaviors with metabolic indices when rating a patient's level of diabetic control (e.g., a child might be labeled well controlled if he or she tested his or her urine for sugar twice a day and 90% of these tests were negative for sugar). The reverse situation occurs as well: Indicators of diabetic control are used as measures of compliance. The pervasiveness of this problem is illustrated in a recent survey of pediatric diabetologists in the United States. Almost 90% of the respondents stated that they used glycosolated hemoglobin (a measure of diabetic control) to assess patient compliance (Clarke, Snyder, & Nowacek, 1985). Unless adherence behaviors and health status are defined and measured separately, their relationship to one another will never be understood.

Specificity and Complexity

Measures of knowledge, adherence behaviors, and health status must be disease-specific. However, even within a particular disease, these constructs appear to be more complex than initially thought. Patient knowledge of one aspect of diabetes does not always predict knowledge of, or skill at, a different aspect of the disease (Harkavy et al., 1983; Johnson et al., 1982). Schafer et al. (1983) and Johnson et al. (1986) have reported that adherence with one component of the diabetic regimen does not predict adherence to different regimen components. These data suggest that global measures of compliance, knowledge, stress, coping, or health may not be adequate. Not only must measures be developed that are specific to specific diseases, but, even within each disease, measures must be sensitive to the different, and sometimes independent, aspects of concepts such as patient knowledge, adherence behavior, and health. This means that a great deal more attention must be given to the specificity and resultant complexity of the constructs selected for study and the design of adequate methods of measurement.

Theoretical Clarity

Investigators often select a psychological variable of interest and test its relationship to patients' health status without specifying and assessing the mechanism by which the psychosocial variable selected should influence metabolic control. Patient knowledge, for example, is often correlated with diabetic control without specifying what relationship should exist between the two. Presumably, patient knowledge should improve patient adherence which, in turn, should influence diabetic control. However, all theoretically relevant variables (e.g., knowledge, adherence, and health status) are rarely assessed. Similarly, measures of psychological stress are often correlated with indices of diabetic control. Although stress could directly effect metabolic control through the stress hormones or indirectly effect it through its influence on adherence, such a priori theoretical models are rarely specified and almost never tested.

Correlation vs. Causality

Because much of the research in this area is correlational, care must be taken with the conclusions drawn. Although it is tempting to conclude that a significant correlation between adherence behaviors and diabetic control, or between psychological stress and diabetic control, means that high adherence "causes" good control or high stress "causes" bad control, this may not be the case. Patients' knowledge, feelings, and behaviors may be the result of the patient's health status. Poor health may lead to feelings of helplessness; the patient may "give up" behaving in a highly compliant manner or develop significant anxiety about the disease. Clearly, the effect of psychological variables on the patient's health, as well as the impact of health or illness on the patient's knowledge, affect, and behavior must be considered. Both longitudinal and intervention studies can be used to explore the directionality of these relationships.

Developmental Issues

Throughout this review, developmental issues have constantly surfaced. Children with diabetes present special problems because of their changing capabilities. Although this has long been recognized, only recently have data been collected that attempt to empirically define when youngsters are capable of various diabetes management tasks (Harkavy et al., 1981; Gilbert et al., 1982; Johnson et al., 1982). The available literature suggests that adolescence is a particularly difficult time. Even in nondiabetic youngsters there is a significant increase in life stress or social readjustment that occurs during this developmental period (Coddington, 1972). For children with diabetes, deterioration in metabolic control is often associated with the adolescent years (Kaar et al., 1984; Schafer et al., 1986). While adolescents know more about diabetes (Johnson et al., 1982) and have more responsibility for managing it (Allen et al., 1983; Ingersoll et al., 1986) then younger patients, they are often less adherent with daily treatment demands (Christensen et al., 1983; Johnson et al., 1986). Recently, investigators have begun to delineate some of the social barriers to adherence that may be particularly important to the teenager. Often these social barriers are recognized by the youngster but not by the parent (LaGreca & Hanna, 1983). Others have argued that, in the interest of encouraging feelings of mastery and control over their disease, health providers may push children to take too much responsibility too fast before they are sufficiently cognitively and socially mature to successfully manage such a complex disease in a complex world (Ingersoll et al., 1986; LaGreca et al., 1982).

Individual Differences

There is a tendency to treat patients with diabetes as a homogeneous group. Educational programs and diabetes management regimens are relatively standardized, presenting the same information and treatment recommendations to all patients. While individual differences are recognized (e.g., different IDDM patients are on different doses of insulin), greater recognition of these differences may prove profitable. As was discussed previously, children with diabetes cannot be effectively educated or managed in a homogeneous fashion because of powerful biological, cognitive, and social differences associated with growth and development. Even with adult patients the importance of individual differences should not be underestimated. Several studies have reported that patients have consistent symptoms associated with hypo- or hyperglycemia, but that these symptoms differ between patients (Freund et al., 1986; Pennebaker et al., 1981). These findings strongly suggest that patients should *not* be taught standard symptoms of hypo- or hyperglycemia. Instead, they should be assisted in determining what their individual symptom patterns associated with these conditions are. It seems reasonable to speculate that different patients' diabetic control may be differently affected by different aspects of the diabetes management regimen. Similarly, stress may influence diabetic control in different ways for different patients. The possibility that patients' adherence behaviors and experience of psychological stress may be consistently related to diabetic control, but in unique and different ways for different patients, needs to be more carefully explored. If such individual differences did exist, large group studies (as are typically conducted) would obscure important but unique associations between the psychological and health status variables selected for study.

REFERENCES

Allen, D. A., Tennen, H., McGrade, B. J., Affleck, G., & Ratzan, S. (1983). Parent and child perceptions of the management of juvenile diabetes. *Journal of Pediatric Psychology, 8,* 129–141.

Anderson, B., Miller, J., Auslander, W., & Santiago, J. (1981). Family characteristics of diabetic adolescents: Relationship to metabolic control. *Diabetes Care, 4,* 586–594.

Ary, D. V., Toobert, D., Wilson, W., & Glasgow, R. E. (1986). Patient perspective on factors contributing to nonadherence to diabetes regimen. *Diabetes Care, 9*(2), 168–172.

Baker, L., Minuchin, S., Milman, L., Leibman, R., & Todd, T. (1975). Psychosomatic aspects of juvenile diabetes mellitus: A progress report. In Z. Laron (Ed.), *Vol. 12. Modern problems in pediatrics. Diabetes in juveniles: Medical and rehabilitation aspects.* New York: Karger.

Barglow, P., Hatcher, R., Berndt, D., & Phelps, R. (1985). Psychosocial childbearing stress and metabolic control in pregnant diabetics. *The Journal of Nervous and Mental Disease, 173*(10), 615–620.

Bedell, J. R., Giordani, B., Amour, J. L., Tavormina, J., & Boll, T. (1977). Life stress and the psychological and medical adjustment of chronically ill children. *Journal of Psychosomatic Research, 21,* 237–242.

Beggan, M. P., Cregan, D., & Drury, M. I. (1982). Assessment of the outcome of an educational programme of diabetes self-care. *Diabetologia, 23,* 246–251.

Belmonte, M. M., Gunn, T., & Gonthier, M. (1981). The problem of "cheating" in the diabetic child and adolescent. *Diabetes Care, 4,* 116–120.

Bennett, P. H. (1983). Classification of diabetes. In M. Ellenberg & H. Rifkin (Eds.), *Diabetes mellitus: Theory and practice* (pp. 409–414). New York: Medical Examination Publishing Co., Inc.

Bistrian, B. R., Blackburn, G. L., Flatt, J.-P., Sizer, J., Scrimshaw, N. S., & Sherman, M. (1976). Nitrogen metabolism and insulin requirements in obese diabetic adults on a protein-sparing modified fast. *Diabetes, 25*(6), 494–504.

Bobrow, E. S., Avruskin, T. W., & Siller, J. (1985). Mother-daughter interaction and adherence to diabetes regimens. *Diabetes Care, 8,* 146–151.

Bowen, R. G., Rich, R., & Schlotfeldt, R. M. (1961). Effects of organized instruction for patients with the diagnosis of diabetes mellitus. *Nursing Research, 10*(3), 151–159.

Bradley, C. (1979). Life events and the control of diabetes mellitus. *Journal of Psychosomatic Research, 23,* 159–162.

Brand, A., Johnson, J., & Johnson, S. B. (1986). Life-stress and diabetic control in children and adolescents. *Journal of Pediatric Psychology, 11,* 481–496.

Bruch, H. (1949). Physiological and psychological interrelationships in diabetes in children. *Psychosomatic Medicine, 11,* 200–210.

Cahill, G., Etzwiler, D., & Freinkel, N. (1976). "Control" and diabetes. *New England Journal of Medicine, 294,* 1004.

Carney, R. M., Schechter, K., & Davis, T. (1983). Improving adherence to blood glucose testing in insulin-dependent diabetic children. *Behavior Therapy, 14,* 247–254.

Chandalia, H. B., & Bagrodia, J. (1979). Effect of nutritional counseling on the blood glucose and nutritional knowledge of diabetic subjects. *Diabetes Care, 2*(4), 353–356.

Chase, H. P., & Jackson, G. G. (1981). Stress and sugar control in children with insulin-dependent diabetes mellitus. *Journal of Pediatrics, 98,* 1011–1013.

Christensen, N. K., Terry, R. D., Wyatt, S., Pichert, J. W., & Lorenz, R. A. (1983). Quantitative assessment of dietary adherence in patients with insulin-dependent diabetes mellitus. *Diabetes Care, 6*(3), 245–250.

Clarke, W. L., Snyder, A. L., & Nowacek, G. (1985). Outpatient pediatric diabetes-I. Current practices. *Journal of Chronic Diseases, 38,* 85–90.

Coddington, R. (1972). The significance of life events as etiologic factors in the diseases of children. II. A study of a normal population. *Journal of Psychosomatic Research, 16,* 205–213.

Cox, D. J., Taylor, A. G., Nowacek, G., Holley-Wilcox, P., Pohl, S. L. & Guthrow, E. (1984). The relationship between psychological stress and insulin-dependent diabetic blood glucose control: Preliminary investigations. *Health Psychology, 3*(1), 63–75.

Davidson, M. B. (Ed.). (1981). *Diabetes mellitus: Diagnosis and treatment.* New York: John Wiley and sons.

Delamater, A. M., Kurtz, S. M. S., Bubb, J., White, N. H., & Santiago, J. V. (1987). Stress and coping in relation to metabolic control of adolescents with Type I diabetes. *Developmental and Behavioral Pediatrics, 8,* 136–140.

Doar, J. W. H., Thompson, M. E., Wilde, C. E., & Sewell, P. F. J. (1975). Influence of treatment with diet alone on oral glucose-tolerance test and plasma sugar and insulin levels in patients with maturity-onset diabetes mellitus. *The Lancet, 1,* 1263–1266.

Dunbar, F. (1954). *Emotions and bodily changes.* New York: Columbia University Press.

Dunn, S. M., Bryson, J. M., Hoskins, P. L., Alford, J. B., Handelsman, D. J., & Turtle, J. R. (1984). Development of the Diabetes Knowledge (DKN) Scales: Forms DKNA, DKNB, and DKNC. *Diabetes Care, 7*(1), 36–41.

Eastman, B. G., Johnson, S. B., Silverstein, J., Spillar, R. P., & McCallum, M. (1983). Understanding of hypo- and hyperglycemia by youngsters with diabetes and their parents. *Journal of Pediatric Psychology, 8*(3), 229–243.

Epstein, L. H., Coburn, P. C., Becker, D., Drash, A., & Siminero, L. (1980). Measurement and modification of the accuracy of the determinations of urine glucose concentration. *Diabetes Care, 3,* 535–536.

Epstein, L. H., Figueroa, J., Farkas, G. M., & Beck, S. (1981). The short-term effects of feedback on accuracy of urine glucose determinations in insulin dependent diabetic children. *Behavior Therapy, 12,* 560–564.

Ernould, C., Graff, M. P., & Bourguignon, J. P. (1982). Incidence of "cheating" in diabetic children and adolescents. In Z. Laron & A. Galatzer (Eds.), *Psychological Aspects of Diabetes in Adolescents, Pediatric and Adolescent Endocrinology* (Vol. 10, pp. 43–46). Barel: Karger.

Etzwiler, D. (1962). What the juvenile diabetic knows about his disease. *Pediatrics, 29,* 135–141.

Etzwiler, D. D., & Robb, J. R. (1972). Evaluation on programmed education among juvenile diabetics and their families. *Diabetes, 21,* 967–971.

Etzwiler, D. D., & Sines, L. K. (1962). Juvenile diabetes and its management: Family, social, and academic implications. *Journal of the American Medical Association, 181,* 94–98.

Fishbein, H. A. (1985). Precipitants of hospitalization in insulin-dependent diabetes mellitus (IDDM): A statewide perspective. *Diabetes Care, 8* (Suppl.), 61–64.

Follansbee, D. J., La Greca, A. M., & Citrin, W. C. (1983). *Coping skills training for adolescents with diabetes.* Paper presented at the annual meeting of the American Diabetes Association, San Antonio, TX.

Fowler, J. E., Budzynski, T. H., & VandenBergh, R. L. (1976). Effects of an EMG Biofeedback Relaxation Program on the Control of Diabetes. *Biofeedback and Self-Regulation, 1,* 105–112.

Frankel, A. (1975). Juvenile diabetes—the look from within. In Z. Laron (Ed.), *Diabetes in juveniles: Medical and rehabilitation aspects. Modern problems in Paediatrics* (Vol. 12, pp. 358–360). Basel: Karger.

Freund, A., Johnson, S. B., Rosenbloom, A., Alexander, B., & Hansen, C. A. (1986). Subjective symptoms, blood glucose estimation, and blood glucose concentrations in adolescents with diabetes. *Diabetes Care, 9*(3), 236–243.

Galatzer, A., Amir, S., Gil, R., Karp, M., & Laron, Z. (1982). Crisis intervention program in newly diagnosed diabetic children. *Diabetes Care, 5*(4), 414–419.

Garner, A., Thompson, C., & Partridge, J. (1969). Who knows best? *Diabetes Bulletin, 45,* 3–4.

Geiger, A., Barta, L., & Hubay, M. (1973). Diabetes and mental state. *Acta Paediatrica Academiae Scientiarum Hungaricae, 14*(2), 119–124.

Gilbert, B. O., Johnson, S. B., Spillar, R., McCallum,. M., Silverstein, J. H., & Rosenbloom, A. (1982). The effects of a peer-modeling film on children learning to self-inject insulin. *Behavior Therapy, 13,* 186–193.

Grant, I., Kyle, G., C., Teichman, A., & Mendels, J. (1974). Recent life events and diabetes in adults. *Psychosomatic Medicine, 36*(2), 121–128.

Gross, A. M. (1982). Self-management training and medication compliance in children with diabetes. *Child & Family Behavior Therapy, 4,* 47–55.

Gross, A. M., Johnson, W. G., Wildman, H., & Mullett, N. (1981). Coping skills training with insulin dependent pre-adolescent diabetics. *Child Behavior Therapy, 3,* 141–153.

Hamburg, B. A., & Inoff, G. E. (1982). Relationships between behavioral factors and diabetic control in children and adolescents: A camp study. *Psychosomatic Medicine, 44*(4), 321–339.

Harkavy, J., Johnson, S. B., Silverstein, J., Spillar, R., McCallum, M., & Rosenbloom, A. (1983). Who learns what at diabetes summer camp. *Journal of Pediatric Psychology, 8,* 143–153.

Hassel, J., & Medved, E. (1975). Group/audiovisual instruction for patients with diabetes. *The Journal of the American Dietetic Association, 66,* 465–470.

Hess, G. E., & Davis, W. K. (1983). The validation of a diabetes patient knowledge test. *Diabetes Care, 6*(6), 591–596.

Heston, J. V., & Lazar, S. J. (1980). Evaluating a learning device for juvenile diabetic children. *Diabetes Care, 3*(6), 668–671.

Hinkle, L. E., & Wolf, S. (1949). Experimental study of life situations, emotions, and the occurrence of acidosis in a juvenile diabetic. *American Journal of the Medical Sciences, 217,* 130–135.

Hinkle, L. E., Conger, C., & Wolf, S. (1950). Studies on diabetes mellitus: Relation of stressful life situations to the concentration of ketone bodies in the blood of diabetic and nondiabetic humans. *Journal of Clinical Investigation, 29,* 513–520.

Hinkle, L. E., & Wolf, S. (1952). Importance of life stress in the course and management of diabetes mellitus. *Journal of the American Medical Association, 148,* 513–520.

Huang, S. W., Plaut, S. M., Taylor, G., & Warehein, L. E. (1981). Effect of stressful stimulation on the incidence of streptozotocin-induced diabetes in mice. *Psychosomatic Medicine, 43*(5), 431–437.

Hulka, B. S., Cassel, J. C., Kupper, L. L., & Burdette, J. A. (1976). Communication, compliance, and concordance between physicians and patients with prescribed medications. *American Journal of Public Health, 66,* 847–853.

Hulka, B. A., Kupper, L. L., Cassel, J. C., & Mayo, F. (1975). Doctor-patient communication and outcomes among diabetic patients. *Journal of Community Health, 1*(1), 15–27.

Ingersoll, G. M., Orr, D. P., Herrold, A. J., & Golden, M. P. (1986). Cognitive maturity and self-management among adolescent with insulin-dependent diabetes mellitus. *Journal of Pediatrics, 108,* 620–623.

Jacobsen, J. M., O'Rourke, P. J., & Wolf, A. E. (1983). Impact of a diabetes teaching program on health care trends in an Air Force Medical Center. *Military Medicine, 148*(1), 46–47.

Johnson, S. B. (1980). Psychosocial factors in juvenile diabetes: A review. *Journal of Behavioral Medicine, 3,* 95–115.

Johnson, S. B., Pollak, T., Silverstein, J. H., Rosenbloom, A. L., Spillar, R., McCallum, M., & Harkavy, J. (1982). Cognitive and behavioral knowledge about insulin dependent diabetes among children and parents. *Pediatrics, 69,* 708–713.

Johnson, S. B., Silverstein, J., Rosenbloom, A., Carter, R., & Cunningham, W. (1986). Assessing daily management in childhood diabetes. *Health Psychology, 5,* 545–564.

Kaar, M. L., Akerblom, H. K., Huttenen, N. P., Knip, M., & Sakkinen, K. (1984). Metabolic control in children and adolescents with insulin-dependent diabetes mellitus. *Acta Paediatrica Scandinavia, 73,* 102–108.

Kaplan, R. M., Chadwick, M. W., & Schimmel, L. E. (1985). Social Learning intervention to promote metabolic control in type I diabetes mellitus: Pilot experiment results. *Diabetes Care, 8,* 152–155.

Karlander, S. G., & Kindstedt, K. (1983). Effects of a formalized diabetes education. *Acta Medica Scandinavia, 213,* 41–43.

Karp, M., Manor, M., & Laron, Z. (1970). What do juvenile diabetics and their family know about diabetes? In Z. Laron (Ed.), *Habilitation and rehabilitation of juvenile diabetics.* Leiden, Holland: H. E. Stenfert Kroese, N. V.

Koch, M., & Molnar, G. (1974). Psychiatric aspects of patients with unstable diabetes mellitus. *Psychosomatic Medicine, 36,* 67–68.

Kohler, E., Hurwitz, L. S., & Milan, D. (1982). A developmentally staged curriculum for teaching self-care to the child with insulin-dependent diabetes mellitus. *Diabetes Care, 5*(3), 300–304.

Korhonen, T., Huttunen, J. K., Aro, A., Hentinen, M., Ihalainen, O., Majander, H., Siitonen, O., Uusitupa, M., & Pyorala, K. (1983) A controlled trial on the effects of patient education in the treatment of insulin-dependent diabetes. *Diabetes Care, 6*(3), 256–261.

Koski, M. L. (1969). The coping processes in childhood diabetes. *Acta Paediatrica Scandinavica,* Supplement, *198,* 7–56.

Kovacs, M., Feinberg, T. L., Paulauskas, S., Finkelstein, R., Pollock, M., &

Crouse-Novak, M. (1985). Initial coping responses and psychosocial characteristics of children with insulin-dependent diabetes mellitus. *The Journal of Pediatrics, 106*(5), 827–834.

LaGreca, A. M., Follansbee, D., & Skyler, J. S. (1982). *Behavioral aspects of diabetes management in children and adolescents.* Paper presented at the meeting of the American Psychological Association, Washington, DC.

LaGreca, A. M., & Hanna, N. C. (1983). *The health beliefs of children with diabetes and their mothers: Implications for treatment.* Paper presented at the meeting of the American Diabetes Association, San Antonio, TX.

Lammers, C. A., Naliboff, B. D., & Straatmeyer, A. J. (1984). The effects of progressive relaxation on stress and diabetic control. *Behavioral Research and Therapy, 22*(6), 641–650.

Lane, D. S., & Evans, D. (1979). Measures and methods in evaluating patient education programs for chronic illness. *Medical Care, 17*(1), 30–42.

LaPorte, R. E., & Cruikshanks, K. J. (1985). Incidence and risk factors for insulin-dependnet diabets. In M. I. Harris & R. F. Hamman (Eds.), *Diabetes in America* (pp. 1–12). Washington, DC: National Institutes of Health.

Laron, Z., Karp, M., & Frankel, J. J. (1972). *A study of the rehabilitation of juvenile and adolescent diabetics in the central region of Israel. Final report.* Unpublished report, Tel Auiv University, Petach-Tiqva, Israel.

Leibman, R., Minuchin, S., & Baker, L. (1974). The use of structural family therapy in the treatment of intractable asthma. *American Journal of Psychiatry, 131*(5), 535–540.

Lowe, K., & Lutzker, J. R. (1979). Increasing compliance to a medical regimen with a juvenile diabetic. *Behavior Therapy, 10,* 57–64.

Ludvigsson, J. (1977). Socio-psychological factors and metabolic control in juvenile diabetes. *Acta Paediatrica Scandinavica, 66,* 431–437.

Maudsley, H. (1899). *The pathology of mind* (3rd ed.). New York: Appleton.

Mazze, R. S., Lucido, D., & Shamoon, H. (1984). Psychological and social correlates of glycemic control. *Diabetes Care, 7*(4), 360–366.

Mazzuca, S. A. (1982). Does patient education in chronic disease have therapeutic value? *Journal of Chronic Diseases, 35,* 521–529.

Mazzuca, S. A., Moorman, N. H., Wheeler, M. L., Norton, J. A., Fineberg, N. S., Vinicor, F., Cohen, S. J., & Clark, C. M., Jr. (1986). The diabetes education study: A controlled trial of the effects of diabetes patient education. *Diabetes Care, 9*(1), 1–11.

McCulloch, D. K., Young, R. J., Steel, J. M., Wilson, E. M., Prescott, R. J., & Duncan, L. J. P. (1983). Effect of dietary compliance on metabolic control in insulin dependent diabetics. *Human Nutrition: Applied Nutrition, 37A,* 287–292.

Merritt, G. J., Hall, N. J., Kobernus, C. A., & Tanenberg, R. J. (1983). Outcome analysis of a diabetic education clinic. *Military Medicine, 148,* 545–547.

Minuchin, S., Rosman, B., & Baker, L. (1978). *Psychosomatic families.* Cambridge, MA: Harvard University Press.

Mirsky, A. (1948). Emotional factors in the patient with diabetes mellitus. *Bulletin of the Menninger Clinic, 12,* 187–194.

Naughten, E., Smith, M. A., & Baum, J. D. (1982). At what age do diabetic children give their own injections? *American Journal of the Diseases of Children, 136*(8), 690–692.

Olefsky, J., Reaven, G. M., & Farquhar, J. W. (1974). Effects of weight reduction on obesity: Studies of lipid and carbohydrate metabolism in normal and hyperlipoproteinemic subjects. *The Journal of Clinical Investigation, 53,* 64–76.

Patridge, J. W., Garner, A. M., Thompson, C. W., & Cherry, T. (1972). Attitudes of adolescents toward their diabetes. *American Journal of the Diseases of Children, 124,* 226–229.

Pennebaker, J. W., Cox, D. J., Gonder-Frederick, L., Wunsch, M. G., Evans, W. S., & Pohl, S. (1981). Physical symptoms related to blood glucose in insulin dependent diabetics. *Psychosomatic Medicine, 43,* 489–500.

Peyrot, M., & McMurry, J. F., Jr. (1985). Psychosocial factors in diabetes control: Adjustment of insulin-treated adults. *Psychosomatic Medicine, 47*(6), 542–557.

Rabkin, S. W., Boyko, E., Wilson, A., & Streja, D. A. (1983). A randomized clinical trial comparing behavior modification and individual counseling in the nutritional therapy of non-insulin-dependent diabetes mellitus: Comparison of the effect on blood sugar, body weight, and serum lipids. *Diabetes Care, 6*(1), 50–56.

Raskin, P. (1983). Open and closed insulin infusion systems: Newer methods of insulin delivery. In M. Ellenberg & H. Rifkin (Eds.), *Diabetes mellitus: Theory and practice* (pp. 941–957). New York: Medical Examination Publishing Co., Inc.

Robinson, N., & Fuller, J. H. (1985). Role of life events and difficulties in the onset of diabetes mellitus. *Journal of Psychosomatic Research, 29*(6), 583–591.

Salans, L. B., Knittle, J. L., & Hirsch, J. (1983). Obesity, glucose intolerance, and diabetes mellitus. In M. Ellenberg & H. Rifkin (Eds.), *Diabetes mellitus: Theory and practice* (3rd ed., pp. 469–479). New York: Medical Examination Publishing Co., Inc.

Schade, D. S., & Eaton, R. P. (1983). Hormonal interrelationships. In M. Ellenberg & H. Rifkin (Eds.), *Diabetes mellitus: Theory and practice* (3rd ed., pp. 255–266). New York: Medical Examination Publishing Co., Inc.

Schade, D. S., Santiago, J. V., Skyler, J. S., & Rizza, R. A. (1983). *Intensive insulin therapy.* Princeton, NJ: Excerpta Medica.

Schafer, L. C., Glasgow, R. E., & McCaul, K. D. (1982). Increasing the adherence of diabetic adolescents. *Journal of Behavioral Medicine, 5*(3), 353–362.

Schafer, L. C., Glasgow, R. E., McCaul, K. D., & Dreher, M. (1983). Adherence to IDDM regimens: Relationship to psychosocial variables and metabolic control. *Diabetes Care, 6,* 493–498.

Schafer, L. C., McCaul, K. D., & Glasgow, R. E. (1986). Supportive and nonsupportive family behaviors: Relationships to adherence and metabolic control in persons with type I diabetes. *Diabetes Care, 9*(2), 179–185.

Seeburg, K. N., & DeBoer, K. F. (1980). Effects of EMG biofeedback on diabetes. *Biofeedback and Self-Regulation, 5,* 289–293.

Simonds, J., Goldstein, D., Walker, B., & Rawlings, S. (1981). The relationship between psychological factors and blood glucose regulation in insulin-dependent diabetic adolescents. *Diabetes Care, 4*(6), 610–615.

Simonds, J. F. (1979). Emotions and compliance in diabetic children. *Psychosomatics, 20,* 544–551.

Spevack, M., Johnson, S. B., Harkavy, J. M., Silverstein, J., Shuster, J., Rosenbloom, A., & Malone, J. (1987). Diabetologists' judgments of diabetic control: Reliability and mathematical simulation. *Diabetes Care, 10,* 217–224.

Stein, S., & Charles, E. (1971). A study of early life experiences of adolescent diabetics. *American Journal of Psychiatry, 128,* 700–704.

Stone, D. G. (1961). A study of the incidence and causes of poor control in patients with diabetes mellitus. *American Journal of the Medical Sciences, 241,* 436–442.

Surwit, R. S., & Feinglos, M. N. (1984). Relaxation-induced improvement in glucose tolerance is associated with decreased plasma cortisol. *Diabetes Care, 7*(2), 203.

Tarnow, J., & Silverman, S. (1981–1982). The psychophysiologic aspects of stress in juvenile diabetes mellitus. *Psychiatry in Medicine, 11,* 25–44.

Tattersall, R. B., & Lowe, J. (1981). Diabetes in adolescence. *Diabetologia, 20,* 517–523.

Vandenbergh, R., Sussman, K., & Titus, C. (1966). Effects of hypnotically induced acute emotional stress on carbohydrate and lipid metabolism in patients with diabetes mellitus. *Psychosomatic Medicine, 28,* 382–390.

Vandenbergh, R. L., Sussman, K. E., & Vaughn, G. D. (1967). Effects of combined physical-anticipatory stress on carbohydrate-lipid metabolism in patients with diabetes mellitus. *Psychosomatics, 8*(1), 16–19.

Watkins, J. D., Roberts, D. E., Williams, T. F., Martin, D. A., & Coyle, V. (1967). Observation of medication errors made by diabetic patients in the home. *Diabetes, 16,* 882–885.

Watkins, J. D., Williams, F., Martin, D. A., Hogan, M. D., & Anderson, E. (1967). A study of diabetic patients at home. *American Journal of Public Health, 57,* 452–459.

Watts, F. N. (1980). Behavioral aspects of the management of diabetes mellitus: Education, self-care, and metabolic control. *Behavior Research and Therapy, 18,* 171–180.

Webb, K. L., Dobson, A. J., Tupling, H. E., Harris, G. W., O'Connell, D. L., Atkinson, J., Sulway, M. J., & Leeder, S. R. (1982). Evaluation of a diabetes education programme. *Australian & New Zealand Journal of Medicine, 12*(2), 153–160.

Weil, W. B., Sussman, M. B., & Crain, A. J. (1967). Social patterns and diabetic glucosuria. *American Journal of Disease in Children, 113,* 454–460.

Wharton, C. L., Wicking, J., Wills, H. R., & Martin, F. I. R. (1972). The diet of insulin-dependent diabetics. *Medical Journal of Australia, 2,* 707–713.

Whitehouse, F. W., Whitehouse, I. J., Smith, J., & Hohl, R. D. (1979). Teaching the person with diabetes: Experience with a follow-up session. *Diabetes Care, 2,* 35–38.

Williams, T. F., Martin, D. A., Hogan, M. D., Watkins, J. D., & Ellis, E. V.

(1967). The clinical picture of diabetic control, studied in four settings. *American Journal of Public Health, 57*(3), 441–451.

Willis, T. (1684). Pharmaceutice rationalis. In *The works of Thomas Willis.* London: Dring, Harper and Leigh.

Wing, R. R., Epstein, L. H., Nowalk, M. P., Koeske, R., & Hagg, S. (1985). Behavior change, weight loss, and physiological improvements in type II diabetic patients. *Journal of Consulting and Clinical Psychology, 53*(1), 111-112.

Wing, R. R., Nowalk, M. P., Epstein, L. H., & Koeske, R. (1986). Calorie-counting compared to exchange system diets in the treatment of overweight patients with type II diabetes. *Addictive Behaviors, 11,* 163–168.

Wing, R. R., Nowalk, M. P., Marcus, M. D., Koeske, R., & Finegold, D. (1986). Subclinical eating disorders and glycemic control in adolescents with type I diabetes. *Diabetes Care, 9*(2), 162–167.

World Health Organization. (1980). *Expert Committee on Diabetes Mellitus, second report* (Tech. Rep. Series 646). Geneva: Author.

Wysocki, M., Czyzyk, A., Slonska, Z., Krolewski, A., & Janeczko, D. (1978). *Diabete & Metabolisme, 4,* 117–122.

Zimmet, P. (1983). Epidemiology of diabetes mellitus. In M. Ellenberg & H. Rifkin (Eds.), *Diabetes mellitus: Theory and practice* (pp. 451–468). New York: Medical Examination Publishing Co., Inc.

14

Behavioral Preparation for Medical Procedures

Lizette Peterson
Vanessa Selby
Lisa Mori

University of Missouri-Columbia

BEHAVIORAL PREPARATION FOR MEDICAL PROCEDURES

There is perhaps no other area in behavioral medicine with a more heterogeneous subject matter than that of behavioral preparation for medical procedures. Preparation techniques range from the provision of procedural and sensory information to instruction in techniques for postsurgical breathing, turning in bed and ambulating, methods of relaxing the body and creating distracting mental imagery, and a large variety of cognitive-behavioral techniques including positive restructuring, self-instruction, and attention focusing. Similar preparation techniques have been employed for relatively painless procedures such as pelvic examinations, for stressful procedures in which the examinee must be conscious such as endoscopy or cardiac catheterization, for minor surgical procedures such as tooth extractions, and for major interventions such as open-heart surgeries. In the course of this brief chapter, it is not possible to exhaustively review all of the studies in any one subarea of this rapidly expanding field. Thus, our tactic will be to offer a sample of the variety of published studies in order to introduce the preparation methods which are currently available. Before we begin our overview, however, we would like to outline some of the major methodological issues that may temper the current findings and that should be addressed to strengthen and clarify future research. This initial consideration will offer a perspective for our later review.

METHODOLOGICAL ISSUES

In an introduction to preparation techniques, perhaps one of the major methodological issues which should be raised is the absence of standardization of research studies in terms of measurement instrumentation and time of measurement, treatment content or treatment application, and general goals for successful treatment. One clear problem is the absence of a standard meaning for treatment labels. For example, techniques termed *coping* may range from physical techniques such as endoscopy patients panting to reduce gagging, or abdominal surgery patients breathing deeply and coughing to improve pulmonary functioning, to detailed EMG desensitization and progressive muscle relaxation or cognitively based techniques such as self-instruction.

Even where clinicians use the same word to label the same technique, the active ingredients included within that technique may differ. For example, some investigators regard positive relabeling, flexible suggestions, and the balancing of aversive sensations with neutral and positive sensations as necessary components of sensory information preparation, while others do not accept these components. Some individuals mix procedural and sensory information, whereas others maintain their effects must be considered separately (see review of this issue by Schultheis, Peterson, & Selby, 1987).

In some cases, the use of a generic label to encompass multiple dependent variables creates confusion, although in some cases it is unavoidable, as will be seen later in this chapter. It is difficult to discuss the multiple behaviors which have been assessed in each study without resorting to some general terms such as *reduced distress, improved adjustment, or enhanced recovery*. Unfortunately, in a field where multiple measures are made within each of the three general classes of physiological variables, observable behavior, and self-report data, generic labels can obscure accurate comparisons of results. The reader must also consider that these multiple measures are made at several differing times, as well. If treatment A reduces self-reported fear before a procedure, treatment B reduces maladaptive physical behavior during the procedure, and treatment C reduces the number of medications required in recovering from the procedure, which is the "most successful"? Are they equally successful? To say they all reduce distress is to obscure their real effects, in the sense that preprocedure self-reported fear, maladaptive responding during the procedure, and postprocedure medications may not be equally important in a given population or for a given medical procedure. Thus, when possible in the present chapter, we will attempt to supply specific labels.

Further problems arise when researchers make large numbers of measurements and then focus on a single positive finding, ignoring the many other findings of no difference. This tactic creates, not only the problems of increased chance findings as alpha level is inflated, but also a conceptual problem in focusing on any measurement showing differences as "more important" than those not showing differences. We have argued elsewhere (Peterson, 1984) that a sensible solution to the problem in future research is the avoidance of generic labels and generic thinking, and the a priori selection of target behaviors which are most important to evaluating treatment impact. Many other variables would be considered as well, but the focus of the findings could thus be kept on the a priori targeted variables as opposed to those which become highlighted post hoc.

In addition to using specific and standardized labels for variables and assigning attention to variables in an a priori fashion, standardization of both the temporal and instrumentation aspects of measures would be useful. For example, it is not uncommon for ratings of behavioral distress in children to range from time samples of 3 minutes for a list of several specific responses to occur to global ratings (which are not behaviorally anchored) of ward adjustment over several days. In another example, coping dispositions have been measured with three short questions, 30-item pencil and paper measures, and in-depth interviews, with predictably different results. Some studies take measures only preprocedure, others postprocedure, and some both times. Even then, the preprocedure data collection may be done the week before surgery, the night before surgery, or the hour in the morning before surgery. It is clear that these times are likely to have differing meanings to a patient. Thus, the wary reader must recognize that even measures as specific as a self-report of anxiety taken before surgery may differ in terms of timing and instrumentation, and thus may yield differing conclusions.

It goes without saying that, even if treatment and measurement techniques were identical, medical procedures which have different psychological and physical stressors and outcomes may create very different patterns of responding. A hysterectomy in a young woman, a cardiac catheterization in a middle-aged man following a myocardial infarct, and a cholecystectomy in an elderly woman will each have different psychological meanings and differing physical sensations, and thus may demand different preparation strategies.

If the reader has not been dissuaded from examining the research in this area by this lengthy list of caveats, we will also acknowledge that, although many questions remain, there are several meaningful conclusions which can be made on the basis of the existing literature. Furthermore, this area is growing rapidly, and the number of studies which can remediate these past deficiencies is growing. Thus, this seems an ideal time to take stock of the behavior preparation methods which exist.

Interestingly, unlike much of clinical psychology in which child treatment methods were downward extensions of adult methods (Gelfand & Peterson, 1985), child and adult methods of preparation for medical procedures have grown in parallel, with surprisingly little shared theory or treatment methodology. Thus, it seems most logical to review the major preparation techniques and issues separately for adult and child patients. We will therefore consider the general need for preparation, the differential need for preparation of persons with differing coping dispositions, the predominant preparation techniques which have been used, variations in the application of techniques which have been studied, comparisons of techniques, and ways in which various techniques may interact with personal coping dispositions, first for child, then for adult, patients.

As will be clear in this presentation, the child and adult literatures have proceeded along very dissimilar paths. For example, there are very few studies on coping dispositions and few comparative treatment studies with children, with many studies having examined single treatments like modeling and variations on the method and timing of treatment applications. In contrast, there are numerous studies with adult patients which have examined the role of coping dispositions and their interaction with treatments, many comparative treatment studies, but very few investigations of treatment application differences. We will begin the discussion of these contrasting fields by considering data on the need for preparation in children.

CHILD PATIENTS

The Need for Preparation

Early reports on child preparation noted that children were often told nothing about the upcoming medical event and were sometimes "grossly deceived" about what was to take place (Chapman, Loeb, &

Gibbons, 1956). Most experts conceded that hospitalization was stressful for children, and in some cases problems like reading difficulties, conduct disorder, and delinquency were linked to the stress of early hospitalization (Douglas, 1975). Paradoxically, unlike the adult literature (reviewed later in this chapter), where there have been several studies conducted which suggested potential sensitizing effects of preparation, the large majority of the child studies reviewed below suggest that sensitive, developmentally appropriate preparation is beneficial. Where sensitizing effects for children have been found, they have typically involved only one small subsection of treatment groups (e.g., young children only when prepared a week before surgery, as in Melamed, Meyer, Gee, & Soule, 1976, or only experienced child surgery patients, as in Faust & Melamed, 1984) and the demonstration of sensitization has been limited to palmar sweating, with no negative effects demonstrated on overt behavior, self-report, or variables such as medications required or medical complications. Thus, although it certainly seems important to be alert to possible negative effects of preparation, the overwhelming proportion of existing empirical data suggest that, when appropriately applied, preparation is very valuable to children. Further, naturalistic studies of children's reactions to hospitalization and surgery suggest that the majority of children in all age groups from toddler and preschool to school age actively engage in information seeking (Caty, Ellerton, & Ritchie, 1984).

We feel a need to underline children's need for preparation, because the current literature is still replete with undocumented suggestions that "overpreparation of children is to be avoided" (Levinson & Ousterhout, 1980), that children can only deal with a single upsetting event at a time (Chan, 1980), and that to attempt to explain more is harmful. Some authors suggest definitely (in the absence of data) that information on the most frightening events should not be included in the general preparation but rather given only directly before an event (e.g., Rushton, 1983). Heffernan and Azarnoff (1971) reported that many physicians and nurses still feel that for potentially painful procedures (e.g., inserting an I.V. or performing a lumbar puncture), any preparation will only agitate the child, and that quick physical restraint with no warning and no preparation is the preferred method. Couple this antipreparation bias with the news that many preparation programs have been eliminated in recent years due to concerns about cost and benefit (Azarnoff, 1982), and the trends for the future become ominous.

In the recent past, there has been widespread consensus in the field that children's preparation for medical and dental procedures should be a primary goal (Ramirez-Johnson, 1979). Such preparation has been recommended by the Association for the Care of Children in Hospitals and by the American Academy of Pediatrics (Azarnoff & Woody, 1981). It has also been included as an integral component of "A Bill of Rights for Children in Medical Settings" (Seagull, 1978). Given the compelling evidence provided by numerous empirical studies of children's preparation for medical procedures (many reviewed in the following section), it would appear that the attitude within medicine, and the modern layperson's belief, that children should be protected from relevant information is seriously in error. Alarmist and largely undocumented assumptions of sensitization due to preparation may perpetuate this error. However, we would hasten to add that the best way to insure continued support of preparation procedures is to continue to carefully evaluate them, searching both for positive and negative effects across a variety of different dependent variables. Such a search should include attention to individual differences in the way in which children respond to medical procedures. The small but growing literature on individual coping dispositions in children will thus be considered next.

Coping Dispositions

Although many different names have been used, the basic differentiation of coping dispositions in adults has been between those who actively welcome information (called *vigilants, sensitizers,* or *copers)* and those who avoid information (called *repressors, avoiders,* or *deniers).* Only recently have investigators posited that young children, despite their relative absence of experience with stressful medical situations, may have already evolved personal or dispositional methods of coping. The few studies based on this presumption have demonstrated a similar information-seeking versus information-avoiding tendency.

In one preliminary study, Knight, Atkins, Eagle, Evans, Finkelstein, Fukushima, Katz, and Weiner (1979) assessed the characteristic coping styles of 25 child surgery patients between ages 7 and 11, using the Rorschach and a clinician rating system. Then, the relationship of this coping style to a physical indicator of anxiety (urinary 17-hydroxy-corticosteroids) was investigated at home after a clinic visit, at the hospital prior to surgery, and the day after surgery. Children received preparation (content undescribed) from the clinician at the clinic visit and prior to surgery. There was no relationship between coping style and anxiety when at home, but a relatively strong relationship between coping style and anxiety ($r = -.49$) prior to surgery. Coping via intellectualization (more information-tolerant coping) was associated with lower anxiety, while coping via denial, displacement, or projection (less information-tolerant coping) was associated with more anxiety. Global ratings, by ward personnel of how well adjusted the children were, validated the use of the anxiety indicator, with better-adjusted children having lower cortisol production rates.

Burstein and Meichenbaum (1979) used very different measures, but produced similar conclusions. They assessed 5- to 9-year-old children's receptivity to information about hospitalization by allowing children to select medical (hospital stress relevant) or nonmedical (nonstress relevant) toys the week before, during, and after hospitalization. No formal preparation was given, but parents apparently prepared their children (the extent or content of preparation was not described). Anxiety was measured by a self-report inventory using an adjective checklist, sentence completion, and open-ended questions. This self-reported anxiety was unrelated to the choice of toys within any measurement period, but choosing hospital relevant toys prior to hospitalization was related to diminished anxiety after hospitalization. Further, a subset of children choosing stress relevant toys prior to hospitalization recalled more medical and hospital related procedures than did children who had selected nonstress relevant toys in a follow-up 7 months after hospitalization.

Peterson and Toler (1986) provided additional data to support this premise and to document the existence of an active coping dimension in children. They assessed children's coping skills via the Coping Strategies Interview (Siegel, 1981) and utilized a special coding system to derive an information-seeking score. Children's high information-seeking scores were positively related to children's actual knowledge of their surgical procedure and to their parents' ratings of how much information the children typically sought out prior to common medical procedures. In addition, high information-seeking scores were related to how well parents reported their children handled stressful medical events; the higher the information-seeking score, the lower the emotional upset. Finally, actual coping behaviors such as discussion of medical procedures and question asking during the blood test (as rated by an objective observer), during the anesthesia induction (as rated by a nurse), and postoperatively, during recovery (as rated by the parent) were related to the interview-assigned information-seeking score. Degree of information seeking also influenced the degree of distress experienced during stressful medical procedures. Children with high information-seeking scores showed fewer maladaptive responses in anticipation of the blood test, rated themselves as less frightened after surgery, and were rated as less distressed after surgery by an objective observer.

The strongest relationship was found between age and information seeking. It is possible to statistically separate the effects of age from coping style (as was done by Peterson and Toler), but the two appear naturally confounded in actual practice. It is logical that older children who can more effectively seek out and understand information would be more likely to do so. There are other attributes about age as well which are discussed later in this chapter, such as memory, world experience, and attachment to parents. These attributes probably influence reactions to medical procedures as well as influencing the child's responsiveness to common methods of preparation. These preparation techniques will be considered next.

Preparation Techniques

There has been a variety of preparation techniques used successively with children in the last two decades. By the late 1970s, three-quarters of U.S. pediatric hospitals employed formal preparation, with a majority using information provision or hospital tours, and others employing modeling preparations or training in coping techniques (Peterson & Ridley-Johnson, 1980). However, the research literature has not entirely reflected the proportion of actual programs offering tours and educational preparations; in fact, the majority of the research literature has focused on modeling (Peterson, Ridley-Johnson, Tracy, & Mullins, 1984a), particularly the use of filmed modeling. Thus, we will begin our discussion by considering the use of modeling films as preventive preparation.

Filmed models. Vernon and Bailey (1974) employed four filmed child models shown reacting appropriately to anesthesia induction. The 4- to 9-year-old subjects who viewed these models were rated as being less upset in the waiting room and while being prepared for induction. There were no differences during actual anesthesia induction, however.

One of the best known modeling procedures for presurgery preparation is Melamed and Siegel's (1975) "Ethan Has an Operation," a film of an actual child surgery patient undergoing all regular hospital and surgery procedures for hernia repair. Children who viewed this film, as opposed to a control condition, had lower palmar sweating, reported fewer hospital related fears, and were rated as less fearful by observers both before and after surgery. Melamed and Siegel (1980) described a variety of studies demonstrating the value of filmed modeling.

Perhaps because this is the area in which the largest amount of controlled research has been conducted, nearly our entire later sections on "Variations in Treatment Application" and "Comparative Studies" describe factors which influence the efficacy of filmed models.

Thus, we will postpone further discussion of filmed models until later in the chapter.

Other modeling preparations. A film of an actual child patient has many clinical advantages, including a desensitizing introduction to many locations in the hospital and many staff members without disrupting hospital routine, and the provision of a clearly adaptively functioning peer. There are also disadvantages, however. A film can become outdated, it can be expensive to purchase and to show, and as will be seen later, it may not be effective with experienced child patients. Thus, it seems important to investigate other modeling preparations as well.

Cassell (1965) performed one of the first interventions using a puppet model which dispensed information and allowed the child to ask questions and clarify misperceptions. Children who received this preparation were rated by the cardiologist as less distressed during cardiac catheterization, and they were more willing to return to the hospital following release.

These early positive effects of a puppet model have been replicated several times in the last 5 years. For example, Schulz, Raschke, Dedrick, and Thompson (1981) demonstrated that children prepared for short-term hospital procedures, using a puppet model, maintained a constant low level of arousal (as measured by palmar sweating) throughout their hospital stay, but control group children experienced a steady increase in arousal across measurement occasions. Similarly, Peterson, Schultheis, Ridley-Johnson, Miller, and Tracy (1984b) found that a puppet model decreased observer-rated maladaptive responding and anxiety in the children, and also reduced self-reported anxiety in the parents both before and after surgery. These findings were later replicated in a second study by Peterson et al. (1984a). Johnson and Stockdale (1975) demonstrated that viewing a puppet model the day before surgery decreased anxiety following surgery. Thus, puppet models also appear to be effective methods of preparation for children, perhaps uniquely so, as only children are likely to identify with a "Big Bird" or "Teddy Bear" model. The developmental appropriateness of the next technique, "Stress Point Preparation," may not be as clear.

Stress-Point Information/Support

The original studies which assessed the impact of procedural information on children distributed the stress-point information to the mothers rather than directly to the children. Interestingly, when the mothers received special information concerning what would happen during the medical procedure and support for only 5 extra minutes on four stressful occasions, their children had lower blood pressures throughout hospitalization, less vomiting, earlier voiding, and more fluid consumption (Skipper & Leonard, 1968). The mothers also reported less anxiety and more confidence (Skipper, Leonard, & Rhymes, 1968).

Wolfer and Visintainer (1975) have demonstrated similar successful use of stress-point preparation (information and supportive care) given at difficult times such as blood tests and transition to surgery to both parents and minor elective surgery child patients. The experimental group was rated as more calm and cooperative at every measurement point, as less resistant to anesthesia and fluid intake, and had earlier postsurgical voiding. Parents in the experimental groups were also less anxious and more satisfied with the nursing care.

Although stress-point preparation and supportive care are apparently very effective, they are also extremely labor intensive and thus very costly, especially when compared to a brief, one-time modeling intervention. One advantage to these costly procedures is that they are maintained throughout hospitalization. It would be useful if the child or child and parent team, independent of a medical staff person, could provide the necessary psychological support during stressful procedures. In fact, this is the goal of the coping techniques outlined in the next section.

Coping techniques. Peterson and Shigetomi (1981) used a puppet model to give child surgery candidates procedural information and to train them in deep muscle relaxation, imagery distraction, and self-instruction. The addition of these coping techniques to the modeled information decreased fearfulness and increased cooperation as rated by parents, treatment-blind observers, and nurses. The largest effects for both coping and modeling were found during the blood test and preoperative injection. There was also a trend ($p < .08$) for the coping prepared children to eat more foods, drink more fluids, and void sooner after surgery. Peterson and Shigetomi (1982) found that a third of the parents receiving the coping training had used the techniques out of the hospital a year later. Other aspects of this study (such as the comparison groups) will be described under "Comparative Research."

Zastowny, Kirschenbaum, and Meng (1981) used a similar multicomponent procedure in which a film on stress was shown, deep breathing and cognitive distraction were taught, and stress-innoculation instruction was employed. They reported that prepared children were more cooperative, particularly at stress points such as the preoperative injection, and were better adjusted following surgery.

Siegel and Peterson (1980, 1981) used a similar set of techniques to prepare naive preschool dental patients for dental restorations. They found that increased cooperation, decreased fearfulness, reduced disruptive behaviors, and lower heart rates were maintained, as compared to an attention-only control group, across several dental visits. Nocella and Kaplan (1982) replicated these effects for experienced child dental patients with a similar coping package. These studies provide some evidence that, properly trained, the child and parent could initiate and perform all of the necessary stress reduction procedures across settings, whenever the need for active coping was present.

Other techniques. There is a gamut of other techniques used successfully with children that deserve brief mention here. Johnson, Kirchoff, and Endress (1975) demonstrated the positive effects of giving children accurate sensory information during orthopedic cast removal. Siegel and Peterson (1980, 1981) found sensory information to be as effective as coping techniques for their preschool dental patients.

There are many reports of the use of play therapy techniques to give information and sensory experience (e.g., Abbott, Hansen, & Lewis, 1970) and of the use of art to explore surgically related fears (e.g., Crowl, 1980). Books are also frequently suggested (e.g., Crocker, 1979). However, all of these latter techniques are not yet supported by empirical research.

Several creative methods have been used with especially frightening procedures like injections. Ayer (1973) demonstrated the utility of vivid mental imagery to reduce fear of injections. Eland (1981) used a skin coolant called "Frigiderm" to reduce the self-reported pain of injections. Finally, Fernald and Corry (1981) reported that empathetic preparation and sensory information (e.g., "I'll bet the alcohol feels cold. In a moment, I'm going to stick you. You're probably feeling scared.") resulted in reduced behavioral distress and self-reports of anger and pain as compared with more directive preparation.

There are thus a large variety of successful child preparation techniques, as well as many issues still deserving of research attention. For most of these preparation techniques, little is known other than their apparent efficacy in comparison with a no-treatment or information-only control for a given medical procedure. However, for a subset of studies (primarily those dealing with filmed modeling) some information is available concerning variations in the application of treatment which influence treatment effectiveness, as will be seen in the next section.

Variations in treatment Application

Mode of information delivery. Peterson et al. (1984b) compared a series of modeling preparations, including "Ethan Has an Operation" (a commercial modeling film with a real child patient), "Nathan Has an Operation" (a videotape created at the local hospital, patterned after the "Ethan" film and using a child actor), and "Teddy Bear Has an Operation" (a live, three-dimensional puppet presentation). Each of these methods produced reduced observer and parent ratings of fearfulness and increased cooperation, as compared to a group receiving regular hospital preparation and experimenter attention, showing their similar modeling quality as the active ingredient. Peterson et al. (1984b) suggested that, for the children in this study, who experienced only 24-hour hospital stays and minor elective surgeries, any of these three types of modeling preparations were equally effective so long as contradictory information is not presented simultaneously. The only difference among the experimental procedures was that parents felt less anxious and more confident after the puppet program (probably because both films portrayed the parents as relatively inactive). Because hospitals have differing resources, this finding has pragmatic as well as theoretical importance for both children and parents.

The first study in the next section examines a question relevant both to mode of information and to parental involvement. Who should narrate hospital relevant information during a modeling film?

Parental involvement. As noted above, most modeling films do not portray much parental involvement. Recently, Pinto and Hollandsworth (1989) examined a modeling film which was narrated either by the filmed child patient or his father, and viewed by either the children alone or the children and parents. The results from these four conditions were quite complicated. Basically, children who viewed the tape with their parents were less anxious just before surgery. On most dependent variables, children who viewed any film were better off than children who did not view a film.

Many other aspects of the parental role have been considered specifically elsewhere (Peterson, Mori, & Carter, 1985) and will be mentioned only briefly here. It is quite clear that having a parent room-in during hospitalization is beneficial (Brain & Maclay, 1968), and that parental anxiety is strongly related to child anxiety (Vardaro, 1978). In general, reducing parental anxiety seems to reduce the child's anxiety as well (Skipper et al., 1968).

In seeming contrast to the positive impact of parental contact, two recent observational studies suggest that children show more overt distress during an injection or venipuncture if the mother is present (Gross, Stern, Levin, Dale, & Wojnilower, 1983; Shaw & Routh, 1982). Gross et al. (1983) suggested that this is because children are exhibiting an extinction burst as their distress signals, which usually elicit maternal support, fail to do so during a medical procedure. Shaw and Routh (1982) cautioned that more overt distress does not necessarily mean more subjective distress, and they noted that the expression of distress may be beneficial. Finally, Peterson and Mori (1988) argued that the display of increased distress by children indicates the need to train parents to assist their children during medical procedures, rather than suggesting the need to remove parents.

Parents who prepare their children with complete prior information tend to report better responses from their children to common medical procedures (Peterson et al., 1984a), especially when the child is responsive to the information (Heffernan & Azarnoff, 1971). Similarly, parents who reward fear-mastery have children who respond to medical procedures with less fear than do parents who allow their children to escape and withdraw (Zabin & Melamed, 1980). The previously cited studies in which parents served as coping coaches for their children suggest coping training as one vehicle for improving the role of the parent in preventive preparation. This is another important and underresearched area which should be a topic of investigation in the future.

Parental support is important for children of all ages, but it seems to be especially critical for the very young toddler or preschooler undergoing medical interventions. The issue of developmental level is a separate one which, surprisingly, has received little experimental attention. It will be considered briefly now.

Developmental level. One of the clearest and most often replicated findings is that young children more than older children are distressed by medical settings (e.g., Prugh, Staub, Sands, Kirschbaum, & Lenihan, 1953), medical routines (Trouten, 1981), and physical restraint (Chan, 1980). Ironically, although preschool children are psychologically most at risk and are also the age group most often admitted to hospitals in the United States (Azarnoff & Woody, 1981), they are also the age group most underserved by preparation programs (Goslin, 1978) and least often the subject of preparation research (Peterson & Brownlee-Duffeck, 1984), yet they seem capable of self-administering treatments such as coping techniques (Siegel & Peterson, 1981).

Although few different treatments have been shown to be differently effective with younger and older children, there have been some suggestions of the need for different timing of treatments based on the child's age. The issue of temporal parameters of treatment will thus be considered next.

Treatment timing. There has been the suggestion in much of the past literature that young children would benefit from preparation immediately preceding the medical event, while older children would be aided more by advance preparation. A study by Melamed et al. (1976) is most frequently cited to substantiate this point. In fact, that study used multiple dependent variables and found on only one of these (palmer sweating) that younger children who viewed the film a week before admission had higher palmer sweating postoperatively than younger children who viewed the film upon admission, while the reverse was true for older children. There were no such results on self-report or observable indices of anxiety, so this result is perhaps best viewed as a suggestion still in need of replication and extension.

More recently, Faust and Melamed (1984) contrasted the effects of preparation for children who were admitted the day before surgery and who received a modeling slide show the evening before their operation with the effects of preparation of children who were admitted the same day as their operation and received the modeling preparation directly before their actual surgery. Subjects viewing the medically oriented slide show the day before their surgery showed a significant reduction in palmar sweating following the film and a decrease in their medical concerns, whereas the same-day surgery patients tended to show an increase in sweating and medical concerns.

This study would seem to indicate that preparation is only effective if delivered some minimal amount of time (at least overnight in this case) prior to surgery. However, these two groups were not randomly assigned to time of surgery and thus may have differed on many other factors. Because so many hospitals are shifting to same-day surgeries for cost reasons, this first study on the topic is of monumental importance and must be followed by additional evaluation of this question.

Finally, Peterson and Shigetomi (1981) found that coping significantly added to the effects of modeling when presented a week before surgery, but Peterson et al. (1984a) found no difference between a modeling and a modeling plus coping treatment. Peterson et al. posited that this was in part due to ceiling effects in the latter study and in part because the coping techniques may require more time following instruction for rehearsal before they can be used successfully. The differential timing requirements for various forms of preparation is only the facet of comparative research considered in the next section.

Comparative Research

Several studies outlined above compared differing aspects of the same type of preparations (variations on modeling techniques) and other studies have compared an active treatment to simple information, but in this section, we will consider only studies utilizing differing types of active preparation in their comparisons. There are far fewer studies comparing two active treatments. Peterson and Shigetomi (1981) attempted to do this by contrasting coping techniques and filmed modeling. However, they distributed developmentally appropriate information to all groups, using a puppet model (arguing that it makes no sense to train the coping group in coping skills without informing them about the experiences with which they will need to cope). As later work (Peterson et al., 1984a,b) showed that a puppet model has similar effects to a filmed model, this initial comparative study probably actually used a hierarchical design, comparing a puppet model only, puppet model + film or + coping techniques, and puppet model + coping techniques + modeling film. Not surprisingly, the group receiving all three techniques had lower distress ratings on almost all of the dependent measures.

Ferguson (1979) conducted one of the only true comparative studies, in which she varied both time of treatment and method of treatment (unfortunately, these were confounded in her design). Some children received a preadmission home visit from a nurse, while others viewed a modeling film after admission to the hospital. Mothers were less anxious both before and after hospitalization, and were more satisfied with their hospital experience if they had received the preoperative visit. Both preparations reduced 3- to 5-year-old and 6- to 7-year-old children's undesirable posthospital behaviors, as compared to a no-treatment control, but the preadmission visit was effective only with the older children. There were no treatment-related differences on child self-report, physiological arousal (EMG scores), or observer-rated anxiety. Thus, it would appear that both techniques have strengths and weaknesses, at least with minor surgery (tonsillectomy) patients. It is unclear whether a dual treatment would have the advantages of both. Because of the cost of a nurse home visit, additional comparisons of these two treatments may not be conducted, as their applicability to general preparation of children for medical procedures may be limited.

Perhaps the ultimate goal of comparative research would be to match each child to the optimal type of preparation for that child. One important factor influencing treatment effectiveness may be the child's characteristic way of coping. As seen earlier in the chapter, there are some indications that children do have characteristic ways of dealing with stress, either information seeking or avoiding. The only findings which do exist regarding coping by treatment interactions in children (and these are suggestive rather than definitive) indicate that preparation is more effective for information-seeking than information-avoiding children (e.g., Melamed, 1982).

We will turn our attention now from the child patient to the adult. As noted earlier, the adult literature has diverged in very different directions from the literature we have just described. For example, there is an absence of research on modeling and an intense interest in comparative studies and treatment by coping disposition interactions. We hope that, by reviewing both literatures in contrast, the aspects that each could contribute to the other will be highlighted.

ADULT PATIENTS

The Need for Preparation

In contrast to the layperson's view of the inadvisability of child preparation, most people seem to believe in routine informed preparation of adults for medical procedures. Adults, unlike children, are expected to be able to "take it" and to be good patients (Kendall, 1982). Further, unlike children whose parents can sign the informed consent documents necessary for invasive medical procedures and for surgery, mentally competent adults must make their own assessment and treatment decisions. They thus require a certain understanding of what will happen, what the potential benefits and risks are, what financial costs are involved, and how long the recovery period is likely to last.

The early literature on preventive preparation for adults also stressed the need of the adult patient to be fully informed and to complete "the work of worrying" prior to the medical procedure (Janis, 1958, p. 374). Further, current data clearly suggest that uncertainty about aspects of medical care such as "not knowing when to expect things will be done to you" and "not having your questions answered by staff" are major stresses (Volicer & Bohannon, 1975). Thus, the need for preparation of adults would seem well established. However, as the following section will illustrate, in some cases preparation may not have purely positive effects. Thus, the adult's coping style should be considered in evaluating the need for preparation.

Coping Dispositions

There are a variety of different personal factors in coping which have been investigated, and all of them cannot be considered in this brief review. Many, like gender (Bruegel, 1971; Cohen & Lazarus, 1973) and trait anxiety (Chaves & Brown, 1978; George, Scott, Turner, & Gregg, 1980), do not consistently show direct influence on coping, although where direct effects are found, they indicate that women report more anxiety than men (e.g., Graham & Conley, 1971), and that high trait anxiety is related to more emotional distress both before and after surgery (e.g., Martinez-Urrutia, 1975). There is a larger literature on locus of control, with some conflicting findings, primarily indicating that individuals with internal locus of control may have less anxiety (e.g., Lowery, Jacobsen, & Keane, 1975) but take more medications and more time to discharge (e.g., Johnson, Leventhal, & Dabbs, 1971). These findings are not mutually incompatible; rather they seem to indicate that internals maintain lower anxiety by taking control over their environment, obtaining more medications and taking more time to recover.

The bulk of the data on coping dispositions, however, has centered upon the dichotomy of information-seeking sensitizers or vigilants, and information-avoiding deniers or repressors, which was presented earlier (Goldstein, 1959) and has shown treatment by coping interactions. However, there are a few studies which have examined the coping dispositions alone and may provide some preliminary conclusions. Interactions will be reported later in this chapter. Cohen and Lazarus (1973) measured coping styles in two different ways, both by pencil-and-paper questionnaires that regarded coping style as a fixed personality variable, and with a structured interview, that looked at coping as an ongoing process rather than a mere fixed disposition. They found that interview-rated vigilants were slower to recover from surgery than other patients, both in terms of days in the hospital and minor complications. Interview-rated avoiders recovered most quickly. There were no differences in individuals when categorized by the pencil-and-paper measures. George et al. (1980) replicated this finding to some extent with an abbreviated experimenter rating and open-ended question categorization. They suggested that vigilants were more likely to report pain, interference of the surgery with daily living, and poor postoperative healing following oral surgery. On the other hand, Sime (1976) also categorized individuals according to an interview, but found no effects of coping style, although she did note that individuals with high preoperative fear had a longer recovery period, had higher levels of negative affect postsurgically, and required more medication for pain. Thus, in these studies in which preparation was not offered, vigilant individuals seemed to fare worse or to not differ from other patients. There are a variety of successful preparation techniques which could be offered to these information-seeking patients, and these will be overviewed next.

Preparation Techniques

Procedural information. There are over a hundred articles which have reported formally or informally on the impact of providing information. Devine and Cook (1983) offered a metaanalysis of 49 empirical studies in this area, in which they examined the single outcome variable of "days in the hospital." They pointed out that there are many different levels of information which can be offered, and that most studies with adults have offered multidimensional types of information, including procedural information, sensory information, necessary skills, cognitive interventions, and so on. There are few studies with adults which have assessed the simplest kind of information, a description of the medical procedure, by itself. However, such procedural information has been shown to improve confidence in the medical staff and to reduce anger in hernia repair patients (Vernon & Bigelow, 1974). It forms the basis (and sometimes the control group!) for other procedures such as sensory information, which have been more often investigated and will be considered next.

Sensory Information. Johnson, Rice, Fuller, and Endress (1978b) presented two experiments which contrasted procedural and sensory information, the first with female cholecystectomy (gall bladder removal) patients and the second with male herniorrhaphy (hernia repair surgery) patients. Johnson et al. found that procedural information improved preoperative mood states in those female patients who were initially fearful, but the sensory information was even more effective in reducing fear and more effective in improving recovery. There were no beneficial effects for either procedural or sensory information for the male patients, however. Johnson, Fuller, Endress, and Rice (1978a) later replicated these findings.

Johnson's research group has also shown the value of sensory information for reducing heart rate variability and the need for tranquilizers in young (not older than 50) endoscopy patients (Johnson & Leventhal, 1974), and for reducing overt distress and pulse rate variability in young women undergoing a routine pelvic examination (Fuller, Endress, & Johnson, 1978).

This preliminary series of studies suggested much promise for sensory information as a treatment strategy. However, later studies do not universally confirm this early promise. For example, Hill (1982) studied the use of sensory information preparation for cataract surgery patients and found no benefit from sensory information alone. However, sensory information plus physical self-care instructions resulted in more rapid transition to leaving the home after surgery. There were no other beneficial effects on the many other dependent variables. Similarly, Ziemer (1983) contrasted a 5-minute audiotaped procedural information preparation with a similar sensory information preparation and found no effects for adult surgery patients on physical symptoms, pain intensity, or self-reported distress.

Langer, Janis, and Wolfer (1975) compared procedural plus sensory information with preparation involving psychological coping procedures. They found, surprisingly, that subjects in the sensory information group were actually more anxious, asked for more major pain medication, and received poorer ratings from the nursing staff on their ability to cope than patients in the control group. Patients in the coping instruction group, however, benefited from their preparation.

There could scarcely be more conflict in the conclusions advanced by these authors, suggesting sensory information is very effective, ineffective, or actually has negative effects. The content of these treatments, including the degree of focus on unpleasant sensations, the number of reassurances offered, the portrayed inevitability of an aversive sensation, the extent to which the sensation is labeled positively but accurately, and the number of suggestions concerning methods to cope with the sensations, may have differed. Although there is no supporting empirical evidence at this point, we believe a balanced focus of sensations, the offering of reassurances that the sensations are not physically harmful, the suggestion that the sensation is common but not inevitable, the positive but accurate labeling of a sensation, and the offering of coping suggestions will all improve the effectiveness of sensory information. These conclusions are compatible with the limited empirical work which has been done on aspects of sensory information (e.g., Mohros, 1977) as well as conceptual advice (Janis, 1971). What is really needed, however, is additional research on this fascinating question.

Coping Techniques. Perhaps because of the intuitive appeal of enhancing an individual's ability to cope with stressful medical procedures, the term *coping* has been applied to a variety of very different procedures. Each of these methods of intervention will be briefly considered below.

(a) Physical coping methods. One of the additional methods compared to sensory information by Johnson et al. (1978a) was a set of coping behaviors which included coughing, early ambulation, leg exercises, and methods for reducing discomfort when turning in bed. They found that patients receiving training in such behaviors increased ambulation and decreased requests for pain medication. King and Tarsitano (1982) came to similar conclusions, and they were able to document improvements in breathing and coughing by pulmonary function tests. Other researchers were able to demonstrate that such physical coping techniques reduced the number of postsurgery days in hospital (Lindeman & Van Aernam, 1971).

Physical coping instructions have been used to decrease problems in patients undergoing diagnostic procedures as well. For example, Johnson and Leventhal (1974) taught endoscopy patients to breath rapidly through their mouths, to pant during the application of anesthetic to their throat, and to make swallowing motions with their mouths open and chins down during entubation. There were trends for this training to reduce gagging and the need for tranquilizers, and to reduce heart rate variability. When such training was combined with sensory information, there was even greater reduction in gagging and increased heart-rate stability. Thus, physical coping techniques, particularly when combined with information concerning the sensations which should cue them, appear to be useful preventive methods.

(b) Relaxation. Relaxation training is a very specific kind of physical coping technique which also has important psychological properties. Several studies have relaxation training in concert with other cognitive preparation techniques, and these studies are described below as "Coping Package Treatments." However, some studies have focused on the use of relaxation alone as a treatment method. For example, Aiken and Henricks (1971) taught systematic relaxation skills to open-heart surgery patients and found that this preparation reduced postoperative impairment of consciousness. However, other authors have reduced postoperative delirium with information alone (e.g., Owens & Hutelmyer, 1982), so it is not clear if relaxation or information concerning when to relax is the active ingredient in delirium reduction. Flaherty and Fitzpatrick (1978) trained patients who were undergoing cholecystectomy, herniorrhaphy, or hemerroidectomy surgery to breathe slowly and rhythmically, relax their jaws, and clear their minds. This training resulted in less reported pain at incision and lower reported distress and need for medications postsurgically, as contrasted with a no-treatment control.

Relaxation is probably most logically applied in concert with procedural information, to ensure that the patient knows when to apply the relaxation. Egbert, Battit, Welch, and Bartlett (1964) conducted one of the first studies on the use of abdominal muscle relaxation and procedural information for surgery patients. This combination resulted in decreased need for pain medication and an improved hospital course. Berggren and Carlsson (1984) gave detailed exposure to procedural information in a series of slides and amplified their relaxation training with biofeedback. They found this treatment to reduce dental fear in previously dental-phobic individuals.

In sum, studies which have employed relaxation generally show it to be a useful preventive technique. However, if the length of instruction is too short or the patients are unmotivated to use the technique, relaxation is likely to be ineffective (Fuller et al., 1978).

(c) Cognitive techniques. In general, studies using cognitive techniques have focused on ways of changing cognitions or on using cognitions as a way of blocking aversive physical sensations. For example, Kaplan, Atkins, and Lenhard (1982) instructed patients who would be undergoing a stressful sigmoidoscopy (rectal exam) in methods of refocusing their attention on positive thoughts about the physician or on positive self-statements. This resulted in increased behavioral cooperation and lowered anxiety during the exam. Ridgeway and Mathews (1982) demonstrated that replacing frightening cognitions (e.g., "I am worried about the anesthetic") with more positive thoughts (e.g., "Many thousands of people have general anaesthesia every year, they do well and so will I," p. 274) effectively reduced both objective and subjective ratings of pain more than did procedural information, a placebo treatment, or no treatment.

Wallace (1984) employed a booklet that combined unspecified "suggestions of how to cope with preoperative fear and postoperative symptoms and recovery" (p. 66) with procedural and sensory information concerning when to use the coping procedures. Patients receiving this booklet reported less pre- and postsurgery anxiety and had better recoveries than patients receiving a minimal information booklet. Langer et al. (1975), as described earlier, utilized a set of cognitive techniques, including calming self-instructions, selective attention, and cognitive restructuring of events from negative to positive. In comparison to a procedural and sensory information treatment, subjects who used the cognitive techniques were rated as less anxious and better able to cope by nurses uninformed as to treatment designation.

(d) Coping package treatments. Several studies have examined simultaneous use of several different kinds of coping techniques. For example, Tarrier and Maguire (1984) used physical relaxation in combination with cognitive restructuring as a psychological treatment, and antidepressant medication as a pharmacological treatment. They

found the combination of both psychological and pharmacological preventive intervention resulted in the lowest rate of negative emotions in postmastectomy patients.

Kendall, Williams, Pechacek, Graham, Shisslak, and Herzoff (1979) described one of the most complete cognitive behavioral packages in their study of male cardiac catheterization patients. A therapist disclosed a real-life stress experience and modeled the strategy used to reduce the stress, and then the patient was urged to make similar self-disclosures, to which the therapist responded with positive cognitive reconstructions. The patient was trained to become more aware of elicitors of his own anxiety and to use these skills to prompt relaxation and cognitive coping. Rehearsal of this process was followed by self-reinforcement for coping. Patients receiving this treatment were rated by physicians as being better adjusted than patients receiving procedural information or no information, and they experienced a greater reduction in self-reported anxiety following treatment which was maintained after the catheterization.

Detailed, combination treatment protocols such as this are sensible state-of-the-art interventions with highly stressful medical procedures, because they optimize the chance of demonstrating significant treatment effects. However, later research examining the active components may be necessary to create the most cost-effective treatment program possible. For example, Kaplan, Metzger, and Jablecki (1983) conducted a comparative study in their treatment of adult patients undergoing a stressful EMG procedure. They found that relaxation alone was as effective as a cognitive coping plus relaxation package.

In any case, it would appear that all of the different types of coping techniques have at least some evidence supporting their efficacy, and that increasing both physical and cognitive aspects of coping has an important place in preprocedure preparation. These findings, in combination with those in the child area, suggest that research on training coping strategies should continue.

In contrast to the child area, there is very little research on either modeling or treatment variations in application. This apparent gap in the literature will be addressed next.

Relative Absence of Modeling and Treatment Variation Studies

As was seen earlier in this chapter, puppet and filmed models compose the most frequently investigated preparations with children. It is thus somewhat surprising to note that modeling has been very infrequently used as a preventive preparation with adults. Occasionally it has been used as a portion of a larger treatment (as in the Kendall et al., 1979, cognitive behavioral program just described), but rarely as the sole method of treatment.

Two recent studies utilized a procedural information film which showed an adult model undergoing endoscopy. These studies will be considered in more detail later in this chapter when person-by-treatment interactions are considered, as the authors suggested their most important effects were interactive. Briefly, Shipley, Butt, Horwitz, and Farbry (1978) showed their modeling film zero, one, or three times and, overall, found that multiple viewing of the film reduced distress over a single or no viewing. However, a later study using experienced patients demonstrated no overall effect for the film (Shipley, Butt, & Horwitz, 1979). As will be recalled, there has been a similar lack of impact of filmed modeling found with experienced child patients.

There is also a relative absence of attention to variations in treatment application, in contrast to the child data. Christopherson and Pfeiffer (1980) point out that no past studies have considered timing of treatment, but they found that the timing of their treatment booklet, which described procedural and sensory information for cardiac surgery patients, failed to influence outcome variables. The booklet, if read, was equally effective regardless of whether it was read 3 to 35 days preoperatively or within 48 hours of surgery.

Similarly, few studies have examined the way in which information is given to patients, despite clear evidence that the interpersonal aspects of medical care are important. Auerbach, Martelli, and Mercuri (1983) varied aspects such as smiles, eye contact, voice tone, nods, body orientation, and hand movements of the information provider. They found no direct effects of these manipulations, but subjects who rated the preparation agent as interpersonally dominant or hostile tended to be rated as responding more poorly by the surgeon.

Finally, there has been very little work with the spouses or families of adult patients to assess the utility of preventive preparation for them. The few studies which exist suggest that information may be helpful for family members as well as the medical patient. For example, Doerr and Jones (1979) found that families who received an information booklet on the cardiac care unit were more likely to ask questions, and there was a clear reduction in the patients' self-reported anxiety due to family preparation. As will be recalled, similar findings are present in the child literature.

There are many areas of treatment variation in the adult literature, including the mode of preparation application (some studies have used 5-minute audiotapes, others multiple in-person sessions) and the past medical experiences of the patient, which have not been the focus of much examination with adults and are only beginning to be examined in children. Hopefully, these will be the focus of some future research. In contrast, the child area has very few comparative treatment studies, while such research has typified the adult area, as will be seen in the next section.

Comparative Research

The bulk of comparative studies has either already been presented in this chapter under the heading corresponding to the most successful treatment considered or will be described in more detail in the next section on interactions of various treatments and personal coping dispositions. However, it may be useful to draw some of the conclusions regarding treatment comparisons together here. As may be recalled from the earlier discussion, procedural information alone seemed to be an effective preparation for some patients (e.g., hernia repair patients; Vernon & Bigelow, 1974), but procedural information is more often used as a control or comparison condition. In general, it would appear that procedural information is helpful, sensory information is better, and other techniques like physical coping may amplify the effects of sensory information.

The coping area seems to yield similar conclusions. Positive restructuring training appears more effective than information alone. Some individuals have found coping package treatments more effective than procedural information or components of the package alone, while others have found a single component to be equivalent to a detailed package. The continuation of hierarchical designs seems very important to ascertaining the components which are both necessary and sufficient to treatment effectiveness. In addition, it seems vitally important to assess the comparative effectiveness of treatments which might be thought to have differing mechanisms influencing their impact. For example, relaxation and imaginal distraction involve retreating from the stimulus situation, whereas sensory information, and, to a limited extent, physical coping, involve approaching the situation. Comparisons between techniques with such differing goals would seem to have both theoretical and pragmatic importance. It would also seem sensible to consider the role of personal coping types when planting such comparisons, as coping disposition and treatment mechanisms for effect may be intimately related.

Treatment by Coping-Style Interactions

The studies reviewed earlier which have examined the role of coping in isolation from treatment have regarded coping as an ongoing process rather than a fixed trait and have reported either that vigilant copers had a more difficult recovery than (e.g., Cohen & Lazarus, 1973; George et al., 1980), or a similar recovery to, avoiders (Sime, 1976). The studies described in this section have more typically used a trait-oriented approach, and pencil-and-paper measures of sensitizing and avoiding, which have not received extensive construct validation. These studies yield conclusions very different from the studies discussed earlier.

Andrew (1970) reported that when no preparation was received, neutrals (those using both approach and avoiding tactics) had the poorest recovery, avoiders the next, and sensitizers the best recovery. When they had heard an 8-minute procedural information audiotape, neutrals demonstrated improved recoveries and reduced medications, sensitizers did not benefit from the treatment (presumably because they had already sought out the relevant information), and avoiders actually required more medications if prepared than if unprepared, although they recovered at the same rate regardless of preparation.

DeLong (1971) replicated some of these results and not others. In her study, sensitizers who received specific information had much better recoveries than sensitizers who received general information. Avoiders who received specific information were worse in only one respect—their rate of complaining—and otherwise did not differ from avoiders who received general information.

Shipley et al.'s (1978) modeling film also influenced repressors and sensitizers differently, but only on the variable of heart rate. Sensitizers showed a decrease in heart rate each time they viewed the film. Repressors, in contrast, had an increased heart rate if they saw the film only once, with lowered rates at zero or three viewings. Shipley et al. suggest that three viewings allowed desensitization to take place. In a second study, Shipley et al. (1979) examined the impact of their film on experienced endoscopy patients. Again, sensitizers clearly benefited from the film, with lower heart rates, gagging, and nurse-rated anxiety. Repressors again showed an increase in heart rate to the film, but none of the other variables were differentially affected. Shipley et al. (1979) reiterated their concern about possible sensitization of repressor-patients, based on this increase in heart rate.

Other investigators using process rather than trait approaches to the coping-by-treatment interaction question have come to dissimilar conclusions. Wilson (1981) used a control tape, a tape on either sensory information or relaxation, or a tape with both types of preparation. He found no interaction of patient levels of denial with treatment, but he did find other person-related differences. Relaxation was better with low- than high-fear patients, for example, and sensory information resulted in decreased reports of pain, physical symptoms, and negative mood in highly aggressive patients but increased these variables in low aggressive patients. He concluded that, "although ignorance may be blissful for some patients, knowledge in the form of accurate expectations about the future and in the form of ability to cope with that future may be even better" (p. 100).

Finally, some investigators have even suggested complementing rather than matching coping styles. Hitchcock (1982) used an interview method to categorize surgery patients who were then treated as controls, with procedural information plus relaxation, or with sensory information plus cognitive reappraisal. Individuals who sought out little surgery information (avoiders) left their homes sooner after surgery if they received the cognitive rather than the control treatment, whereas there were no such differences for vigilant patients. However, individuals rated as vigilants on their appraisal or surgery took fewer pain medications if they received relaxation training, whereas interview-coded avoiders took more sleeping pills if so prepared. These were the only variables showing a coping-by-treatment interaction. Hitchcock summarizes these findings by noting that "subjects benefited most from treatments complementary rather than congruent with their preoperative mode of coping" (p. ix).

One thing is clear from these conflicting results. Coping dispositions differ depending on the degree to which they are viewed as process measures, specific to the given medical setting and obtained typically through flexible interview techniques, or are viewed as fixed personality traits typically obtained from coping inventories. The process measure studies seem to suggest that repressors/deniers recover well in the absence of treatment (Cohen & Lazarus, 1973) but the also benefit from treatment (e.g., Hitchcock, 1982; Wilson, 1981). The trait measure studies suggest that repressor/deniers may actually become worse if treated, but these findings are often obtained only for one of many dependent variables and range from requests for more medication (Andrew, 1970) to having elevated heart rates (Shipley et al., 1978). We might argue that the press should be toward finding a successful way to prepare such individuals rather than a fearful withdrawal from preparing them at all, especially since the "sensitizing" effects seem quite circumscribed.

The findings from both process-oriented and trait-based studies agree that sensitizers are not harmed and most often derive much benefit from preparation. Most treatments examined in this section have used a base of procedural information with additional procedures, and thus it should not be surprising that those individuals who seek out information characteristically would benefit from these treatments.

There are many additional methods of categorizing coping which cannot be considered in detail here. For example, Miller (1980) discusses *monitors* (who seek information only when it allows them to better control the situation) and *blunters* (who tend to prefer unpredictability in aversive events). She argues that individuals benefit most from preparations which complement individual coping styles. Other researchers have argued that a larger variety of coping dispositions exist and should be studied (Copp, 1974; Chaves & Brown, 1978). Finally, other person factors may influence reaction to treatment as well. Individuals with an internal locus of control seem to do better with specific information, while the reverse or no difference is true for externals (Auerbach, Kendall, Cuttler, & Levitt, 1976; Pickett & Clum, 1982). On the other hand, factors such as gender and trait anxiety very rarely interact with treatment. Future research on the role of person variables in determining treatment effectiveness will need to consider all of this disparate data. A flexible, multimodal conceptualization of person variables would seem warranted at this point and worthy of exploration.

SUMMARY

As this review has repeatedly noted, summary statements made within this area must cut across dissimilar preparation methods and measures and must represent the majority rather than the totality of the data. As has been seen, the areas of child and adult preparation differ extensively, and yet both have techniques and conceptualizations relevant to the other. The modeling data in the child area suggest the strength and flexibility of this method. The single adult study cited here used a matter-of-fact filmed demonstration model rather than a coping model, and yet the film achieved an overall positive effect. The positive influence of modeling has been neglected too long in the adult area, and continues to promote useful work with children.

Both areas have a few studies on sensory information, with the child area suggesting only positive effects and the adult area suggesting mostly positive effects, especially when amplified by coping instructions. However, in the adult area, there have also been some reports of no benefit and one report of actual harm. Future work utilizing the positive facets of sensory information outlined in this chapter may clarify these mixed results and produce a superior sensory information preparation procedure.

There are many types of coping techniques, ranging from purely physical acts such as coughing, to relaxation or cognitive techniques. All have shown some degree of success, and none have been indicated as having sensitizing properties. Thus, this group of techniques may show the most promise for treating experienced patients or information-avoiding individuals who do not seem to profit from modeling or information-based preparations.

We began the review of each area by documenting the need for preparation for both children and adults. It seems fitting to end the chapter the same way, by reiterating that both children and adults profit in numerous ways from appropriate behavioral preparation for medical procedures. As has been seen, internal fear and depression can be reduced, as can maladaptive behaviors, negative physiological reactions, and excessive need for medication. Confidence, a sense of control, adaptive coping, early ambulation, and enhanced recovery can all result from appropriate preparation. The task for the future will be to continue to examine individual characteristics such as information seeking versus avoiding, which may influence treatment effectiveness and to ultimately produce the best match of treatment method, timing, and mode of delivery for any given individual undergoing a specific medical procedure. The literature suggests that we are far from such a goal currently, but that we are going in the right direction.

REFERENCES

Abbott, N. C., Hansen, P., & Lewis, K. (1970). Dress rehearsal for the hospital. *American Journal of Nursing, 70,* 2360.

Aiken, L. H., & Henricks, T. F. (1971). Systematic relaxation as a nursing intervention technique with open heart surgery patients. *Nursing Research, 20,* 212–217.

Andrew, J. (1970). Recovery from surgery, with and without preparatory instruction for three coping styles. *Journal of Personality and Social Psychology, 15,* 223–226.

Auerbach, S., Kendall, P., Cuttler, H., & Levitt, N. (1976). Anxiety, locus of control, type of preparatory information, and adjustment to dental surgery. *Journal of Consulting and Clinical Psychology, 44,* 809–818.

Auerbach, S. M., Martelli, M. F., & Mercuri, L. G. (1983). Anxiety, information, interpersonal impacts, and adjustment to a stressful health care situation. *Journal of Personality and Social Psychology, 44,* 1284–1296.

Ayer, W. A. (1973). Use of visual imagery in needle phobic children. *Journal of Dentistry for Children, 28,* 41–43.

Azarnoff, P. (1982). Hospital tours for school children ended. *Pediatric Mental Health, 1,* 2.

Azarnoff, P., & Woody, P. D. (1981). Preparation of children for hospitalization in acute care hospitals in the United States. *Pediatrics, 66,* 361–368.

Berggren, U., & Carlsson, S. G. (1984). A psychophysiological therapy for dental fear. *Behavioural Research and Therapy, 22,* 487–492.

Brain, D. J., & Maclay, I. (1968). Controlled study of mothers and children in hospital. *British Medical Journal, 1,* 278–280.

Bruegel, M. A. (1971). Relationship of preoperative anxiety to perception of post-operative pain. *Nursing Research, 20,* 26–31.

Burstein, S., & Meichenbaum, D. (1979). The work of worrying in children undergoing surgery. *Journal of Abnormal Child Psychology, 7,* 121–132.

Cassell, S. (1965). Effects of brief puppet therapy upon the emotional responses of children undergoing cardiac catheterization. *Journal of Consulting Psychology, 29,* 1–8.

Caty, S., Ellerton, M. L., & Ritchie, J. A. (1984). Coping in hospitalized children: An analysis of published case studies. *Nursing Research, 33,* 277–282.

Chan, J. M. (1980). Preparation for procedures and surgery through play. *Paediatrician, 9,* 210–219.

Chapman, A. H., Loeb, D. G., & Gibbons, M. J. (1956). Psychiatric aspects of hospitalization of children. *Archives of Pediatrics, 73,* 77–88.

Chaves, J. F., & Brown, J. M. (1978, August). *Self-generated strategies for the control of pain and stress.* Paper presented at the meeting of the American Psychological Association, Toronto, Canada.

Christopherson, B., & Pfeiffer, C. (1980). Varying the timing of information to alter preoperative anxiety and postoperative recovery in cardiac surgery patients. *Heart and Lung, 9,* 854–861.

Cohen, F., & Lazarus, R. S. (1973). Active coping processes, coping dispositions, and recovery from surgery. *Psychosomatic Medicine, 35,* 375–389.

Copp, L. A. (1974). The spectrum of suffering. *American Journal of Nursing, 74,* 491–495.

Crocker, E. (1979). Hospital books for children. *Canadian Nurse, 75,* 33.

Crowl, M. (1980). Case study: The basic process of art therapy as demonstrated by efforts to allay a child's fear of surgery. *American Journal of Art Therapy, 19,* 49–51.

DeLong, D. R. (1971). Individual differences in patterns of anxiety arousal, stress-relevant information and recovery from surgery. *Dissertation Abstracts International, 32,* 554B.

Devine, E. C., & Cook, T. D. (1983). A meta-analytic analysis of effects of psychoeducational interventions on length of postsurgical hospital stay. *Nursing Research, 32,* 267–274.

Doerr, B. C., & Jones, J. W. (1979). Effect of family preparation on the state anxiety level of the CCU patient. *Nursing Research, 28,* 315–316.

Douglas, J. W. B. (1975). Early hospital admission and later disturbances of behaviour and learning. *Developmental Medicine and Child Neurology, 17,* 456–480.

Egbert, L., Battit, G., Welch, C., & Bartlett, W. (1964). Reduction of postoperative pain by encouragement and instruction of patients. *New England Journal of Medicine, 270,* 825–827.

Eland, J. M. (1981). Minimizing pain associated with prekindergarten intramuscular injections. *Issues in Comprehensive Pediatric Nursing, 5,* 361–372.

Faust, J., & Melamed, B. G. (1984). Influence of arousal, previous experience, and age on surgery preparation of same day of surgery and in-hospital pediatric patients. *Journal of Consulting and Clinical Psychology, 52,* 359–365.

Ferguson, B. F. (1979). Preparing young children for hospitalization: A comparison of two methods. *Pediatrics, 64,* 656–664.

Fernald, C. D., & Corry, J. J. (1981). Empathic versus directive preparation of children for needles. *Journal of the Association for the Care of Children's Health, 10,* 44–47.

Flaherty, G. G., & Fitzpatrick, R. (1978). Relaxation technique to increase comfort level of postoperative patients. *Nursing Research, 27,* 352–355.

Fuller, S. S., Endress, M. P., & Johnson, J. E. (1978). The effects of cognitive and behavioral control on coping with an aversive health examination. *Journal of Human Stress, 4,* 18–25.

Gelfand, D. M., & Peterson, L. (1985). *Child development and child psychopathology.* Beverly Hills, CA: Sage.

George, J. M., Scott, D. S., Turner, S. P., & Gregg, J. M. (1980). The effects of psychological factors and physical trauma on recovery from oral surgery. *Journal of Behavioral Medicine, 3,* 291–310.

Goldstein, M. J. (1959). The relationship between coping and avoiding behavior and response to fear-arousing propaganda. *Journal of Abnormal and Social Psychology, 58,* 247–252.

Goslin, E. R. (1978). Hospitalization as a life crisis for the preschool child: A critical review. *Journal of Community Health, 3,* 321–346.

Graham, L. E., & Conley, E. M. (1971). Evaluation of anxiety and fear in adult surgical patients. *Nursing Research, 20,* 113–122.

Gross, A. M., Stern, R. M., Levin, R. B., Dale, J., & Wojnilower, D. A. (1983). The effect of mother-child separation on the behavior of children experiencing a diagnostic medical procedure. *Journal of Consulting and Clinical Psychology, 51,* 783–785.

Heffernan, M., & Azarnoff, P. (1971). Factors in reducing children's anxiety about clinic visits. *Health Services and Mental Health Administration Health Reports, 86,* 1131–1135.

Hill, B. J. (1982). Sensory information, behavioral instructions, and coping with sensory alteration surgery. *Nursing Research, 31,* 17–21.

Hitchcock, L. S. (1982). *Improving recovery from surgery: The interaction of preoperative interventions, coping processes, and personality variables.* Unpublished doctoral dissertation, The University of Texas at Austin.

Janis, I. L. (1958). *Psychological stress.* New York: Wiley.

Janis, I. L. (1971). *Stress and frustration.* New York: Harcourt, Brace, & Jovanovich.

Johnson, J. E., Fuller, S. S., Endress, M. P., & Rice, V. H. (1978a). Altering patients responses to surgery: An extension and replication. *Research in Nursing and Health, 1,* 111–121.

Johnson, J. E., Kirchoff, K., & Endress, M. P. (1975). Altering children's distress behavior during orthopedic cast removal. *Nursing Research, 24,* 404–410.

Johnson, J. E., & Leventhal, H. (1974). Effects of accurate expectations and behavioral instructions on reactions during a noxious medical examination. *Journal of Personality and Social Psychology, 29,* 710–718.

Johnson, J. E., Leventhal, H., & Dabbs, J. M. (1971). Contributions of emotional and instrumental response processes in adaptation to surgery. *Journal of Personality and Social Psychology, 20,* 55–64.

Johnson, J. E., Rice, V. H., Fuller, S. S., & Endress, M. P. (1978b). Sensory information, instruction in a coping strategy, and recovery from surgery. *Research in Nursing and Health, 1,* 4–17.

Johnson, P. A., & Stockdale, D. F. (1975). Effects of puppet therapy on palmar sweating of hospitalized children. *The Johns Hopkins Medical Journal, 137,* 1–5.

Kaplan, R. M., Atkins, C. J., & Lenhard, L. (1982). Coping with a stressful sigmoidoscopy: Evaluation of cognitive and relaxation preparations. *Journal of Behavioral Medicine, 5,* 67–82.

Kaplan, R. M., Metzger, G., & Jablecki, C. (1983). Brief cognitive and relaxation training increases tolerance for a painful electromyographic examination. *Psychosomatic Medicine, 45,* 155–162.

Kendall, P. C. (1982). Stressful medical procedures: Cognitive-behavioral strategies for stress management and prevention. In D. Meichenbaum & M. Jaremko (Eds.), *Stress prevention and management: A cognitive-behavioral approach* (pp. 159–190). New York: Plenum.

Kendall, P. C., Williams, L., Pechacek, T. F., Graham, L. E., Shisslak, C., & Herzoff, N. (1979). Cognitive-behavioral and patient education interventions in cardiac catheterization procedures: The Palo Alto medical psychology project. *Journal of Consulting and Clinical Psychology, 47,* 49–58.

King, I., & Tarsitano, B. (1982). The effect of structured and unstructured preoperative teaching: A replication. *Nursing Research, 31,* 324–329.

Knight, R. B., Atkins, A., Eagle, C., Evans, N., Finkelstein, J. W., Fukushima, D., Katz, J., & Weiner, H. (1979). Psychological stress, ego defenses, and cortisol production in children hospitalized for elective surgery. *Psychosomatic Medicine, 41,* 40–49.

Langer, E., Janis, I., & Wolfer, J. (1975). Reduction of psychological stress in surgical patients. *Journal of Experimental Social Psychology, 11,* 155–165.

Levinson, P., & Ousterhout, D. K. (1980). Art and play therapy with pediatric burn patients. *Journal of Burn Care and Rehabilitation, 1,* 42–46.

Lindeman, C. A., & Van Aernam, B. (1971). Nursing interventions with the presurgical patient: The effects of structured and unstructured preoperative teaching. *Nursing Research, 20,* 319–331.

Lowery, B., Jacobsen, B., & Keane, A. (1975). Relationship of locus of control to preoperative anxiety. *Psychological Reports, 37,* 1115–1121.

Martinez-Urrutia, A. (1975). Anxiety and pain in surgical patients. *Journal of Consulting and Clinical Psychology, 43,* 437–442.

Melamed, B. G. (1982). Reduction of medical fears: An information processing analysis. In J. Boulougouris (Ed.), *Learning theory approaches to psychiatry.* New York: John Wiley & Sons.

Melamed, B. G., Meyer, R., Gee, C., & Soule, L. (1976). The influence of time and type of preparation on children's adjustment to hospitalization. *Journal of Pediatric Psychology, 1,* 31–37.

Melamed, B. G., & Siegel, L. J. (1975). Reduction of anxiety in children facing surgery by modeling. *Journal of Consulting and Clinical Psychology, 43,* 511–521.

Melamed, B. G., & Siegel, L. J. (1980). *Behavioral medicine: Practical application in health care.* New York: Springer.

Miller, S. M. (1980). When is a little information a dangerous thing? Coping with stressful events by monitoring versus blunting. In S. Levine & H. Ursin (Eds.), *Coping and health* (pp. 145–169). New York: Plenum Press.

Mohros, K. L. L. (1977). Effects of reassuring information and sensory information on emotional response during a threatening medical examination. (Doctoral dissertation, University of Minnesota, 1976). *Dissertation Abstracts International, 38,* 1304–1305A.

Nocella, J., & Kaplan, R. M. (1982). Training children to cope with dental treatment. *Journal of Pediatric Psychology, 7,* 175–178.

Owens, J. F., & Hutelmyer, C. M. (1982). The effect of preoperative intervention on delirium in cardiac surgical patients. *Nursing Research, 31,* 60–62.

Peterson, L. (1984). A brief methodological comment on possible inaccuracies induced by multimodal measurement and reporting. *Journal of behavior Medicine, 7,* 307–313.

Peterson, L., & Brownlee-Duffeck, M. (1984). Prevention of anxiety and pain due to medical and dental procedures. In M. C. Roberts & L. Peterson (Eds.), *Prevention of problems in childhood: Psychological research and applications* (pp. 266–310). New York: Wiley-Interscience.

Peterson, L., & Mori, L. (1988). Preparation for hospitalization. In D. Routh (Ed.), *Handbook of pediatric psychology.* Beverly Hills: Sage.

Peterson, L., Mori, L., & Carter, P. (1985). The role of the family in children's responses to stressful medical procedures. *Journal of Clinical Child Psychology, 14,* 98–104.

Peterson, L., & Ridley-Johnson, R. (1980). Pediatric hospital response to survey on prehospital preparation for children. *Journal of Pediatric Psychology, 5,* 1–7.

Peterson, L., Ridley-Johnson, R., Tracy, K., & Mullins, L. J. (1984a). Developing cost-effective presurgical preparation: A comparative analysis. *Journal of Pediatric Psychology, 9,* 274–296.

Peterson, L., Schultheis, K., Ridley-Johnson, R., Miller, D., & Tracy, K. (1984b). Comparison of three modeling procedures in the presurgical and postsurgical responses of children. *Behavior Therapy, 15,* 79–83.

Peterson, L., & Shigetomi, C. (1981). The use of coping techniques to minimize anxiety in hospitalized children. *Behavior Therapy, 12,* 1–14.

Peterson, L., & Shigetomi, C. (1982). One-year follow-up of elective surgery child patients receiving preoperative preparation. *Journal of Pediatric Psychology, 7,* 43–48.

Peterson, L., & Toler, S. (1986). An information seeking disposition in child surgery patients. *Health Psychology, 5,* 343–358.

Pickett, C., & Clum, G. A. (1982). Comparative treatment strategies and their interaction with locus of control in the reduction of postsurgical pain and anxiety. *Journal of Consulting and Clinical Psychology, 50,* 439–441.

Pinto, R. P., & Hollandsworth, J. G., Jr. (1989). Using videotape modeling to prepare children psychologically for surgery: Influence of parents and cost versus benefits of providing preparation services. *Health Psychology, 8,* 79–95.

Prugh, D. G., Staub, E. M., Sands, H. H., Kirschbaum, R. M., & Lenihan, E. A. (1953). A study of the emotional reactions of children and families to hospitalization and illness. *American Journal of Orthopsychiatry, 23,* 70–106.

Ramirez-Johnson, M. (1979). Mental health interventions with medically ill children: A review of the literature 1970–1977. *Journal of Pediatric Psychology, 4,* 147–165.

Ridgeway, V., & Mathews, A. (1982). Psychological preparation for surgery: A comparison of methods. *British Journal of Clinical Psychology, 21,* 271–280.

Rushton, C. H. (1983). Preparing children and families for cardiac surgery: Nursing interventions. *Issues in Comprehensive Pediatric Nursing, 6,* 235–248.

Schultheis, K., Peterson, L., & Selby, V. (1987). Preparation for stressful medical procedures and person x treatment interactions. *Clinical Psychology Review, 7,* 329–352.

Schulz, J. B., Raschke, D., Dedrick, C., & Thompson, M. (1981). The effects of a preoperational puppet show on anxiety levels of hospitalized children. *Journal of the Association for the Care of Children's Health, 9,* 118–120.

Seagull, E. A. W. (1978). The child's rights as medical patient. *Journal of Clinical Child Psychology, 7,* 202–205.

Shaw, E. G., & Routh, D. K. (1982). Effect of mother presence on children's reaction to aversive procedures. *Journal of Pediatric Psychology, 7,* 33–42.

Shipley, R., Butt, J. H., & Horwitz, B. (1979). Preparation to reexperience a stressful medical examination: Effect of repetitious videotape exposure and coping style. *Journal of Consulting and Clinical Psychology, 47,* 485–492.

Shipley, R. H., Butt, J. H., Horwitz, B., & Farbry, J. E. (1978). Preparation for a stressful medical procedure: Effect of amount of stimulus preexposure and coping style. *Journal of Consulting and Clinical Psychology, 46,* 499–507.

Siegel, L. J. (1981, April). *Naturalistic study of coping strategies in children facing medical procedures.* Paper presented at the meeting of the Southeastern Psychological Association, Atlanta, GA.

Siegel, L. J., & Peterson, L. (1980). Stress reduction in young dental patients through coping skills and sensory information. *Journal of Consulting and Clinical Psychology, 48,* 785–787.

Siegel, L. J., & Peterson, L. (1981). Maintenance effects of coping skills and sensory information on young children's response to repeated dental procedures. *Behavior Therapy, 12,* 530–535.

Sime, A. M. (1976). Relationship of preoperative fear, type of coping and information received about surgery to recovery from surgery. *Journal of Personality and Social Psychology, 34,* 716–724.

Skipper, J., & Leonard, R. (1968). Children, stress and hospitalization: A field experiment. *Journal of Health and Social Behavior, 9,* 275–287.

Skipper, J., Leonard, R. C., & Rhymes, J. (1968). Child hospitalization and social interaction: An experimental study of mothers' feelings of stress, adaptation, and satisfaction. *Medical Care, 6,* 496–506.

Tarrier, N., & Maguire, P. (1984). Treatment of psychological distress following mastectomy: An initial report. *Behaviour Research and Therapy, 22,* 81–84.

Trouten, F. (1981). Psychological preparation of children for surgery. *Dimensions of Health Service, 58,* 9–10; 12–13.

Vardaro, J. A. (1978). Preadmission anxiety and mother-child relationships. *Journal of the Association for the Care of Children in Hospitals, 7,* 8–15.

Vernon, D. T., & Bailey, W. C. (1974). The use of motion pictures in the psychological preparation of children for induction of anesthesia. *Anesthesiology, 40,* 68–72.

Vernon, D. T., & Bigelow, D. (1974). Effect of information about a potentially stressful situation on response to stress impact. *Journal of Personality and Social Psychology, 29,* 50–59.

Volicer, B. J., & Bohannon, M. W. (1975). A hospital stress rating scale. *Nursing Research, 24,* 352–359.

Wallace, L. M. (1984). Psychological preparation as a method of reducing the stress of surgery. *Journal of Human Stress, 10,* 62–77.

Wilson, J. F. (1981). Behavioral preparation for surgery: Benefit or harm? *Journal of Behavioral Medicine, 4,* 79–101.

Wolfer, J. A., & Visintainer, M. A. (1975). Pediatric surgical patients' and parents' stress responses and adjustment. *Nursing Research, 24,* 244–255.

Zabin, M. A., & Melamed, B. G. (1980). Relationship between parental discipline and children's ability to cope with stress. *Journal of Behavioral Assessment, 2,* 17–38.

Zastowny, T. R., Kirschenbaum, D. S., & Meng, A. L. (1981, December). *Coping skills training for children: Effects on distress before, during, and after hospitalization for surgery.* Paper presented at the meeting of the Association for the Advancement of Behavior Therapy, Toronto, Canada.

Ziemer, M. M. (1983). Effects of information on postsurgical coping. *Nursing Research, 32,* 282–287.

Author Index

C

D

E

L

M

S

Subject Index

www.ingramcontent.com/pod-product-compliance
Ingram Content Group UK Ltd.
Pitfield, Milton Keynes, MK11 3LW, UK
UKHW020219041026
15470UKWH00012B/451